Clinical Perspectives on Prostate Diseases

Clinical Perspectives on Prostate Diseases

Editor: Blake Xavier

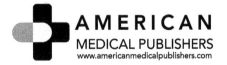

AMERICAN
MEDICAL PUBLISHERS
www.americanmedicalpublishers.com

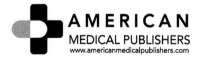
AMERICAN
MEDICAL PUBLISHERS
www.americanmedicalpublishers.com

Cataloging-in-Publication Data

Clinical perspectives on prostate diseases / edited by Blake Xavier.
  p. cm.
Includes bibliographical references and index.
ISBN 979-8-88740-004-4
1. Prostate--Diseases. 2. Prostate--Diseases--Treatment. 3. Prostate--Diseases--Diagnosis. I. Xavier, Blake.
RC899 .C55 2023
616.65--dc23

© American Medical Publishers, 2023

American Medical Publishers,
41 Flatbush Avenue,
1st Floor, New York,
NY 11217, USA

ISBN 979-8-88740-004-4 (Hardback)

Contents

Permissions

List of Contributors

Index

Preface

The prostate is a male gland responsible for producing fluid containing the sperm. Prostate diseases are a group of conditions or diseases that affect the prostate gland or its function. There are three major types of prostate diseases, namely, prostatitis, enlarged prostate or benign prostatic hyperplasia (BPH), and prostate cancer. Prostatitis is classified as bacterial prostatitis and non-bacterial prostatitis. Some common symptoms of prostate diseases are painful urination, blood in the urine, and frequent urge to urinate, particularly during the night. The diagnosis of prostate diseases includes physical examination, prostate biopsies, ultrasound scans, blood tests, and mid-stream urine (MSU) tests. Prostatitis treatment varies according to the type of prostatitis. The treatments for prostate cancer include hormone treatment, chemotherapy, ablative treatments and prostatectomy. It consists of medications such as antibacterial drugs and supportive treatments. This book provides a detailed explanation of the clinical perspectives on prostate diseases. It is a vital tool for all researching and studying these diseases.

Various studies have approached the subject by analyzing it with a single perspective, but the present book provides diverse methodologies and techniques to address this field. This book contains theories and applications needed for understanding the subject from different perspectives. The aim is to keep the readers informed about the progresses in the field; therefore, the contributions were carefully examined to compile novel researches by specialists from across the globe.

Indeed, the job of the editor is the most crucial and challenging in compiling all chapters into a single book. In the end, I would extend my sincere thanks to the chapter authors for their profound work. I am also thankful for the support provided by my family and colleagues during the compilation of this book.

Editor

Preoperative predictors of enucleation time during en bloc 'no-touch' holmium laser enucleation of the prostate

Chun-Hsuan Lin[1], Wen-Jeng Wu[1,2,3], Ching-Chia Li[1,2,3] and Sheng-Chen Wen[1,2,3]*

Abstract

Background: To evaluate preoperative predictors of enucleation time during en bloc 'no-touch' holmium laser enucleation of the prostate (HoLEP)

Methods: We enrolled 135 patients with symptomatic benign prostatic hyperplasia (BPH) treated with en bloc 'no-touch' HoLEP from July 2017 to March 2019 by a single surgeon. Preoperative, perioperative, and postoperative clinical variables were examined. Stepwise linear regression was performed to determine clinical variables associated with enucleation times.

Result: The average (range) enucleation time was 46.1 (12–220) minutes, and the overall operation time was 71 (18–250) minutes. History of antiplatelet agents, history of urinary tract infection (UTI), and increasing specimen weight were each significantly associated with increasing enucleation time. No category IV complications were recorded, and all complications were evenly distributed among the groups according to the HoLEP specimen weight.

Conclusion: En bloc 'no-touch' HoLEP was found to be an efficient and reproducible surgical method for treating BPH. Prostatic gland size was significantly associated with increased enucleation times. Similarly, history of UTI and antiplatelet agents were correlated with increased operative time.

Keywords: Holmium laser enucleation of the prostate, Enucleation time, Benign prostatic hyperplasia, En bloc 'no-touch' enucleation, Preoperative predictors

Background

Since the first clinical report on holmium laser enucleation of the prostate (HoLEP) by Gilling et al. [1], multiple randomized controlled trials have been conducted. In many of those trials, compared with open prostatectomy and transurethral resection of the prostate (TURP), HoLEP has been proven to have advantages in size independence and minimal invasiveness for treatment of obstructive symptoms from benign prostatic hyperplasia

(BPH), with excellent long-term results [2–6]. A recent study revealed that the cost to inpatients was lower for HoLEP than for open prostatectomy [7]. Despite having been introduced into clinical operative practice two decades ago, the HoLEP technique is still not as widely applied as it deserves given its proven advantages (low morbidity, minimal invasiveness, size independence, long-term durability) [8–10]. Because of the potentially long operative times and steep learning curve, the first frustrating attempts often deter many endo-urologists from continuing to use this method [11].

The initial description of the HoLEP technique has been repeatedly modified over the past 20 years. More recent studies of en bloc procedures could prove the

*Correspondence: carl0815@gmail.com
[1] Department of Urology, Kaohsiung Medical University Hospital, Kaohsiung Medical University, No. 100, Tzyou 1st Road, Kaohsiung 807, Taiwan
Full list of author information is available at the end of the article

advantages of improving efficiency of enucleation, better visualization on the correct plane, and optimal safety to preserve the sphincter compared to the three-lobe method [18–20]. We started using a holmium laser to reproduce the en bloc 'no-touch' technique reported by Scoffone [18] in enucleation of the prostate at our department in 2015. Performance and efficiency of HoLEP relies on the most critical step: transitional zone enucleation. Enucleation time and efficiency depend on several critical factors, such as tissue quality and prostatic volume. Because of the potentially prolonged operative times and arduous learning curve of en bloc HoLEP, the study aim was to evaluate a time predictive model and identify preoperative predictors of enucleation time during en bloc 'no-touch' HoLEP to improve patient selection.

Methods

Subjects

Between July 2017 and March 2019, 135 consecutive patients who received en bloc 'no-touch' HoLEP by the same experienced surgeon (SCW) were admitted to the Department of Urology, Kaohsiung Medical University Hospital, Kaohsiung, Taiwan. Inclusion criteria were as follows: International Prostate Symptom Score (IPSS) > 8, postvoid residual urine volume (PVR) > 50 mL, maximum urinary flow rate (Q max) < 15 mL/s, or men with BPH that causes acute urinary retention. Exclusion criteria were voiding disorders not associated with BPH or clinical medicine history not recorded.

Study variables and primary outcome

The following factors were analyzed: pre-HoLEP prostate-specific antigen (PSA), age, history of urinary retention requiring Foley catheter, history of 5-alpha-reductase inhibitor (5ARi) use, history of antiplatelet agents with aspirin which not discontinue prior to surgery, history of recurrent urinary tract infections (UTIs) which was defined as urine culture positive more than 3 times in the 3 most recent months without Foley indwelling, prostate volume measured by transrectal ultrasound (TRUS), TURP treatment, and incidental prostatic malignancy in the HoLEP specimen. Patients with the suspicion of prostate carcinoma were ruled out by prostate biopsy if the PSA value or digital rectal examination results were abnormal. All operations were performed by a single surgeon (SCW). Intraoperatively, overall operative time including applied resectoscope until catheter placed, enucleation time, and morcellation time were documented. Enucleation and Morcellation efficiencies were defined as resected adenoma weight divided by enucleation time and morcellation time respectively. The final pathological HoLEP specimen weight was recorded as measured in operation room before sent for formalin

fixation. The clinical perioperative variables were analyzed. The primary outcome was enucleation time.

Description of the procedure

Prostatic adenoma was enucleated by using the en bloc 'no-touch' technique. The equipment used included a 100-W holmium laser (Lumenis, Santa Clara, California), 550-μm end-firing fiber, 26-Fr continuous-flow laser resectoscope (Olympus, Hamburg, Germany), and a morcellator (VersaCut, Lumenis) introduced through the working channel of the Storz nephroscope. The first step was started near the verumontanum by finding the bilateral surgical plane. Then, the surgeon turned laterally and ventrally to make the bilateral plane close to the anterior commissure. The median lobe and the rest of the bilateral lobe were dissected by using a retrograde approach, and then the whole adenoma was lifted. The only remaining connection of the adenoma and prostate capsule was the mucosal strip, which was carefully incised by laser without forceful traction. After meticulous hemostasis by holmium laser was achieved, the prostate adenoma was evacuated by morcellation.

Occasionally, unusually tough and difficult-to-dissect prostatic tissue (termed "beach balls") may be encountered during enucleation, which may prolong the operative time. A 20-Fr 3-way Foley catheter using normal saline for continuous bladder irrigation was inserted at the end of the surgery. Generally, the irrigation fluid flow was gradually tapered down and terminated the morning after the operation. All patients received perioperative antibiotic treatment. After confirming cessation of hematuria, the Foley catheter was removed.

Statistical analyses

General data were analyzed by using descriptive statistics. For the present study we divided excised specimen weight and prostate volume into groups (W: < 15 g, 15–50 g, 50–80 g, > 80 g; V: < 50 mm^3, 50–80 mm^3, > 80 mm^3) and performed ANOVA between groups to determine significant differences at $P < 0.05$. A simple linear regression analysis of enucleation efficiency measures was performed, and the specimen weight and prostate volume were recorded separately. To identify potential predictors of enucleation time, we used a P value of < 0.2 as our criteria for model inclusion, and backward and forward stepwise linear regression models were constructed. All variables in the analysis were included in the initial stepwise linear regression models, and only variables identified as significant ($P < 0.2$) were included in the final presented multiple linear regression models. Prostate weight of < 15 g is used as a reference then dummy variable regression was used between progressive resected specimen weight category in the final presented multiple linear regression models. A P value of < 0.05 was accepted as indicative of statistical significance for the final multiple linear regression models. Analyses were performed by using SPSS version 19.0 (IBM SPSS Statistics for Windows, Version 19.0; IBM Corp., Armonk, NY).

Results

Patient characteristics

A total of 135 patients were enrolled in this retrospective study. The clinical preoperative characteristics of our study pool are shown in Table 1. The median age was 71.7 (47–95) years. Of the 135 patients, 21 (16%) patients had a history of 5ARi use. Fourteen (10.3%) patients presented with catheter-dependent urinary retention. Twelve (9%) patients had a history of recurrent UTI. Thirteen (10%) patients were receiving ongoing antiplatelet treatment (Aspirin).

Perioperative data

Table 2 shows the perioperative data. The median overall operative time was 71 (18–250) min. The median enucleation and morcellation times were 46.1 (12–220) and 13.3 (4–130) min, respectively. The median enucleation and morcellation efficiencies were 0.9 (0.8) and 4.4 (2.6) g/min, respectively. The overall operative efficiency was 0.5 (0.3) g/min. The advantage of the en bloc 'no-touch' technique was especially obvious in large excised adenoma weight that enucleation efficiency increases with large specimen weight (see Fig. 1). Correspondingly, a coherent correlation between prostate volume on TRUS and operation efficiencies was observed.[Pearson's correlation

Table 1 Characteristic of patients undergoing HoLEP

Characteristic	Data
Total patients, n	135
Age (year), mean (SD)	71.7 (9.3)
History of 5ARi use, n (%)	21 (16)
Requiring Foley catheter at the time of HoLEP, n (%)	14 (10.3)
History of UTI, n (%)	12 (9)
History of anticoagulation, n (%)	13 (10)
Pre-HoLEP PSA (ng/mL), mean (range)	6.2 (0.07–1380)
Previous TURP, n (%)	12 (9)
TRUS-P volume (g), mean (SD)	71.1 (42.8)
< 50 ml, n (%)	51 (37.7)
50–80 ml, n (%)	51 (37.7)
> 80 ml, n (%)	33 (24.4)

5ARi 5-alpha-reductase inhibitor, *HoLEP* holmium laser enucleation of the prostate, *PSA* prostate-specific antigen, *SD* standard deviation, *TRUS-P* transrectal ultrasound of the prostate, *UTI* urinary tract infection

Table 2 Enucleation-associated variables

Variable	Value
Enucleation time (min), mean (range)	46.1 (12–220)
Morcellation time (min), mean (range)	13.3 (4–130)
Overall operation time (min), mean (range)	71 (18–250)
Enucleation efficiency (g/min), mean (SD)	0.9 (0.8)
Morcellation efficiency (g/min), mean (SD)	4.4 (2.6)
Overall operation efficiency (g/min), mean (SD)	0.5 (0.3)
HoLEP specimen weight (g)	
< 15 g, n (%)	38 (28.2)
15–50 g, n (%)	63 (47)
50–80 g, n (%)	16 (11.7)
> 80 g, n (%)	18 (12.9)
Beach ball identified, n (%)	19 (14)
Presence of prostate cancer, n (%)	9 (6.6)

coefficient (R) for excised prostate weight = 0.718; R for transrectal PV = 0.603].

Enucleation time

To further predict the enucleation time, we analyzed the factors identified as correlating with enucleation time from the stepwise linear regression models, which were HoLEP specimen weight, history of antiplatelet agents, and history of UTI (Table 3). In the final model, history of antiplatelet agents was associated with a 19-min increase in enucleation time ($P = 0.021$). History of UTI was associated with an estimated 24-min increase in enucleation time ($P = 0.023$). Each progressive resected specimen weight category had obvious increases in enucleation time ranging from 17 to 80 min relative to the enucleation time for a specimen weight of < 15 g (Table 3).

Complications

Table 4 presents detailed information on all treatment modalities and complications that developed during the first 30 postoperative days. Clavien grades 1 and 2 complications developed in eight patients [Clavien grade 1, 11 (8.1%) patients; Clavien grade 2, three (2.2%) patients] including urinary retention after catheter removal (n = 2), clot retention (n = 9), and postoperative hematuria requiring blood transfusion (n = 3). Clavien grade 3b complications developed in one (0.7%) patient who presented with prostate fossa secondary hemorrhage after HoLEP and needed bipolar coagulation.

Discussion

BPH is a common disease in aged men that affects quality of life. In the Baltimore Longitudinal Study of Aging, > 60% of men aged ≥ 60 years have some degree of obstructive symptoms caused by BPH [12]. TURP is

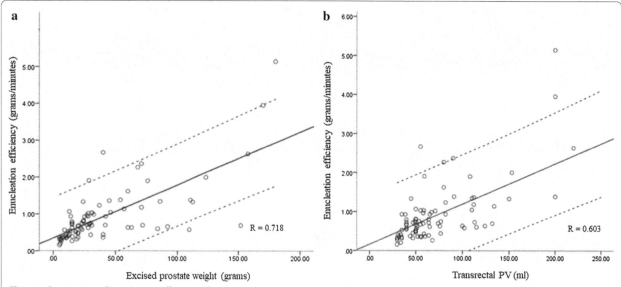

Fig. 1 a Comparison of enucleation efficiency of HoLEP and specimen weight. **b** Comparison of enucleation efficiency of HoLEP and prostate volume. *The 2 parallel lines was 95% CI

Table 3 Predictors of enucleation time from multiple linear regression model

Characteristic	Coefficient (min)	95% CI	P value
History of UTI	24.23	2.48–45.97	.023
History of antiplatelet agents	19.51	− 3.16 to 42.19	.021
HoLEP specimen weight			
<15 g	Reference		
15–50 g	17.28	1.01–33.56	.024
50–80 g	36.37	8.33–64.4	.012
>80 g	80.97	50.66–111.29	<.001
Constant	18.34	4.25–32.43	.011

Other abbreviations as in Table 1. Interpretation of linear regression model: for a patient with a history of UTI and antiplatelet agents, who had a HoLEP specimen weight of 35 g, the estimated enucleation time is 79.36 min (24.23 + 19.51 + 17.28 + 18.34 = 79.36)

CI confidence interval

regarded as the reference standard in the surgical treatment of BPH [13]. Lately, surgical extirpative techniques using lasers, such as holmium and thulium lasers, have been gaining attention as a treatment option for symptomatic BPH. Since Gilling et al. [1] first reported on HoLEP in 1996, it has been proven to be one of the most strictly analyzed surgical treatments for the obstructive symptoms of BPH. More than four randomized controlled trials on this modality have been published [14–17]. More recent descriptions of various approaches to en bloc procedures have been published, mainly to address the goals of improving the effectiveness of enucleation, better visualization on the surgical plane, and optimal safety relative to those of the traditional three-lobe method [18–20]. However, the arduous surgical learning curve and potential long operative times of en bloc HoLEP have been obstacles to its extensive use, despite

Table 4 Detailed analysis of Clavien grade 1–3b complication within the 30-day perioperative period

Complication	Treatment	HoLEP (n = 135)
Clavien grade 1 (n = 11; 8.1%)		
Urinary retention after catheter removal	Bedside recatheterization	2 (1.5)
Clot retention without surgical revision	Tamponade evacuation through catheter	9 (6.7)
Clavien grade 2 (n = 3; 2.2%)		
Postoperative hematuria	Transfusion	3 (2.2)
Clavien grade 3b (n = 1; 0.7%)		
Postoperative hemorrhage	Coagulation of prostate fossa	1 (0.7)

its obvious advantages. Thus, identifying patient groups and tissue characteristics that may increase operative times may help in appropriate patient selection, proper scheduling of the operating room time, and matching the surgeons' experience level to the expected difficulty.

Generally, en bloc 'no-touch' enucleation involves an "outside-in" procedure that starts at the apex and completely uses a Ho:YAG laser to remove the transitional zone of the prostate. Moreover, the Ho:YAG laser in the vaporization procedure is manipulated as a cutting device. Enucleation time significantly depends on visualization, gland size, and recognition of the dissection plane. Enucleated adenoma weight is predicted to largely affect enucleation times. Several previous studies have reported that the HoLEP operative efficiency increases with larger prostate volumes [21, 23]. In our current series, as expected, regardless of enucleated tissue weight or prostate volume on TRUS, the increase in efficiency was shown by a positive slope on the plots of efficiency versus prostate volume.

Giorgio et al. [24] evaluated the effect of chronic inflammation of the prostate and found that patients with a history of chronic prostatic inflammation have an apparent higher risk of retention. Chronic urinary catheterization and recurrent UTI can hypothetically increase prostate inflammation, which may change the natural morphological architecture, increase gland volume, and obscure the natural plane between the prostate capsule and adenoma. These inflamed prostate tissues may also cause bleeding or oozing during surgery, resulting in poorer visualization and more complicated dissection during en bloc 'no-touch' enucleation. In our study, history of UTI history was associated with a 24-min increase in enucleation time (Table 3). However, a Foley in-dwelling catheter at the time of HoLEP was not associated with increased time in the surgical steps of enucleation.

Recent studies have assessed the safety of HoLEP in patients who were taking antiplatelet agents long term and concluded that HoLEP was not a danger to this particular population [25]. This conclusion is expected because the Ho:YAG laser coagulates the bleeding of enucleated tissue with efficiency [8]. We examined whether long-term antiplatelet agents would influence enucleation time and initially hypothesized that because long-term antiplatelet agents could increase bleeding and negatively influence visualization of the operative field, it may increase enucleation time. As expected, our study found that history of long-term chronic antiplatelet agents was related to an apparent increase in enucleation time (Table 3).

Monn. et al. [22] published a retrospective cohort analysis which included a total of 960 patients between 1998 and 2013 illustrating predictor of enucleation and morcellation time during conventional three-lobe HOLEP method. The authors concluded that a history of UTI is associated with an increase in operative time whereas anticoagulation is related to decrease in operative time. The difference impact on the role of antiplatelet agents in surgical time between our present study and the previous published report, in our opinion, is based on difference techniques. The application of en bloc method allows complete adenoma enucleation following surgical capsule at any time, and non-optimal visibility by oozing in patients of long-term antiplatelet agents might lead to increase enucleation time. However, the overall efficiency in the present study (0.5 g/min) indicated no obvious inferior difference compared with earlier randomized clinical trials on the efficiency of retrieval (0.48 g/min) [23]. We believed laminar irrigation between the capsule and enucleated adenoma in en bloc 'no-touch' technique help to maintain visualization throughout the procedure compared with chaotic irrigation in the classic 3-lobe method.

The influence of 5ARi use on prostate tissue quality is known to alter the glandular-to-stromal ratio and reduce the volume of overall glandular tissue [26, 27]. For this reason, hypothetically, long-term 5ARi use might increase the prostate fibrous content, which could lead to more difficult enucleation. However, Sandfeldt et al. [28] found that blood loss volume decreased during TURP after using finasteride for 3 months preoperatively. This might decrease bleeding and positively effect visualization during surgery, leading to a faster enucleation rate. Nevertheless, in our study, we found that history of 5ARi use was not actually related to faster enucleation rate. Warner et al. [29] reported the influence of 5ARi use on HoLEP and found that it did not affect HoLEP operative times or outcomes, which is consistent with our study results. In the current study, we found no clear evidence of a relationship between overall HoLEP surgical time and 5ARi use.

We examined whether presence of "beach ball" and previous TURP would impact enucleation operative time. It is believed that beach balls are easy to enucleate relatively. However, multiple beach balls located diffusely in the peripheral edges of adenoma might cause difficult recognition of the dissection plane, and prolong the operative time. The factor of previous TURP might result in hard to identify the correct plane because of natural anatomical structure undermined. We assumed that each factor mentioned above might have a potential role in the prostatic tissue histological architecture and natural plane. Interestingly, neither previous TURP nor presence of beach ball during surgery had a notable effect on enucleation efficiency. Identification of factors associated with development of these difficult prostate tissues is worth studying in the future. We speculate that because of anticipated concerns regarding the effect of dense tissue or a complicated plane, surgeon's great surgical experience could reduce the effect of difficult recognition of the plane between the capsule and enucleated adenoma on overall operative time.

In the current study, all complications after en bloc 'no-touch' HoLEP were evenly distributed among the groups according to the HoLEP specimen weight. A prospective larger randomized trial of 61 men with prostate sizes of 40–200 g was reported by Tan et al. [14] in which 30 and 31 patients underwent TURP had HoLEP, respectively. This randomized trial reported that mean Foley in-dwelling time and hospital stay were shorter in HoLEP than in TURP. Outcomes and complication rates were similar in both procedures. The above study supports the statement of Kuntz et al. [30] that HoLEP voiding improvement and perioperative morbidity are not based on prostate gland size. There were rather high range of enucleation time(up to 220 min) and morcellation time (up to 130 min) been noted in the present study. Although relative longer operation time, we didn't divided procedure into stages or delayed morcellation, since we believe that this will ultimately accelerate patient recovery. No elevated urethral stricture rate in long operation time group of en bloc 'no-touch' HoLEP. At the time of the study, our en bloc 'no-touch' HoLEP method had been applied for only 1.5 years. Consequently, no long-term follow up data were practicable for interpretation.

This study had some limitations. First, because of its retrospective design, it was intrinsically limited despite inclusion of consecutive patients to avert potential selection bias. Subsequently, we did not consider whether energy usage changed according to the different patient characteristics, but enucleation efficiency may vary depending on the amount of laser energy used. Kim et al. [31] reported a new parameter combining enucleation time and energy consumption to estimate enucleation skills of the operators. It demonstrate that energy consumption decreases as the enucleation technique of a surgeon develops. This trend suggests that as the surgeon's surgical enucleation skill progresses, less energy is used and efficiency is increased. Lastly, surgeries in the study patient group were performed by a single surgeon. Therefore, we recommend that this enucleation time prediction model of en bloc 'no-touch' HoLEP should be examined by multiple surgeons hereafter to determine if it is generally reproducible and acceptable. Despite these limitations, this study examined how preoperative characteristics may affect enucleation times in patients undergoing en bloc 'no-touch' HoLEP for BPH and provided a possible enucleation time prediction model.

Additionally, the study also found that prostate gland size was not associated with increases in complications after HoLEP.

Conclusion

This study showed that the operation time of this technique depends on patient characteristic and prostate size. Aside from adenoma size, a history of UTI and antiplatelet agents were associated with an increase in operative time. This useful enucleation time prediction model and significant information could allow surgeons to schedule suitable surgical times for use of an operating room, choose patients based on their characteristics who are most suitable for the procedure, and match a surgeon's level of experience with the expected degree of surgical difficulty and operative time.

Supplementary information

Additional file 1: Efficacy of holmium laser enucleation of the prostate in patients with a small prostate ($\leq$30 mL).

Abbreviations

BPH: Benign prostatic hyperplasia; PSA: Prostate-specific antigen; TRUS: Transrectal ultrasound; TURP: Transurethral resection of the prostate; UTI: Urinary tract infection; 5ARi: 5-Alpha-reductase inhibitor; HoLEP: Holmium laser enucleation of the prostate; IPSS: International Prostate Symptom Score; PVR: Postvoid residual urine volume; Qmax: Maximum urinary flow rate; PV: Prostate volume.

Acknowledgements

The authors would like to thank everyone who participated in the research and for taking care of the patients.

Authors' contributions

CHL wrote the original draft. WJW performed data curation. CCL was involved in visualization. SCW was responsible for project administration. All authors read and approved the final manuscript.

Author details

[1] Department of Urology, Kaohsiung Medical University Hospital, Kaohsiung Medical University, No. 100, Tzyou 1st Road, Kaohsiung 807, Taiwan. [2] Department of Urology, School of Medicine, College of Medicine, Kaohsiung Medical University, Kaohsiung, Taiwan. [3] Graduate Institute of Clinical Medicine, College of Medicine, Kaohsiung Medical University, Kaohsiung, Taiwan.

References

1. Gilling PJ, et al. Holmium laser resection of the prostate: preliminary results of a new method for the treatment of benign prostatic hyperplasia. Urology. 1996;47:48–51.
2. Naspro R, et al. Holmium laser enucleation of the prostate versus open prostatectomy for prostates > 70 g: 24-month follow-up. Eur Urol. 2006;50:563–8.

3. Salonia A, et al. Holmium laser enucleation versus open prostatectomy for benign prostatic hyperplasia: an inpatient cost analysis. Urology. 2006;68:302–6.
4. Fraundorfer MR, Gilling PJ. Holmium: YAG laser enucleation of the prostate combined with mechanical morcellation: preliminary results. Eur Urol. 1993;33:69–72.
5. Gilling PJ, et al. Long-term results of a randomized trial comparing holmium laser enucleation of the prostate and transurethral resection of the prostate: results at 7 years. BJU Int. 2012;109:408–11.
6. Cornu JN, et al. A systematic review and meta-analysis of functional outcomes and complications following transurethral procedures for lower urinary tract symptoms resulting from benign prostatic obstruction: an update. Eur Urol. 2015;67:1066–96.
7. Kuntz RM, Lehrich K. Ahyai SA Holmium laser enucleation of the prostate versus open prostatectomy for prostates greater than 100 grams: 5-year follow-up results of a randomised clinical trial. Eur Urol. 2008;53:160–8.
8. Krambeck AE, Handa SE, Lingeman JE. Experience with more than 1,000 holmium laser prostate enucleations for benign prostatic hyperplasia. J Urol. 2013;189:S141–5.
9. Dusing MW, et al. Holmium laser enucleation of the prostate: efficiency gained by experience and operative technique. J Urol. 2010;184:635–40.
10. Vavassori I, et al. Three-year outcome following holmium laser enucleation of the prostate combined with mechanical morcellation in 330 consecutive patients. Eur Urol. 2008;53:599–606.
11. Shah HN, et al. Prospective evaluation of the learning curve for holmium laser enucleation of the prostate. J Urol. 2007;177:1468–74.
12. Arrighi HM, et al. Natural history of benign prostatichyperplasia and risk of prostatectomy: the Baltimore Longitudinal Study of Aging. Urology. 1991;38:4–8.
13. Committee APG. AUA guideline on management of benign prostatic hyperplasia. J Urol. 2003;170:530–47.
14. Tan A, et al. A randomized trial comparing holmium laser enucleation of the prostate with transurethral resection of the prostate for the treatment of bladder outlet obstruction secondary to benign prostatic hyperplasia in large glands (40 to 200 grams). J Urol. 2003;170:1270–4.
15. Montorsi F, et al. Holmium laser enucleation versus transurethral resection of the prostate: results from a 2-center, prospective, randomized trial in patients with obstructive benign prostatic hyperplasia. J Urol. 2004;172:1926–9.
16. Kuntz RM, Lehrich K, Ahyai S. Transurethral holmium laser enucleation of the prostate compared with transvesical open prostatectomy: 18-month follow-up of a randomized trial. J Endourol. 2004a;18:189–91.
17. Kuntz RM, et al. Transurethral holmium laser enucleation of the prostate versus transurethral electrocautery resection of the prostate: a randomized prospective trial in 200 patients. J Urol. 2004;172:1012–6.
18. Scoffone CM, Cracco CM. The en-bloc no-touch holmium laser enucleation of the prostate (HoLEP) technique. World J Urol. 2016;34(8):1175–81.
19. Minagawa S, Okada S, Morikawa H. Safety and effectiveness of holmium laser enucleation of the prostate using a lowpower laser. Urology. 2017;110:51–5.
20. Kuo RL, Paterson RF, Kim SC, Siqueira TM Jr, Elhilali MM, Lingeman JE. Holmium laser enucleation of the prostate (HoLEP): a technical update. World J Surg Oncol. 2003;1(1):6.
21. Matlaga BR, et al. Holmium laser enucleation of the prostate for prostates of > 125 mL. BJU Int. 2006;97:81–4.
22. Monn MF, et al. Predictors of enucleation and morcellation time during holmium laser enucleation of the prostate. Urology. 2015;86:338–42.
23. Shah HN, et al. Influence of prostate size on the outcome of holmium laser enucleation of the prostate. BJU Int. 2008;101:1536–41.
24. Gandaglia G, et al. The role of chronic prostatic inflammation in the pathogenesis and progression of benign prostatic hyperplasia (BPH). BJU Int. 2013;112:432–41.
25. Elzayat E, Habib E, Elhilali M. Holmium laser enucleation of the prostate in patients on anticoagulant therapy or with bleeding disorders. J Urol. 2006;175:1428–32.
26. Marks LS, et al. Prostate tissue composition and response to finasteride in men with symptomatic benign prostatic hyperplasia. J Urol. 1997;157:2171–8.
27. Marks LS, et al. Long-term effects of finasteride on prostate tissue composition. Urology. 1999;53:574–80.
28. Sandfeldt L, Bailey DM, Hahn RG. Blood loss during transurethral resection of the prostate after 3 months of treatment with finasteride. Urology. 2001;58:972–6.
29. Warner JN, et al. A multiinstitutional study of the effects of medical therapy for lower urinary symptoms on the perioperative outcomes of holmium laser enucleation of the prostate. Urology. 2011;78:1385–90.
30. Kuntz RM, Lehrich K, Ahyai S. Does perioperative outcome of transurethral holmium laser enucleation of the prostate depend on prostate size? J Endourol. 2004b;18:183–8.
31. Khae HK, et al. Enucleated weight/enucleation time, is it appropriate for estimating enucleation skills for holmium laser enucleation of the prostate? A consideration of energy consumption. World J Mens Health. 2018;36(1):79–86.

2

Facklamia hominis bacteremia after transurethral resection of the prostate

Miriam Gahl[1], Thomas Stöckli[2] and René Fahrner[1]* ⓘ

Abstract

Background: Transurethral resection of the prostate (TUR-P) is one of the most frequent routine procedures in urology. Because of the semisterile environment, postoperative infections, including sepsis, are a common complication, with *Escherichia coli*, *Klebsiella* spp., *Proteus mirabilis* or *Enterococcus faecalis* as frequently isolated pathogens. *Facklamia hominis* is a gram-positive, facultatively anaerobic, alpha-hemolytic, catalase-negative coccus that was first described in 1997. To date, only a few cases of infectious complications have been described. We report the first case of postoperative bacteremia due to *Facklamia hominis* after TUR-P.

Case presentation: An 82-year-old man developed fever only a few hours after elective TUR-P because of benign prostate syndrome. After cultivation of blood cultures, antibiotic therapy with ceftriaxone was intravenously administered and changed to oral cotrimoxazole before discharge of the afebrile patient. One anaerobic blood culture revealed *Facklamia hominis*. Under antibiotic therapy, the patient remained afebrile and showed no signs of infections during follow-up.

Conclusions: Fever and bacteremia are frequent complications after TUR-P. This study is the first report of *Facklamia hominis* in a postoperative blood culture after TUR-P. To date, there are only a few reports of patients with infectious complications and isolation of *Facklamia hominis* in various patient samples. Because *Facklamia hominis* resembles viridans streptococci on blood agar analysis, this pathogen may often be misidentified. In this case identification of *Facklamia hominis* was possible with matrix-assisted laser desorption/ionization time-of-flight mass spectrometry. It has been postulated that *Facklamia hominis* might be a facultative pathogen and that its incidence will increase in the future.

Keywords: Bacteremia, *Facklamia hominis*, Transurethral resection of the prostate, Genital flora

Background

Transurethral resection of the prostate (TUR-P) is one of the most frequent routine procedures in urology. Because of the semisterile environment and continuous rinsing with water, postoperative infections, including sepsis, are a common complication [1, 2]. Despite this

*Correspondence: r.fahrner@web.de
Department of General, Visceral and Thoracic Surgery, Bürgerspital Solothurn, Schöngrünstrasse 42, 4500 Solothurn, Switzerland
Full list of author information is available at the end of the article

fact, prophylactic antibiotics are still controversial, and applied substances vary in regard to the local spectrum of bacteria [1–4]. As a sign of procedural bacteremia, postoperative fever is often encountered early after surgical intervention. The most frequently isolated pathogens are *Escherichia coli*, *Klebsiella* spp., *Proteus mirabilis* and *Enterococcus faecalis*, which are also often detected during simple cystitis [5]. To cover these pathogens, preoperative prophylaxis with a single dose of oral ciprofloxacin is usually given in our department. In a case of postoperative urinary tract infection, daily ceftriaxone is administered intravenously, with a change to oral treatment before discharge. The antibiotic prophylaxis regarding the guidelines of the European Association of Urology should include the local pathogen prevalence and might thus differ from center to center [6].

To the best of our knowledge, we present the first case of *Facklamia hominis* bacteremia during the postoperative course after urological surgery.

Case presentation

An 82-year-old man underwent elective TUR-P because of a symptomatic benign prostate syndrome. Preoperatively, no urinary sample was analyzed regarding bacterial colonization. He had a past history of cerebrovascular insult with minimal residuals, curative surgery for an adenocarcinoma of the rectum and cervical discus hernia. In addition, he suffered from hypertensive cardiopathy with a normal ejection fraction.

One hour after an uneventful operation, he developed chills that were successfully treated with pethidine. Three hours later, he developed a fever up to 38.7 °C so that two pairs of blood cultures were taken before initiating intravenous antibiotic therapy with ceftriaxone. Because of postoperative continuous rinsing of the bladder, it was impossible to cultivate the urine. The further course was uneventful, the patient remained afebrile and was in good condition so that the antibiotic therapy was changed to oral cotrimoxazole, and the patient was discharged. To our surprise, one out of four blood cultures turned positive for *Facklamia hominis* after the discharge of the patient. As the patient remained afebrile and in good clinical condition under the current antibiotic treatment, the therapy was continued for 14 days, although cotrimoxazole has not been described as a therapy so far. During 6 months of follow-up, the patient did not develop fever or signs of an urinary tract infection and had no need for antibiotic therapy again. During follow-up, there

were urine and blood cultures without detection of *Facklamia hominis*.

Discussion and conclusions

In our case, bacteremia with *Facklamia hominis* was detected in blood cultures of a patient after TUR-P only a few hours after the intervention. *Facklamia hominis* is a gram-positive, facultative anaerobic, alpha-hemolytic, catalase-negative coccus [7]. It was first described in 1997 [8], and for six clinical isolates, previously nonclassified cocci were characterized by phenotypic and phylogenetic methods as *Facklamia hominis* [9]. Since then, *Facklamia hominis* has been isolated in several specimens, such as urine, vaginal swabs, abscesses, joints, mitral valves, placentas, gastric aspirates, cerebrospinal fluid, preputial swabs, and blood [10–15]. Moreover, *Facklamia hominis* is thought to be a resident of the bacterial flora of the vaginal and urinary tracts [14]. Interestingly, *Facklamia hominis* has been so far isolated predominantly from females. In total, 16 cases of *Facklamia hominis* infections have been reported worldwide (Table 1). Furthermore, five other species of the genus Facklamia have been described, namely, *Facklamia ignava* [17], *Facklamia sourekii* [18], *Facklamia languida* [19], *Facklamia miroungii* [20] and *Facklamia tabaciasalis* [21]. Except for *Facklamia tabaciasalis* [21] and *Facklamia miroungii* [20], all Facklamia species have been isolated from human clinical specimens. It is postulated that, as *Facklamia* spp. resemble viridans streptococci on 5% sheep blood agar, they might have been confounded in the past with this group of organisms [9, 16].

This study is the first case reported with *Facklamia hominis* bacteremia after TUR-P. There have been reports about isolations from patients with abscesses, joint infections, endocarditis with positive blood cultures, cerebrospinal fluid, urine and vaginal swabs (Table 1). It has been postulated that *Facklamia*

Table 1 Overview of *Facklamia hominis* infections in the current literature

Author	Year	Number of patients	Type of sample	Outcome
Collins [8]	1997	6	Urine, vaginal swab, blood, abscess	Not reported
Healy [10]	2005	2	Blood, placental tissue, gastric aspirate	Cured
Safavi [11]	2010	1	Blood	Died
Ananthakrishna [16]	2012	1	Blood	Cured
Corona [7]	2014	1	Joint	Cured
Parvataneni [9]	2015	1	Cerebrospinal fluid	Cured
Abat [15]	2016	1	Abscess	Not reported
Schlipkoter [12]	2017	1	Abscess	Cured
Gomez-Luque [13]	2019	1	Preputial swab	Cured
Mostafa [14]	2019	1	Urine	Cured

hominis might be a resident of the vaginal and urinary tract floras and a facultative pathogen inducing urinary tract infections [14]. In the reported case, the source of *Facklamia hominis* is speculative and might be displaced during surgery from the urinary tract or urine. Furthermore, the prostate might be colonized, but microscopy of the surgical tissue failed to detect large amount of bacteria. Fever or infections after TUR-P are frequently seen complications, as the intervention is semisterile, and microorganisms located within the urinary tract are often opportunistic. These facultative pathogens are common sources of postoperative bacteremia or urinary tract infections [1, 2]. Accordingly, it is not surprising that *Facklamia hominis* was now isolated in blood cultures after TUR-P. The treatment includes immediate antibiotic therapy depending on the prevalent resistance pattern after cultivation of blood and urine. To obtain an optimal antibiotic therapy, the isolation of the underlying pathogens is mandatory.

Traditional microbiological methods are often ineffective in correctly detecting pathogens such as *Facklamia hominis* [15]. Current methods of identification include matrix-assisted laser desorption/ionization time-of-flight mass spectrometry (MALDI-TOF) [13, 15], genome sequencing [14], rRNA PCR [7], VITEK 2 system [9, 16] and characterization by the API Rapid ID32 and API ZYM method [8]. Comparable to previous reports, in our case, *Facklamia hominis* was detected by MALDI-TOF.

Several treatment regimens have been described so far. They include penicillin derivatives, beta-lactamase inhibitors, metronidazole, cephalosporins, carbapenems, aminoglycosides, and glycopeptide antibiotics [7, 10–12, 16]. In our case, the intravenous treatment with ceftriaxone for 3 days and cotrimoxazole for a total of 14 days was successful. Whether the intravenous administration of ceftriaxone alone would have been sufficient as treatment is unclear. However, the patient rapidly recovered and remained afebrile without signs of bloodstream or urinary tract infection.

It is possible that due to the morphologic resemblance to viridans streptococci and ineffectiveness of traditional microbiological testing, *Facklamia hominis* has probably been often misdiagnosed in the past [15]. Whether *Facklamia hominis* will be an emerging pathogen in the future needs to be confirmed, but additional reports on antibiotic therapy are needed.

Abbreviations

C: Celcius; MALDI-TOF: Matrix-assisted laser desorption/ionization time-of-flight mass spectrometry; spp.: species; TUR-P: Transurethral resection of the prostate.

Acknowledgements

Not applicable for this study.

Authors' contributions

Study conception and design: M. G., T. S., and R. F. Acquisition of data: M. G., T. S., and R. F. Analysis and interpretation of data: M. G., T. S., and R. F. Drafting of manuscript: M. G., and R. F. Critical revision of manuscript: T. S. All authors have read and approved the final version of this manuscript.

Author details

[1] Department of General, Visceral and Thoracic Surgery, Bürgerspital Solothurn, Schöngrünstrasse 42, 4500 Solothurn, Switzerland. [2] Department of Internal Medicine, Bürgerspital Solothurn, Schöngrünstrasse 42, 4500 Solothurn, Switzerland.

References

1. Schneidewind L, Kranz J, Schlager D, Barski D, Muhlsteadt S, Grabbert M, Queissert F, Frank T, Pelzer AE. Mulitcenter study on antibiotic prophylaxis, infectious complications and risk assessment in TUR-P. Central Eur J Urol. 2017;70(1):112–7.
2. Wagenlehner FM, Wagenlehner C, Schinzel S, Naber KG, Working group "urological infections" of German Society of U. Prospective, randomized, multicentric, open, comparative study on the efficacy of a prophylactic single dose of 500 mg levofloxacin versus 1920 mg trimethoprim/sulfamethoxazole versus a control group in patients undergoing TUR of the prostate. Eur Urol. 2005;47(4):549–56.
3. Schmiedl S, Thurmann PA, Roth S. Antibiotic prophylaxis for patients with transurethral resection of the prostate (TUR-P). Der Urol Ausg A. 2009;48(1):66–72.
4. Berry A, Barratt A. Prophylactic antibiotic use in transurethral prostatic resection: a meta-analysis. J Urol. 2002;167(2 Pt 1):571–7.
5. Hautmann R, Gschwend JE. Urologie. Springer Medizin Verlag. 2014. https://doi.org/10.1007/978-3-642-34319-3.
6. https://uroweb.org/guideline/urological-infections/. Accessed 07 Nov 2020.
7. Corona PS, Haddad S, Andres J, Gonzalez-Lopez JJ, Amat C, Flores X. Case report: first report of a prosthetic joint infection caused by Facklamia hominis. Diagn Microbiol Infect Dis. 2014;80(4):338–40.
8. Collins MD, Falsen E, Lemozy J, Akervall E, Sjoden B, Lawson PA. Phenotypic and phylogenetic characterization of some Globicatella-like organisms from human sources: description of Facklamia hominis gen. Nov., sp. nov. Int J Syst Bacteriol. 1997;47(3):880–2.
9. Parvataneni KC, Iyer S, Khatib R, Saravolatz LD. Facklamia Species and *Streptococcus pneumoniae* Meningitis: A Case Report and Review of the Literature. Open forum Infect Dis. 2015;2(2):ofv029.
10. Healy B, Beukenholt RW, Tuthill D, Ribeiro CD. Facklamia hominis causing chorioamnionitis and puerperal bacteraemia. J Infect. 2005;50(4):353–5.
11. Safavi S, Tufnell M, Bhalla A. Multi-territory ischaemic strokes and subacute bacterial endocarditis. BMJ Case Rep. 2010;2010.
12. Schlipkoter M, Grieser T, Forst H. Unusual complication following placement of an epidural catheter. Anaesthesist. 2017;66(7):506–10.
13. Gomez-Luque JM, Foronda-Garcia-Hidalgo C, Gutierrez-Fernandez J. Balanopostitis by Facklamia hominis in pediatrics. Revista espanola de quimioterapia. 2019;32(3):278–80.
14. Mostafa HH, Taffner SM, Wang J, Malek A, Hardy DJ, Pecora ND. Genome sequence of a Facklamia hominis isolate from a patient with Urosepsis. Microbiol Resource Announcements. 2019;8(17).
15. Abat C, Garcia V, Rolain JM. Facklamia hominis scapula abscess, Marseille, France. New Microbes New Infect. 2016;9:13–4.
16. Ananthakrishna R, Shankarappa RK, Jagadeesan N, Math RS, Karur S, Nanjappa MC. Infective endocarditis: a rare organism in an uncommon setting. Case Rep Infect Dis. 2012;2012:307852.
17. Collins MD, Lawson PA, Monasterio R, Falsen E, Sjoden B, Facklam RR. Facklamia ignava sp. nov., isolated from human clinical specimens. J Clin Microbiol. 1998;36(7):2146–8.
18. Collins MD, Hutson RA, Falsen E, Sjoden B. Facklamia sourekii sp. nov., isolated from human sources. Int J Syst Bacteriol. 1999;49(Pt 2):635–8.
19. Lawson PA, Collins MD, Falsen E, Sjoden B, Facklam RR. Facklamia languida sp. nov., isolated from human clinical specimens. J Clin Microbiol. 1999;37(4):1161–4.

20. Hoyles L, Foster G, Falsen E, Thomson LF, Collins MD. Facklamia miroun-
    gae sp. nov., from a juvenile southern elephant seal (Mirounga leonina).
    Int J Syst Evol Microbiol. 2001;51(Pt 4):1401–3.
21. Collins MD, Hutson RA, Falsen E, Sjoden B. Facklamia tabacinasalis sp. nov.,
    from powdered tobacco. Int J Syst Bacteriol. 1999;49(Pt 3):1247–50.

3

The use of hyperbaric oxygen to treat actinic rectal fistula after SpaceOAR use and radiotherapy for prostate cancer

Tairo Kashihara[1]*[iD], Koji Inaba[1], Motokiyo Komiyama[2], Hiroki Nakayama[1], Kotaro Iijima[1], Shie Nishioka[1], Hiroyuki Okamoto[1], Nao Kikkawa[3], Yuko Kubo[3], Satoshi Shima[1], Satoshi Nakamura[1], Ayaka Takahashi[1], Kana Takahashi[1], Kae Okuma[1], Naoya Murakami[1], Hiroshi Igaki[1], Yuko Nakayama[1], Arinobu Fukunaga[2], Yoshiyuki Matsui[2], Hiroyuki Fujimoto[2] and Jun Itami[1]

Abstract

Background: In definitive radiation therapy for prostate cancer, the SpaceOAR® System, a hydrogel spacer, is widely used to decrease the irradiated dose and toxicity of rectum. On the other hand, periprostatic abscesses formation and rectal perforation are known as rare adverse effects of SpaceOAR. Nevertheless, there is a lack of reports clarifying the association between aggravation of abscesses and radiation therapy, and hyperbaric oxygen therapy (HBOT) is effective for a peri-SpaceOAR abscess and rectal perforation.

Case presentation: We report a case of a 78-year-old high-risk prostate cancer patient. After SpaceOAR insertion into the correct space, he started to receive external beam radiation therapy (EBRT). He developed a fever, perineal pain and frequent urination after the completion of EBRT, and the magnetic resonance imaging (MRI) revealed a peri-SpaceOAR abscess. Scheduled brachytherapy was postponed, administration of antibiotics and opioid via intravenous drip was commenced, and transperineal drainage was performed. After the alleviation of the abscess, additional EBRT instead of brachytherapy was performed with MRI-guided radiation therapy (MRgRT). On the last day of the MRgRT, perineal pain reoccurred, and MRI and colonoscopy detected the rectal perforation. He received an intravenous antibiotics drip and HBOT, and fully recovered from the rectal perforation.

Conclusions: Our report indicates that EBRT can lead to a severe rectum complication by causing inflammation for patients with a peri-SpaceOAR abscess. Furthermore, HBOT was effective for the peri-SpaceOAR abscess and rectal perforation associated with EBRT.

Keywords: Radiotherapy, Hydrogel spacer, Side effects, Hyperbaric oxygen therapy, MR-guided radiation therapy

*Correspondence: tkashiha@ncc.go.jp
[1] Department of Radiation Therapy, National Cancer Center Hospital, Tsukiji 5-1-1, Chuo-ku, Tokyo, Japan
Full list of author information is available at the end of the article

Background

A hydrogel spacer is used in radiation therapy (RT) for a variety of cancers to decrease the irradiated dose to the organs at risk (OARs) [1–5]. Furthermore, in pelvic radiation therapy, a hydrogel spacer is used to decrease the rectal dose [6–9]. In definitive RT for prostate cancer, The SpaceOAR® System (Boston Scientific, Marlborough,

MA, USA), a hydrogel spacer, is widely used to decrease the rectal dose and toxicity [10, 11]. A prospective randomised study revealed that insertion of SpaceOAR significantly reduced the rectal dose and toxicity and improved bowel/urinary quality of life [12–14]. On the other hand, a patient who developed periprostatic abscess formation after SpaceOAR insertion was reported [15]; however, it was not clear whether SpaceOAR insertion was successful, although the infection improved after percutaneous drainage. Periprostatic abscess is a rare adverse effect of SpaceOAR, and the association between aggravation of abscesses and radiotherapy has not been clarified. Furthermore, the effectiveness of hyperbaric oxygen therapy (HBOT) for peri-SpaceOAR has not been reported. Here, we have presented a case of rectal perforation after peri-SpaceOAR abscess that was successfully treated with HBOT.

Case presentation

The patient was a 78-year-old prostate cancer patient who had no medical history, except surgical history of goiter and nasal haemangioma. A prostate-specific antigen (PSA) level was 13.89 ng/mL in a routine evaluation. The clinical stage was T3a. Ultrasound-guided transperineal prostate biopsy revealed Grade Group 4 adenocarcinoma in 1 of 24 specimens. Two months after the biopsy, administration of a luteinizing hormone-releasing hormone agonist was initiated. He opted for external beam RT (EBRT) 46 Gy in 23 fractions combined with high-dose-rate (HDR) brachytherapy 15 Gy in 1 fraction as a definitive treatment. Four months after initiating hormone therapy, SpaceOAR was inserted into the space between the prostate and the rectum, and fiducial markers were inserted into the prostate under local

anaesthesia with lidocaine (day 0). The insertion was completed without any side effects, and magnetic resonance imaging (MRI) confirmed that the SpaceOAR was inserted in the correct position (Fig. 1, left). Three weeks after inserting SpaceOAR (day 21), EBRT with computed tomography linear accelerator was initiated. The clinical target volume (CTV) included the prostate, all seminal vesicles, and whole pelvic lymph node regions. The planning target volume (PTV) margin of the whole pelvis was 3 mm, 7 mm, and 8 mm in the RL, SI, and AP directions, respectively. Six days after initiating EBRT (day 27), he developed perineal pain. Owing to increased perineal pain and a diagnosis of urinary tract infection on day 40, antibiotic treatment was initiated. Perineal pain gradually subsided, and he completed oral antibiotic treatment in 1 week (day 47). Four days later (day 51), he experienced perineal pain and frequent urination again; hence, antibiotic treatment was reinitiated. On day 60, oral administration of opioids was initiated due to increasing perineal pain. The next day (day 61), he developed high fever; thus, MRI was performed for detailed examination. A peri-SpaceOAR abscess was detected on MRI (Fig. 1, middle). Thus, HDR brachytherapy was postponed, administration of antibiotics and opioids via intravenous drip was initiated, and transperineal drainage was performed. Subsequently, the pain gradually subsided and the abscess shrunk slightly on MRI; therefore, intravenous administration of antibiotics changed to oral administration (day 76). Three weeks later (day 97), shrinkage of the abscess and decrease in inflammatory response were confirmed by MRI. Therefore, on day 112, additional RT was initiated. At our conference, EBRT of 20 Gy in 4 fractions was recommended as additional RT instead of HDR monotherapy to decrease the dose

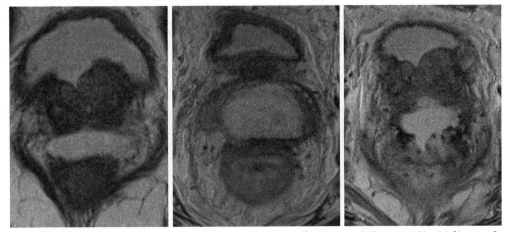

Fig. 1 The changes of MRI findings after the SpaceOAR insertion. MRI taken 1 week after the SpaceOAR insertion (day 7, left). A peri-SpaceOAR abscess (day 61, middle) and a rectal perforation were detected on MRI (day 120, right)

per fraction. Magnetic resonance-guided RT (MRgRT) with ^{60}Co MRIdian under a magnetic field of 0.345 T (ViewRay MRIdian System, Oakwood Village, OH) was selected to accurately assess intrafractional and interfractional motion of the prostate, seminal vesicles, and OARs (rectum and bladder). The CTV included the prostate and seminal vesicles. The PTV margin was 5 mm, 4 mm, and 3 mm in the RL, SI, and AP directions, respectively. On the last day of MRgRT (day 119), he experienced perineal pain again, and MRI was performed. MRI on day 120 showed aggravated peri-SpaceOAR inflammation and penetration to the rectum was suspected (Fig. 1, right). Colonoscopy was subsequently performed, and penetration of SpaceOAR into the rectum was detected (Fig. 2). To treat rectal perforation, he was kept nothing per os and administration of antibiotics via intravenous drip and intravenous hyperalimentation initiated. He was also transferred to another hospital for HBOT (day 131). HBOT was initiated on day 131. After 24 HBOT sessions for 5 weeks, recovery from rectal perforation was confirmed by colonoscopy, and administration of antibiotics was discontinued. Ten weeks after termination of HBOT, disappearance of a peri-SpaceOAR abscess was confirmed on MRI (day 243).

Discussion and conclusions

A 78-year-old patient with prostate cancer developed rectal perforation caused by a peri-SpaceOAR abscess and MRgRT (cured by HBOT). To the best of our knowledge, this is the first report showing that HBOT was effective for rectal perforation associated with a peri-SpaceOAR abscess.

Radiotherapy is one of the most significant treatment modalities in prostate cancer [16–18]. The National Comprehensive Cancer Network guidelines recommend EBRT + androgen deprivation therapy (ADT) and EBRT + brachytherapy + ADT for the treatment of high-risk prostate cancer [19]. Our patient was scheduled to receive EBRT + HDR brachytherapy + ADT. However, the treatment plan was changed to EBRT + ADT because HDR brachytherapy could cause infection [20] and a large dose per fraction could cause strong inflammation. Furthermore, MRgRT was selected because of its several potential advantages. Murray J et al. [21] reported three advantages of MRgRT—improvement in prostate visibility, monitoring of intrafractional prostate position, and daily adaptive replanning. Owing to these advantages, the margin size of MRgRT in our patient was smaller than that of CT-based RT, as mentioned above.

Radiation-induced intestinal side effects such as bleeding and ulcer are occasionally observed [22–24], but rectal perforation associated with RT is rarely observed. A case of rectal ulceration due to insertion of SpaceOAR into the anterior rectal wall was reported by Teh et al. [25]. However, in our case, SpaceOAR was inserted into the correct space between the prostate and the rectum, confirmed by MRI. A peri-prostate abscess is a rare side effect of SpaceOAR [15]. In our study, after improvement of the peri-SpaceOAR abscess, rectal perforation was detected after EBRT. Rectal perforation could have been caused by not only a peri-SpaceOAR abscess but also inflammation due to EBRT.

HBOT has been reported to be effective for the treatment of abscesses [26–29]. In addition, HBOT is also reported to be effective for the treatment of RT side effects [30–34]. We, therefore, recommended HBOT for the treatment of peri-SpaceOAR abscess and radiation-induced rectal perforation.

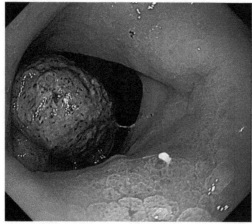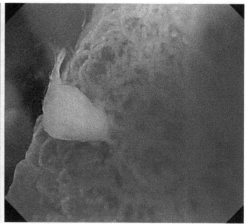

Fig. 2 SpaceOAR penetration into rectum wall detected by colonoscopy. After the penetration of peri-SpaceOAR abscess into rectum wall was suspected on MRI, colonoscopy was performed. SpaceOAR penetrating rectum wall was detected on colonoscopy

The exacerbation of peri-SpaceOAR abscess and rectal perforation occurred after the resumption of radiotherapy in our patient, but the abscess and rectal perforation resolved after initiating HBOT. The resumption of radiotherapy probably caused decreased blood flow and increased hypoxia, which could reduce endothelial progenitor cell (EPC) homing to the injured rectum area. However, HBOT is known to facilitate EPC trafficking/homing, thereby promoting wound repair due to angiogenesis [35, 36]. In addition, HBOT elevates hypoxia inducible factor (HIF)-1 and HIF-2 levels in vasculogenic stem/progenitor cells due to increases in reactive oxygen species [36], and this mechanism would also facilitate neovascularization. Furthermore, increasing the oxygen partial pressure can inhibit the growth of anaerobic bacteria and control the infection. HBOT may have helped our patient recover from the abscess and rectal perforation by these mechanisms.

In the management of radiation-induced haemorrhagic cystitis, early initiation of HBOT has been reported to lead to better outcomes [37]. In this previous report, HBOT within 6 months from the onset of haematuria resulted in a better response rate. In our patient, HBOT was initiated within 4 months from the onset of perineal pain, and within 2 weeks from the onset of rectal perforation. It was feared that HBOT had a cancer-promoting effect and enhanced tumour progression. However, three review articles [38–40] have reported that HBOT does not promote cancer growth. Hence, HBOT was a good treatment option in our case.

Our case report indicates that EBRT can lead to severe rectal complications by causing inflammation in patients with a peri-SpaceOAR abscess. Furthermore, it indicates that HBOT is effective for the treatment of peri-SpaceOAR abscess and rectal perforation associated with EBRT.

Abbreviations

ADT: Androgen deprivation therapy; CT: Computed tomographic; CTV: Clinical target volume; EBRT: External beam radiation therapy; HBOT: Hyperbaric oxygen therapy; HDR: High-dose-rate; HIF: Hypoxia inducible factors; LHRH: Leutinizing hormone-releasing hormone; MRgRT: Magnetic resonance imaging-guided radiation therapy; MRI: Magnetic resonance imaging; NCCN: National Comprehensive Cancer Network; OAR: Organ at risk; PTV: Planning target volume; PSA: Prostate-specific antigen; RT: Radiation therapy.

Acknowledgements

We would like to thank Editage (www.editage.jp) for English language editing.

Authors' contributions

Conception and design of the work: TK, KI, MK, HN, KI, SN, HO, NK, YK, SS, SN, AT, KT, KO, NM, HI, YN, AF, YM, HF, JI. Supervision and wrote the paper: TK. All authors read and approved the final manuscript.

Author details

[1] Department of Radiation Therapy, National Cancer Center Hospital, Tsukiji 5-1-1, Chuo-ku, Tokyo, Japan. [2] Department of Urological Oncology, National Cancer Center Hospital, Tokyo, Japan. [3] Department of Radiology, National Cancer Center Hospital, Tokyo, Japan.

References

1. Feng Z, Rao AD, Cheng Z, et al. Dose prediction model for duodenum sparing with a biodegradable hydrogel spacer for pancreatic cancer radiation therapy. Int J Radiat Oncol Biol Phys. 2018;102(3):651–9.
2. Rao AD, Feng Z, Shin EJ, et al. A novel absorbable radiopaque hydrogel spacer to separate the head of the pancreas and duodenum in radiation therapy for pancreatic cancer. Int J Radiat Oncol Biol Phys. 2017;99(5):1111–20.
3. Kerdsirichairat T, Narang AK, Thompson E, et al. Feasibility of using hydrogel spacers for borderline-resectable and locally advanced pancreatic tumors. Gastroenterology. 2019;157(4):933–5.
4. Struik GM, Pignol JP, Kolkman-Deurloo IK, et al. Subcutaneous spacer injection to reduce skin toxicity in breast brachytherapy: a pilot study on mastectomy specimens. Brachytherapy. 2019;18(2):204–10.
5. Rao AD, Coquia S, De Jong R, et al. Effects of biodegradable hydrogel spacer injection on contralateral submandibular gland sparing in radiotherapy for head and neck cancers. Radiother Oncol. 2018;126(1):96–9.
6. Trifiletti DM, Garda AE, Showalter TN. Implanted spacer approaches for pelvic radiation therapy. Expert Rev Med Devices. 2016;13(7):633–40.
7. Kashihara T, Murakami N, Tselis N, et al. Hyaluronate gel injection for rectum dose reduction in gynecologic high-dose-rate brachytherapy: initial Japanese experience. J Radiat Res. 2019;60(4):501–8.
8. Murakami N, Shima S, Kashihara T, et al. Hyaluronic gel injection into the vesicovaginal septum for high-dose-rate brachytherapy of uterine cervical cancer: an effective approach for bladder dose reduction. J Contemp Brachyther. 2019;11(1):1–7.
9. Murakami N, Nakamura S, Kashihara T, et al. Hyaluronic acid gel injection in rectovaginal septum reduced incidence of rectal bleeding in brachytherapy for gynecological malignancies. Brachytherapy. 2020;19(2):154–61.
10. Hwang ME, Mayeda M, Liz M, et al. Stereotactic body radiotherapy with periprostatic hydrogel spacer for localized prostate cancer: toxicity profile and early oncologic outcomes. Radiat Oncol. 2019;14(1):136.
11. Wu SY, Boreta L, Wu A, et al. Improved rectal dosimetry with the use of SpaceOAR during high-dose-rate brachytherapy. Brachytherapy. 2018;17(2):259–64.
12. Mariados N, Sylvester J, Shah D, et al. Hydrogel spacer prospective multicenter randomized controlled pivotal trial: dosimetric and clinical effects of perirectal spacer application in men undergoing prostate image guided intensity modulated radiation therapy. Int J Radiat Oncol Biol Phys. 2015;92(5):971–7.
13. Hamstra DA, Mariados N, Sylvester J, et al. Continued benefit to rectal separation for prostate radiation therapy: final results of a phase III trial. Int J Radiat Oncol Biol Phys. 2017;97(5):976–85.
14. Shaikh T, Li T, Handorf EA, et al. Long-term patient-reported outcomes from a phase 3 randomized prospective trial of conventional versus hypofractionated radiation therapy for localized prostate cancer. Int J Radiat Oncol Biol Phys. 2017;97(4):722–31.
15. Hoe V, Yao HH, Huang JG, et al. Abscess formation following hydrogel spacer for prostate cancer radiotherapy: a rare complication. BMJ Case Rep. 2019;12(10):e229143.
16. D'Amico AV, Whittington R, Malkowicz SB, et al. Biochemical outcome after radical prostatectomy, external beam radiation therapy, or interstitial radiation therapy for clinically localized prostate cancer. JAMA. 1998;280(11):969–74.
17. Parker CC, James ND, Brawley CD, et al. Radiotherapy to the primary tumour for newly diagnosed, metastatic prostate cancer (STAMPEDE): A randomised controlled phase 3 trial. Lancet. 2018;392(10162):2353–66.
18. Kashihara T, Nakamura S, Wakita A, et al. Importance of the site of positive surgical margin in salvage external beam radiation therapy for biochemical recurrence of prostate cancer after radical prostatectomy. Cancer Med. 2018;7(5):1723–30.
19. Mohler JL, Antonarakis ES, Armstrong AJ, et al. Prostate Cancer, Version 2.2019, NCCN clinical practice guidelines in oncology. J Natl Compr Cancer Netw. 2019;17(5):479–505.

20. Emory CL, Montgomery CO, Potter BK, et al. Early complications of high-dose-rate brachytherapy in soft tissue sarcoma: a comparison with traditional external-beam radiotherapy. Clin Orthop Relat Res. 2012;470(3):751–8.

21. Murray J, Tree AC. Prostate cancer—advantages and disadvantages of MR-guided RT. Clin Transl Radiat Oncol. 2019;18:68–73.

22. Fuccio L, Guido A, Andreyev HJ. Management of intestinal complications in patients with pelvic radiation disease. Clin Gastroenterol Hepatol. 2012;10(12):1326–34.

23. Kashihara T, Murakami N, Iizumi S, et al. Hemorrhage from ascending colon and gluteal muscle associated with Sorafenib and radiation therapy: radiation dose distribution corresponded with colonoscopy findings and computed tomography images. Pract Radiat Oncol. 2019;9(4):214–9.

24. Weiner JP, Wong AT, Schwartz D, et al. Endoscopic and non-endoscopic approaches for the management of radiation-induced rectal bleeding. World J Gastroenterol. 2016;22(31):6972–86.

25. Teh AY, Ko HT, Barr G, et al. Rectal ulcer associated with SpaceOAR hydrogel insertion during prostate brachytherapy. BMJ Case Rep. 2014;2014:bcr2014206931.

26. Sahin A, Kilic M, Dalgic N. A case report of a 4-year-old boy with intradural spinal cord abscess successfully treated with adjuvant hyperbaric oxygen therapy. Turk Neurosurg. 2019;29(5):789–92.

27. Kutlay M, Colak A, Yildiz S, et al. Stereotactic aspiration and antibiotic treatment combined with hyperbaric oxygen therapy in the management of bacterial brain abscesses. Neurosurgery. 2008;62(Suppl 2):540–6.

28. Cimşit M, Uzun G, Yildiz S. Hyperbaric oxygen therapy as an anti-infective agent. Expert Rev Anti Infect Ther. 2009;7(8):1015–26.

29. Ciodaro F, Gazia F, Galletti B, et al. Hyperbaric oxygen therapy in a case of cervical abscess extending to anterior mediastinum, with isolation of Prevotella corporis. BMJ Case Rep. 2019;12(7):e229873.

30. Hartmann A, Almeling M, Carl UM. Hyperbaric oxygenation (HBO) in the treatment of radiogenic side effects. Strahlenther Onkol. 1996;172(12):641–8.

31. Peusch-Dreyer D, Dreyer KH, Müller CD, et al. Management of postoperative radiation injury of the urinary bladder by hyperbaric oxygen (HBO). Strahlenther Onkol. 1998;174(Suppl 3):99–100.

32. Corman JM, McClure D, Pritchett R, et al. Treatment of radiation induced hemorrhagic cystitis with hyperbaric oxygen. J Urol. 2003;169(6):2200–2.

33. Cardinal J, Slade A, McFarland M, et al. Scoping review and meta-analysis of hyperbaric oxygen therapy for radiation-induced hemorrhagic cystitis. Curr Urol Rep. 2018;19(6):38.

34. Ashamalla HL, Thom SR, Goldwein JW. Hyperbaric oxygen therapy for the treatment of radiation-induced sequelae in children. Univ Pa Exp Cancer. 1996;77(11):2407–12.

35. Hsu SL, Yin TC, Shao PL, et al. Hyperbaric oxygen facilitates the effect of endothelial progenitor cell therapy on improving outcome of rat critical limb ischemia. Am J Transl Res. 2019;11(4):1948–64.

36. Thom SR. Hyperbaric oxygen—its mechanisms and efficacy. Plast Reconstr Surg. 2011;127(Suppl 1):131S-141S.

37. Chong KT, Hampson NB, Corman JM. Early hyperbaric oxygen therapy improves outcome for radiation-induced hemorrhagic cystitis. Urology. 2005;65(4):649–53.

38. Feldmeier J, Carl U, Hartmann K, et al. Hyperbaric oxygen: does it promote growth or recurrence of malignancy? Undersea Hyperb Med. 2003;30:1–18.

39. Daruwalla J, Christophi C. Hyperbaric oxygen therapy for malignancy: a review. World J Surg. 2006;30:2112–31.

40. Moen I, Stuhr LE. Hyperbaric oxygen therapy and cancer—a review. Target Oncol. 2012;7(4):233–42.

4

Dermatomyositis associated with prostate adenocarcinoma with neuroendocrine differentiation

Hideyuki Minagawa[1,2], Taketo Kawai[2*], Akihiko Matsumoto[2], Katsuhiro Makino[1,2], Yusuke Sato[2], Kenji Nagasaka[3], Masami Tokura[3], Nao Tanaka[3], Eisaku Ito[4], Yuta Yamada[2], Masaki Nakamura[2], Daisuke Yamada[2], Motofumi Suzuki[2], Takashi Murata[1] and Haruki Kume[2]

Abstract

Background: Although it is known that malignancies can be associated with dermatomyositis, there are few reports on dermatomyositis associated with prostate cancer with neuroendocrine differentiation.

Case presentation: A 63-year-old man visited our hospital due to pollakiuria. High levels of PSA and NSE were observed, and prostate biopsy revealed an adenocarcinoma with neuroendocrine differentiation. Multiple metastases to the lymph nodes, bones, and liver were identified, and androgen deprivation therapy (ADT) was started immediately. Following 2 weeks of treatment, erythema on the skin, and muscle weakness with severe dysphagia appeared. The patient was diagnosed with dermatomyositis, and high-dose glucocorticoid therapy was initiated. ADT and subsequent chemotherapy with etoposide and cisplatin (EP) were performed for prostate cancer, which resulted in decreased PSA and NSE and reduction of all metastases. After the initiation of EP therapy, dermatomyositis improved, and the patient regained oral intake function. Although EP therapy was replaced by docetaxel, abiraterone, and enzalutamide because of adverse events, no cancer progression was consistently observed. Dermatomyositis worsened temporarily during the administration of abiraterone, but it improved upon switching from abiraterone to enzalutamide and dose escalation of glucocorticoid.

Conclusions: We successfully treated a rare case of dermatomyositis associated with prostate adenocarcinoma with neuroendocrine differentiation.

Keywords: Dermatomyositis, Prostate cancer, Neuroendocrine differentiation, Dysphagia, Glucocorticoid, ADT, EP, Docetaxel, Abiraterone, Enzalutamide

Background

Approximately 20% of all dermatomyositis cases are accompanied by malignancies [1–3]. Furthermore, among patients with dermatomyositis, those with malignancies have a poor prognosis [1, 2]. Although there are several reports of prostate cancer with dermatomyositis [1, 3, 4], we are aware of only one case of neuroendocrine prostate cancer with dermatomyositis [5], who responded poorly to treatment and died within 4 months after initiation of treatment. Here, we report a case of long-term survival of dermatomyositis with severe dysphagia which was associated with prostate adenocarcinoma with neuroendocrine differentiation.

*Correspondence: taketokawai@yahoo.co.jp
Department of Urology, Graduate School of Medicine, The University of Tokyo, 7-3-1, Hongo, Bunkyo-ku, Tokyo 1138655, Japan
Full list of author information is available at the end of the article

Case presentation

A 63-year-old man visited our hospital complaining of frequent urination and hesitancy, which had worsened a year prior to the visit. He also complained of muscle weakness and pain in the upper arms. Blood tests revealed abnormally high PSA (147.7 ng/mL), NSE (60.9 ng/mL), and CK (647 IU/L) (Fig. 1). Prostate biopsy revealed adenocarcinoma with Gleason score 4+5 accompanied by neuroendocrine differentiation, which was positive for PSA, synaptophysin, and NCAM1/CD56 by immunohistochemistry (Fig. 2). Contrast-enhanced computed tomography (CT) revealed prostate cancer which showed invasion to the bladder, seminal vesicles, and rectum. Multiple metastases to the liver (Fig. 3a), pelvic lymph nodes, and bone were observed. The patient was diagnosed with prostate adenocarcinoma with neuroendocrine differentiation, cT4N1M1. At the time of diagnosis, the use of abiraterone and docetaxel for high-risk metastatic hormone-sensitive prostate cancer (HSPC) was not yet approved in medical insurance in Japan. Therefore, combined androgen blockade (CAB) therapy with surgical castration and bicalutamide was initiated as the most intense treatment available in Japan at that time for high-risk metastatic HSPC. Chemotherapy with etoposide and cisplatin (EP) was not performed at this time because pure adenocarcinoma components dominated, few with neuroendocrine differentiation in the prostate biopsy.

Two weeks later, dysphagia, edema of both upper limbs, and erythema on the skin were identified. Bicalutamide

was discontinued and high-dose glucocorticoid therapy with methylprednisolone (mPSL) was initiated at a dose of 125 mg/day intravenously (IV) for the first 3 days, 80 mg/day IV for the next 3 days, and 40 mg/day IV for the next 3 days. At this time, the symptoms were suspected to be bicalutamide-induced adverse events. One week after the initiation of mPSL, dysphagia and erythema of the skin and muscle weakness of both arms did not improve. Physical examination revealed erythema on the back of the finger joints (Gottron's sign) (Fig. 4a), from the shoulder to the upper back (shawl sign) (Fig. 4b) and around the neck (V-neck sign) (Fig. 4c), and edematous erythema on the bilateral eyelids (heliotrope rash) (Fig. 4d). Blood tests revealed abnormally high values of CK (1727 IU/L, Fig. 1), aldolase (14.5 U/L), and myoglobin (435.8 ng/mL). Anti-nuclear antibody was positive at titers of 1:640, anti-ARS antibody was negative, and anti-TIF1-γ antibody was positive. Based on these findings, the patient was diagnosed with malignancy-associated dermatomyositis. He was presented with dysphagia, which was severe and required temporary fasting and central parenteral nutrition. Glucocorticoid administration was changed from mPSL to prednisolone (PSL) at a dose of 60 mg/day IV.

Four weeks after the start of androgen deprivation therapy (ADT), CT showed residual multiple liver metastases (Fig. 3b), although PSA and NSE decreased to 7.0 ng/mL and 21.9 ng/mL, respectively (Fig. 1). Then, EP therapy (etoposide 100 mg/m^2 and cisplatin 20 mg/m^2, every 3 weeks) was commenced, resulting in a rapid decrease of

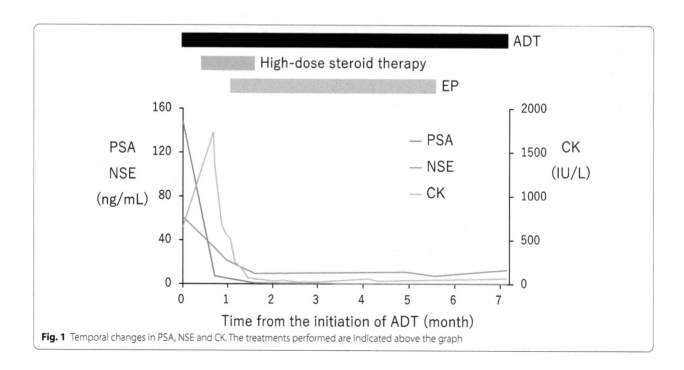

Fig. 1 Temporal changes in PSA, NSE and CK. The treatments performed are indicated above the graph

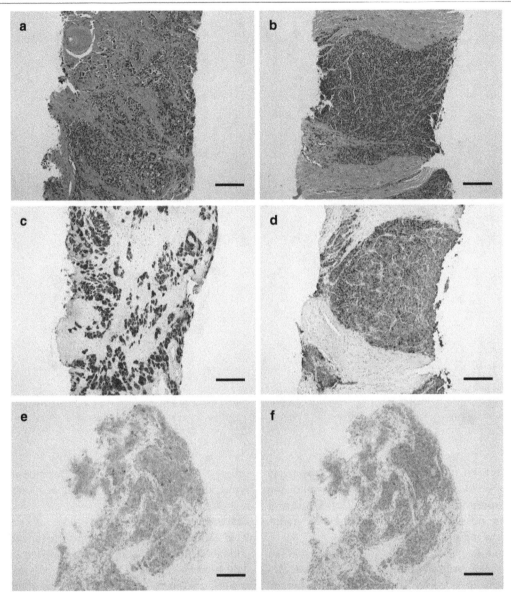

Fig. 2 Immunohistochemical findings of prostate biopsy; hematoxylin and eosin (**a, b**), PSA (**c, d**), synaptophysin (**e**), and NCAM1/CD56 (**f**). Hematoxylin and eosin staining reveals adenocarcinoma with Gleason score 4 + 5 (**a**) and components of neuroendocrine differentiation (**b**). The components of typical adenocarcinoma (**c**) and neuroendocrine differentiation (**d**) are highly and weakly positive for PSA, respectively. The components of neuroendocrine differentiation are positive for synaptophysin (**e**) and NCAM1/CD56 (**f**). The bar indicates 100 μm

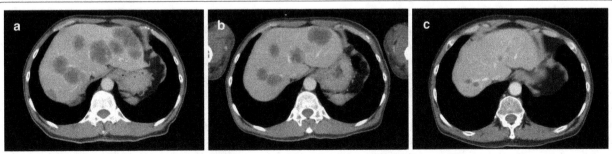

Fig. 3 CT findings of liver metastases before ADT (**a**), before EP therapy (**b**), and after 4 courses of EP therapy (**c**)

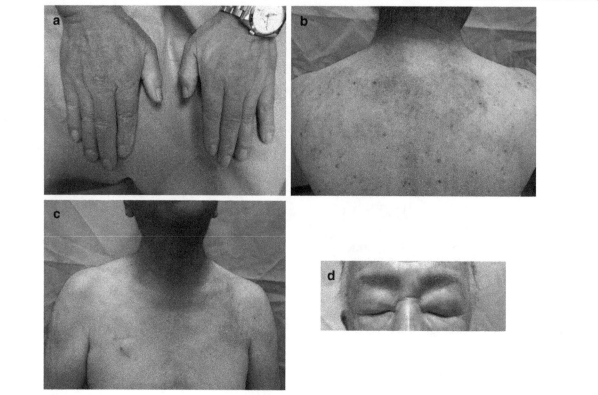

Fig. 4 Various skin symptoms observed in the patient. Erythema on the back of the finger joint (Gottron's sign) (**a**), erythema from shoulder to upper back (shawl sign) (**b**), erythema around the neck (V-neck sign) (**c**), and edematous erythema on the bilateral eyelids (heliotrope rash) (**d**)

PSA and NSE to < 1 ng/mL and < 13 ng/mL, respectively (Fig. 1). Two weeks after EP therapy started, swallowing function improved with a decrease in CK (Fig. 1) and oral intake became possible. PSL administration was gradually tapered to 5 mg/day.

After 4 courses of EP therapy, CT showed marked reduction of the primary tumor and all metastases including those in the liver (Fig. 3c), but EP therapy was discontinued due to grade 3 malaise. Although the metastases had shrunk, they did not disappear, and we supposed that a small amount of cancer progression could lead to a relapse of dermatomyositis. The patient was therefore switched to docetaxel therapy (70 mg/m², every 3 weeks). After 4 courses, docetaxel was also discontinued due to grade 3 malaise, and abiraterone acetate treatment was initiated. Abiraterone acetate treatment was ceased after one month because erythema on his face and extremities and serum CK level worsened (246 IU/L). Enzalutamide treatment and dose escalation of PSL to 30 mg/day were started, and dermatomyositis improved. PSA and NSE were consistently low, and no progressions were observed during the administration of docetaxel, abiraterone, and enzalutamide. At present, 31 months after the start of enzalutamide administration, no cancer

progression has been observed. Dermatomyositis is in remission, and the patient is on PSL at 10 mg/day.

Discussion and conclusions

It is difficult to obtain a good therapeutic effect in patients with dermatomyositis complicated by malignant tumors, as long as the tumor is present; conversely, radical treatment of malignancy may improve muscle and skin symptoms. Therefore, treatment of malignancy is prioritized in order to improve dermatomyositis [3]. In the present case, dermatomyositis was improved by treatment for prostate cancer in addition to high-dose glucocorticoid therapy. ADT was initially performed to treat prostate cancer with neuroendocrine differentiation and the treatment had limited effects on dermatomyositis, and dysphagia became apparent. Although dermatomyositis tends to improve with high-dose glucocorticoid therapy, oral intake was possible after EP therapy was commenced. These findings suggest that EP therapy was required to address the component of neuroendocrine differentiation.

Pure neuroendocrine prostate cancer (including small cell carcinoma and large cell carcinoma) has a poor prognosis. However, it is controversial whether neuroendocrine differentiation in adenocarcinomas worsens the prognosis [6, 7]. In the present case, multiple liver metastases were observed from the first visit, suggesting that the cancer was aggressive. ADT was followed by EP therapy and other strong treatments with docetaxel, abiraterone, and enzalutamide before the onset of castration resistance. We believe that the ability to control aggressive cancers with these treatments may have led to an improvement in disease activity of dermatomyositis.

In conclusion, we encountered a rare case of dermatomyositis associated with prostate adenocarcinoma with neuroendocrine differentiation. The patient was successfully treated with ADT and subsequent EP therapy for prostate cancer and high-dose glucocorticoid therapy for dermatomyositis.

Abbreviations

PSA: Prostate specific antigen; NSE: Neuron specific enolase; CK: Creatinine kinase; NCAM1: Neural cell adhesion molecule 1.

Acknowledgements

Not applicable.

Authors' contributions

HM collected data and wrote the manuscripts. TK contributed to concept of this paper, interpreted the data, and prepared the manuscripts. AM, KM, and YS contributed to concept of this paper. KN, MT, and NT collected data regarding the dermatomyositis, and reviewed the manuscripts. EI performed the histological examination. YY, MN, DY, MS, TM, and HK reviewed the manuscripts. All authors read and approved the final manuscript.

Author details

[1] Department of Urology, Ome Municipal General Hospital, 4-16-5, Higashiome Ome, Ome, Tokyo 1980042, Japan. [2] Department of Urology, Graduate School of Medicine, The University of Tokyo, 7-3-1, Hongo, Bunkyo-ku, Tokyo 1138655, Japan. [3] Department of Rheumatology, Ome Municipal General Hospital, 4-16-5, Higashiome Ome, Ome, Tokyo 1980042, Japan. [4] Department of Pathology, Ome Municipal General Hospital, 4-16-5, Higashiome Ome, Ome, Tokyo 1980042, Japan.

References

1. Motomura K, Yamashita H, Yamada S, Takahashi Y, Kaneko H. Clinical characteristics and prognosis of polymyositis and dermatomyositis associated with malignancy: a 25-year retrospective study. Rheumatol Int. 2019;39(10):1733–9.
2. Liu Y, Xu L, Wu H, Zhao N, Tang Y, Li X, Liang Y. Characteristics and predictors of malignancy in dermatomyositis: analysis of 239 patients from northern China. Oncol Lett. 2018;16(5):5960–8.
3. Zerdes I, Tolia M, Nikolaou M, Tsoukalas N, Velentza L, Hajiioannou J, Mitsis M, Kyrgias G. How can we effectively address the paraneoplastic dermatomyositis: diagnosis, risk factors and treatment options. J BUON. 2017;22(4):1073–80.
4. Yang Z, Lin F, Qin B, Liang Y, Zhong R. Polymyositis/dermatomyositis and malignancy risk: a metaanalysis study. J Rheumatol. 2015;42(2):282–91.
5. Papagoras C, Arelaki S, Botis I, Chrysafis I, Giannopoulos S, Skendros P. Co-occurrence of dermatomyositis and polycythemia unveiling rare *de novo* neuroendocrine prostate tumor. Front Oncol. 2018;8:534.
6. Epstein JI, Amin MB, Beltran H, Lotan TL, Mosquera JM, Reuter VE, Robinson BD, Troncoso P, Rubin MA. Proposed morphologic classification of prostate cancer with neuroendocrine differentiation. Am J Surg Pathol. 2014;38(6):756–67.
7. Shariff AH, Ather MH. Neuroendocrine differentiation in prostate cancer. Urology. 2006;68(1):2–8.

5

Prostatic abscess with infected aneurysms and spondylodiscitis after transrectal ultrasound-guided prostate biopsy

Shunichiro Nomura*⬥, Yuka Toyama, Jun Akatsuka, Yuki Endo, Ryoji Kimata, Yasutomo Suzuki, Tsutomu Hamasaki, Go Kimura and Yukihiro Kondo

Abstract

Background: Transrectal ultrasonography (TRUS)-guided prostate biopsy is the conventional method of diagnosing prostate cancer. TRUS-guided prostate biopsy can occasionally be associated with severe complications. Here, we report the first case of a prostate abscess with aneurysms and spondylodiscitis as a complication of TRUS-guided prostate biopsy, and we review the relevant literature.

Case presentation: A 78-year-old man presented with back pain, sepsis, and prostate abscesses. Twenty days after TRUS-guided prostate biopsy, he was found to have a 20-mm diameter abdominal aortic aneurysm that expanded to 28.2 mm in the space of a week, despite antibiotic therapy. Therefore, he underwent transurethral resection of the prostate to control prostatic abscesses. Although his aneurysm decreased to 23 mm in size after surgery, he continued to experience back pain. He was diagnosed as having pyogenic spondylitis and this was managed using a lumbar corset. Sixty-four days after the prostate biopsy, the aneurysm had re-expanded to 30 mm; therefore, we performed endovascular aneurysm repair (EVAR) using a microcore stent graft 82 days after the biopsy. Four days after the EVAR, the patient developed acute cholecystitis, and he underwent endoscopic retrograde biliary drainage. One hundred and sixty days after the prostate biopsy, all the complications had improved, and he was discharged. A literature review identified a further six cases of spondylodiscitis that had occurred after transrectal ultrasound-guided prostate biopsy.

Conclusions: We have reported the first case of a complication of TRUS-guided prostate biopsy that involved prostatic abscesses, aneurysms, and spondylodiscitis. Although such complications are uncommon, clinicians should be aware of the potential for such severe complications of this procedure to develop.

Keywords: Spondylodiscitis, Aneurysm, Prostate biopsy

Background

Transrectal ultrasonography (TRUS)-guided prostate biopsy is the standard method of diagnosing prostate cancer [1]. TRUS-guided prostate biopsy is a relatively safe method that is usually well-tolerated by patients, although minor complications (such as pain, hematuria, hematospermia, and rectal hemorrhage) or, rarely, significant complications (such as sepsis, macroscopic hematoma, and urinary retention) can develop [2]. Here, we report the first case of prostatic abscess with aneurysms and spondylodiscitis after TURS-guided prostate biopsy, and contextualize this with a review of the literature.

*Correspondence: s-nomura@nms.ac.jp
Department of Urology, Nippon Medical School, 1-1-5 Sendagi, Bunkyo-ku, Tokyo 113-8603, Japan

Case presentation

A 78-year-old man was hospitalized to undergo TRUS-guided prostatic biopsy because he had a serum prostate-specific antigen (PSA) concentration of 15.86 ng/ml. The TRUS-measured prostate volume was 41 ml. His medical history included coronary artery disease with previous intracoronary stenting. He received intravenous (IV) cefazolin 2 g daily as antimicrobial prophylaxis prior to the biopsy. The day after the biopsy, he had a fever (temperature 39.5 °C), but his vital signs were otherwise normal. Blood analyses revealed a white blood cell (WBC) count of 7100/μl. After 3 days, he was started on intravenous ceftriaxone and gamma-globulin 5 g because of a continuous fever and a high serum C-reactive protein (CRP) concentration (Fig. 1). After 5 days, a gram-negative bacillus was grown on blood culture. A digital rectal examination revealed an enlarged prostate. Computed tomography (CT) of the pelvis showed mild enlargement of the prostate. Therefore, the patient's antibiotics were changed to meropenem 1.5 g and clindamycin to treat the sepsis of prostatitis, and a transabdominal catheter was placed into his urinary bladder. However, his condition worsened 6 days later and he had difficulty breathing, with an oxygen saturation of 85%, according to pulse oximetry, and a low pO2 (32.4 mmHg), according to arterial blood gas measurement. A chest X-ray showed air-space consolidation. Therefore, he was transferred to the intensive care unit for the diagnosis of acute respiratory distress syndrome (ARDS).

At this time, a further blood culture showed the presence of extended-spectrum-lactamase (ESBL)-producing *Escherichia coli* (*E. coli*), which was sensitive to imipenem; therefore, his antibiotics were changed accordingly. Twelve days later, rectal examination revealed a tender, fluctuant prostate consistent with a prostatic abscess. The CT images were consistent with the presence of three prostatic abscesses (< 1.5 cm each). Thirteen days after the prostate biopsy, his bacteremia had improved and his ARDS had resolved; therefore, he was transferred to the general ward. Twenty days after the prostate biopsy, an abdominal/pelvic CT scan was performed to identify any remaining prostatic abscesses. However, instead, the scan revealed the presence of an abdominal aortic aneurysm with surrounding periaortic inflammatory changes (Fig. 2a). Therefore, IV doripenem was administered. CT examination after 26 days showed no change in the prostatic abscesses, but the aneurysm had expanded to a diameter of 28.2 mm.

Transurethral resection of the prostate was planned as a means of controlling prostatic abscesses for day 27 after the prostate biopsy. During the surgery, a whitish purulent substance discharged from the prostate. After

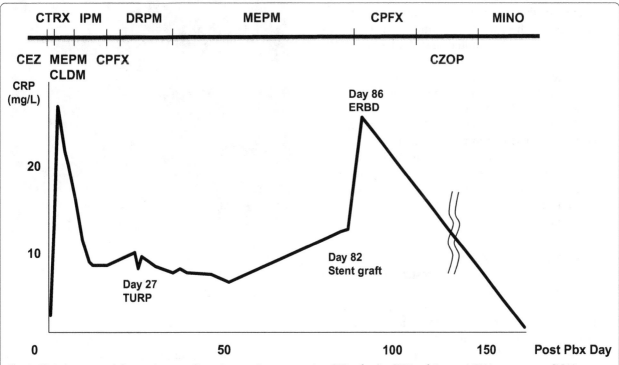

Fig. 1 Clinical course and changes in serum C-reactive protein concentration. CEZ: cefazolin, CTRX: ceftriaxone, MEPM: meropenem, CLDM: clindamycin, IPM: imipenem, CPFX: ciprofloxacin, DRPM: doripenem, CZOP: cefozopran, MINO: minocycline

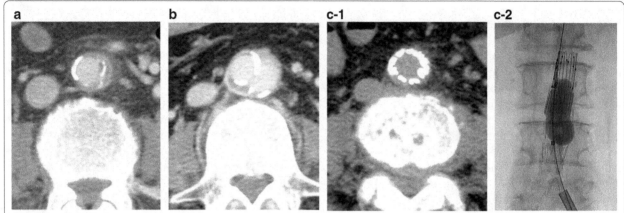

Fig. 2 Images of the aortic aneurysm. **a** Initial computed tomography (CT) image of the abdomen/pelvis, demonstrating a 20-mm abdominal aortic aneurysm, with evidence of inflammatory changes, 20 days after prostate biopsy. **b** Repeat CT image revealing that the abdominal aortic aneurysm diameter has increased to 30 mm, 64 days after the prostate biopsy. **c** CT and angiography showing the successful exclusion of the aortic rupture by endovascular stent grafting

surgery, the patient made excellent progress. Postoperative CT (31 days after prostate biopsy) showed that the aneurysm had a satisfactory appearance (23 mm diameter). However, he had also been experiencing back pain for 4 weeks, from day 11 after the prostate biopsy. Contrast-enhanced magnetic resonance imaging of the lumbar spine revealed contrast enhancement of the L2, L4, and L5 vertebral bodies (Fig. 3). Therefore, he was diagnosed as having pyogenic spondylitis and this was managed using a lumbar corset. Sixty-four days after the original biopsy, the aneurysm had re-expanded to 30 mm (Fig. 2b), but as the patient's condition was unsatisfactory, surgery was not attempted. Instead, he underwent endovascular aneurysm repair (EVAR) using a microcore stent graft at our hospital 82 days after the prostate biopsy (Fig. 2c). Four days after the endovascular treatment, he developed a stomach ache and CT revealed acute cholecystitis. Therefore, endoscopic retrograde biliary drainage (ERBD) was performed and the patient's antibiotic was changed to ciprofloxacin. By day 160 after the prostate biopsy, all the complications had improved, and the patient was discharged. He then underwent active surveillance for prostate cancer 1 year after the original diagnosis.

Discussion and conclusions

To the best of our knowledge, prostate abscess with infected aneurysms and spondylodiscitis has not been reported in the literature as a complication of transrectal prostate biopsy. Furthermore, infected aneurysm alone is an extremely rare complication of TURS-guided prostate biopsy: only two cases have been reported previously [3].

Infected aneurysms can arise because of the hematogenous spread of bacteria, which cause aneurysmal changes

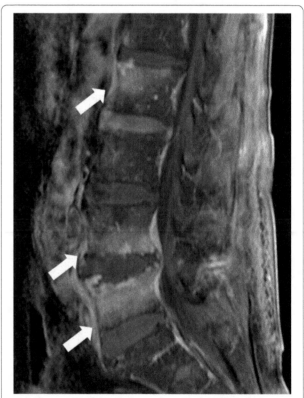

Fig. 3 Lumbar images obtained 40 days after prostate biopsy. Contrast-enhanced T1-weighted magnetic resonance image of the lumbar spine shows contrast-enhancement of the L2, L4, and L5 vertebral bodies

in the arterial wall, and a pathogen can be further disseminated by this route to cause a prostate abscess. The gold-standard treatment of the disease remains surgical resection and debridement of the infected aorta,

Table 1 Review of the reported cases of spondylodiscitis after transrectal ultrasound-guided prostate biopsy

References	Age	Symptoms	Antimicrobial prophylaxis	Location	Susceptibility	Bacteremia
Taşdemiroğlu et al. [12]	53	Fever, backache	None	L2–3	E. coli	No
Karapolat et al. [13]	70	Fever, backache	Ciprofloxacin, Gentamicin	T6–7	E. coli	No
Kaya et al. [14]	59	Fever, backache	Ciprofloxacin	L4–5	E. coli	No
Dobson et al. [15]	69	Fever, backache	Ciprofloxacin	L2–3	Fluoroquinolone resistant E. coli	Yes
Hiyama et al. [16]	59	Fever, backache	Cefotiam	C7/T1	Enterococcus faecalis	Yes
Li et al. [17]	71	Fever, backache	Levofloxacin	L3–5	Multiple drug resisitant E. coli	Yes
Present case	78	Fever, backache	Cefazolin	L2, 4, 5	ESBL E. coli	Yes

Reference	Risk factor	Surgery	Complications	Outcome
Taşdemiroğlu et al. [12]	DM	Hemilaminectomy	Epidural abscess	Resolution
Karapola et al. [13]	BPH	Bone graft reconstruction	None	Resolution
Kaya et al. [14]	None	Hemilaminectomy	Epidural and intradiscal abscess	Resolution
Dobson et al. [15]	None	Aspiration	Epidural abscess	Resolution
Hiyama et al. [16]	None	Aortic valve displacement	Endocarditis	Resolution
Li et al. [17]	BPH	Laminectomies	Epidural and psoas muscle abscess	Resolution
Present case	None	TURP, EVAR	Prostate abscesses, infected aneurysm	Resolution

E. coli Escherichia coli, ESBL extended-spectrum lactamase, DM diabetes mellitus, BPH benign prostatic hypertrophy, TURP transurethral resection of the prostate, EVAR endovascular aneurysm repair involving the placement of an interposition graft or extra-anatomic bypass, and long-term antibiotic therapy. However, this procedure is associated with high mortality of 13.3–40% [4, 5]. Therefore, EVAR has been developed as an elective open method of repair of an infected aneurysm, especially for high-risk surgical patients. Because the present patient was high-risk, we chose to treat the aneurysm using EVAR, and although he developed acute cholecystitis 4 days after the EVAR, his condition was improved by ERBD.

Spondylodiscitis is also an extremely rare complication of TURS-guided prostate biopsy. The incidence of spondylodiscitis ranges from 0.4 to 2.4/100,000 in Europe [6]. Six cases of spondylodiscitis following TRUS-guided prostate biopsy have been previously described in the English-speaking literature, (Table 1) and in all these cases the clinical symptoms were fever and backache. *E. coli* was the dominant cause of the spondylodiscitis, being identified in five of the cases, three of which were antibiotic-resistant. *Enterococcus faecalis* was identified as the causative agent in the remaining case. Here, we report the first case of spondylodiscitis that was caused by ESBL *E. coli*. Four of the seven reported cases had positive blood culture results. Lumbar vertebrae are most frequently affected in spondylodiscitis, as in five of the reported cases, including the present case. Risk factors to infection include immunosuppression, diabetes mellitus, and benign prostatic hypertrophy. Although three of the reported cases had risk factors, our patient had none of the risk factors. Five of the cases were treated using a surgical intervention, but the spondylodiscitis in the present case was treated by antibiotic therapy and spinal immobilization. Four of the cases also had an epidural abscess. However, all the identified lesions resolved, suggesting that such lesions have good prognoses.

Fluoroquinolones, and particularly ciprofloxacin, are widely used prophylactically alongside TRUS-guided prostate biopsy. However, the incidence of infectious complications associated with prostate biopsy has significantly increased in recent years [7]. Recent studies have shown that approximately half of post-biopsy infections are resistant to fluoroquinolone, and many are also resistant to other antibiotics [8]. Therefore, to prevent post-biopsy infection, we should consider selectively targeting antibiotic prophylaxis by performing a pre-biopsy rectal culture. Taylor et al. reported that targeted antimicrobial prophylaxis is associated with a notable reduction, in the incidence of infectious complications associated with TRUS-guided prostate biopsy that were caused by fluoroquinolone-resistant organisms, as well as a reduction in the overall cost of care. No infectious complications arose in the 112 men who received targeted antimicrobial prophylaxis, whereas there were nine cases (including

one of sepsis) among the 345 men who were on empirical therapy [9]. Other proposed procedures include transperineal prostate biopsy and selectively augmented prophylaxis with two antibiotics in higher risk patients [10, 11].

In conclusion, we have reported the first case of prostatic abscess with aneurysm and spondylodiscitis after TRUS-guided prostate biopsy. Although this combination of complications is extremely rare, we should be aware of the possibility that severe complications can arise following this procedure.

Abbreviations

TRUS: Transrectal ultrasonography; IV: Intravenous; CRP: C-reactive protein; CT: Computed tomography; EVAR: Endovascular aneurysm repair.

Acknowledgements

We thank Mark Cleasby, PhD, from Edanz Group (https://en-author-services.edanzgroup.com/ac) for editing a draft of this manuscript. We also thank Megumi Nomura for your support.

Authors' contributions

SN contributed to the acquisition of the history, performed the imaging, and wrote the manuscript. YT and JA administered the treatment. YE and RK reviewed the manuscript and gave their opinions. YS supervised the research and helped write the manuscript. TH revised the manuscript. GK reviewed the manuscript. YK acted as a supervisor and reviewed the manuscript. All the authors read and approved the final manuscript.

References

1. Rodriguez LV, Terris MK. Risks and complications of transrectal ultrasound guided prostate needle biopsy: a prospective study and review of the literature. J Urol. 1998;160(6 Pt 1):2115–20.
2. de Jesus CM, Correa LA, Padovani CR. Complications and risk factors in transrectal ultrasound-guided prostate biopsies. Sao Paulo Med J = Revista paulista de medicina. 2006;124(4):198–202.
3. Al-Ani HH, Khashram M, Dean A, Bourchier R, Bhamidipaty V, Hill A. Infected abdominal aortic aneurysm after transrectal ultrasound-guided biopsy of the prostate: a report of two cases. Ann Vasc Surg. 2019;61:469.e461-469.e464.
4. Muller BT, Wegener OR, Grabitz K, Pillny M, Thomas L, Sandmann W. Mycotic aneurysms of the thoracic and abdominal aorta and iliac arteries: experience with anatomic and extra-anatomic repair in 33 cases. J Vasc Surg. 2001;33(1):106–13.
5. Kyriakides C, Kan Y, Kerle M, Cheshire NJ, Mansfield AO, Wolfe JH. 11-year experience with anatomical and extra-anatomical repair of mycotic aortic aneurysms. Eur J Vasc Endovasc Surg. 2004;27(6):585–9.
6. Grammatico L, Baron S, Rusch E, Lepage B, Surer N, Desenclos JC, Besnier JM. Epidemiology of vertebral osteomyelitis (VO) in France: analysis of hospital-discharge data 2002–2003. Epidemiol Infect. 2008;136(5):653–60.
7. Loeb S, Carter HB, Berndt SI, Ricker W, Schaeffer EM. Complications after prostate biopsy: data from SEER-medicare. J Urol. 2011;186(5):1830–4.
8. Zaytoun OM, Vargo EH, Rajan R, Berglund R, Gordon S, Jones JS. Emergence of fluoroquinolone-resistant Escherichia coli as cause of postprostate biopsy infection: implications for prophylaxis and treatment. Urology. 2011;77(5):1035–41.
9. Taylor AK, Zembower TR, Nadler RB, Scheetz MH, Cashy JP, Bowen D, Murphy AB, Dielubanza E, Schaeffer AJ. Targeted antimicrobial prophylaxis using rectal swab cultures in men undergoing transrectal ultrasound guided prostate biopsy is associated with reduced incidence of postoperative infectious complications and cost of care. J Urol. 2012;187(4):1275–9.

10. Grummet JP, Weerakoon M, Huang S, Lawrentschuk N, Frydenberg M, Moon DA, O'Reilly M, Murphy D. Sepsis and 'superbugs': should we favour the transperineal over the transrectal approach for prostate biopsy? BJU Int. 2014;114(3):384–8.

11. Liss MA, Chang A, Santos R, Nakama-Peeples A, Peterson EM, Osann K, Bilimek J, Szabo RJ, Dash A. Prevalence and significance of fluoroquinolone resistant *Escherichia coli* in patients undergoing transrectal ultrasound guided prostate needle biopsy. J Urol. 2011;185(4):1283–8.

12. Taşdemiroğlu E, Sengöz A, Bagatur E. Iatrogenic spondylodiscitis. Case report and review of literature. Neurosurg Focus. 2004;16(6):Ecp1.

13. Karapolat H, Akkoç Y, Arda B, Sesli E. Spondylodiscitis caused by sudden onset back pain following transrectal ultrasonography-guided prostate biopsy: a case report. Agri. 2009;21(3):121–5.

14. Kaya M, Kösemehmetoğlu K, Yildirim CH, Orman G, Çelebi Ö, Taşdemiroğlu E. Spondylodiscitis as a spinal complication of transrectal ultrasound-guided needle biopsy of the prostate. Spine. 2012;37(14):E870-872.

15. Dobson G, Cowie CJ, Holliman D. Epidural abscess with associated spondylodiscitis following prostatic biopsy. Ann R Coll Surg Engl. 2015;97(5):e81-82.

16. Hiyama Y, Takahashi S, Uehara T, Ichihara K, Hashimoto J, Masumori N. A case of infective endocarditis and pyogenic spondylitis after transrectal ultrasound guided prostate biopsy. J Infect Chemother. 2016;22(11):767–9.

17. Li CC, Li CZ, Wu ST, Cha TL, Tang SH. Spondylodiscitis with epidural and psoas muscle abscesses as complications after transrectal ultrasound-guided prostate biopsy: report of a rare case. Eur J Case Rep Intern Med. 2017;4(8):000694.

6

Effect of prior cancer on survival outcomes for patients with advanced prostate cancer

Yechen Wu[1†], Xi Chen[2†], Duocheng Qian[3†], Wei Wang[4], Yiping Zhang[1], Jinxin Hu[1], Jun Zhu[1], Qiang Wu[2*] and Tinghu Cao[1*]

Abstract

Background: A history of prior cancer commonly results in exclusion from cancer clinical trials. However, whether a prior cancer history has an adversely impact on clinical outcomes for patients with advanced prostate cancer (APC) remains largely unknown. We therefore aimed to investigate the impact of prior cancer history on these patients.

Methods: We identified patients with advanced prostate cancer diagnosed from 2004 to 2010 in the Surveillance, Epidemiology, and End Results (SEER) database. Propensity score matching (PSM) was used to balance baseline characteristics. Kaplan–Meier method and the Cox proportional hazard model were utilized for survival analysis.

Results: A total of 19,772 eligible APC patients were included, of whom 887 (4.5%) had a history of prior cancer. Urinary bladder (19%), colon and cecum (16%), melanoma of the skin (9%) malignancies, and non-hodgkin lymphoma (9%) were the most common types of prior cancer. Patients with a history of prior cancer had slightly inferior overall survival (OS) (AHR = 1.13; 95% CI [1.02–1.26]; P = 0.017) as compared with that of patients without a prior cancer diagnosis. Subgroup analysis further indicated that a history of prior cancer didn't adversely impact patients' clinical outcomes, except in patients with a prior cancer diagnosed within 2 years, at advanced stage, or originating from specific sites, including bladder, colon and cecum, or lung and bronchus, or prior chronic lymphocytic leukemia.

Conclusions: A large proportion of APC patients with a prior cancer history had non-inferior survival to that of patients without a prior cancer diagnosis. These patients may be candidates for relevant cancer trials.

Keywords: Advanced prostate cancer, Prior cancer, Survival, SEER, Trial eligibility

Background

Prostate cancer represents the most common malignancy in men, accounting for estimated 164,690 new cases in the United States, in 2018 [1]. According to the latest statistical report, prostate cancer still represents the second most common cause of death in men (9%

of all cancer deaths) [2]. Although great advances have been made in the past several years, huge challenges still exist in patients with advanced prostate cancer, which is still associated with substantial morbidity and mortality, particularly in patients who develop resistance after multiple lines of therapy. The National Comprehensive Cancer Network hold the opinion that the best management for those patients with advanced disease is clinical trials, because well-designed clinical trials are pivotal for exploring new treatments and improving patients' clinical outcomes. Unfortunately, patients who had a prior cancer history are often excluded by strict eligibility criteria in cancer trial. Given the dramatical increase in the number of cancer survivors as well as the decreasing cancer mortality rate, the exclusion criterion may limit the

†

*Correspondence: qiang_wu0988@163.com; tinghu_cao@126.com

Yechen Wu, Xi Chen and Duocheng Qian contributed equally to this work

Department of Urology, Baoshan Branch, Shuguang Hospital Affiliated to Shanghai University of Traditional Chinese Medicine, Shanghai 201900, People's Republic of China

Department of Urology, Tongji Hospital, Tongji University School of Medicine, Shanghai 200065, People's Republic of China

Full list of author information is available at the end of the article

accrual and generalizability of clinical trials, and thus leaves many pivotal clinical issues unanswered [3, 4].

It was reported that up to 18% of lung cancer patients were unconditionally excluded by over 80% of lung cancer trials due to a history of prior cancer [5]. This practice is mainly due to concerns regarding to prior treatment interference and its survival impact, though little evidence clearly support this assumption. However, a previous retrospective study made by Laccetti et al. reported that a prior cancer history did not adversely affect survival of patients with advanced lung cancer, regardless of different stage or types of prior cancer [6]. Another study also suggested that the prognosis of patients with uterine papillary serous carcinoma was not affected by a prior breast cancer and tamoxifen exposure [7]. On the contrary, it was also reported that the overall survival were significantly lower in breast cancer patients as the second primary cancer than in that of patients with breast cancer as the primary cancer [8]. These different results implied that the survival impact of a prior cancer may vary among different cancer types. However, until recently, it remain unknown whether a history of prior cancer affects the clinical outcomes of APC patients.

Therefore, we conducted this study to assess the prevalence, types, timing, and prognostic impact of a prior cancer diagnosis on patients who developed advanced prostate cancer as a second primary malignancy by using the SEER database. Our finding may provide implications for exclusion criteria of relevant clinical trial.

Methods

Data source and case selection

The SEER*Stat software (v. 8.3.6.1) was utilized to extract data from the custom SEER database [Incidence- SEER 18 Regs Custom Data (with additional treatment fields), Nov 2018 Sub (1975–2016 varying)], which covers approximately 28% of the United States population [9]. We included patients who were diagnosed with advanced prostate cancer (site code C) from 2004 to 2010 in order to ensure a 5-year follow-up at least. Patients were eligible if they had stage IV prostate cancer (N1M0 or M1) according to the 8th edition of the AJCC Cancer Staging Manual. Only patients with a single primary tumor or patient who had exactly one prior tumor were included. Other exclusion criteria were listed as follows: (1) patients whose prior cancer was prostate cancer; (2) patients with incomplete follow-up; (3) patients with only death certificates or autopsy records; (4) patients whose diagnosis time of malignancy was not known.

Covariates

Multiple variables including demographic characteristics (diagnosed year, age, race, and marital status), disease

characteristics (Seer stage, histologic grade, and prior cancer type), and treatment modalities (surgery, chemotherapy and radiotherapy). Marital status was categorized as single, married and other status (divorced, widowed, separated and domestic partner). The record of SEER sequence number was used to determine the prior cancer diagnosis. For example, patients who had only one primary tumor were recorded as "00". For patients with multiple malignancies, the sequence number of "01" represented the first tumor, and "02" represented the second one, and so forth. We then calculated the timing, namely the time interval between two cancer record, by subtracting the diagnosis date of the prior cancer from that of index prostate cancer. Detections of vital status and cause-specific death classification were used to define the primary outcomes including overall survival (OS) and cancer-specific survival (CSS).

Statistical analysis

Pearson chi-square test was utilized to compare clinicopathologic characteristics between patients with or without prior cancer. The propensity score matching (PSM) method was used to reduce the bias in baseline characteristics. Propensity scores were calculated based on variables including age, diagnosed year, race, marital status, histological grade, surgery, chemotherapy, and

Table 1 Summary description of demographic and clinical factors

At prior cancer diagnosis		At advanced prostate cancer diagnosis	
Variable	Value	Variable	Value
Age, years		Age, years	
Mean	69.5	Mean	75.6
Median (IQR)	70 (27–78)	Median (IQR)	77 (68–84)
Marital status, n (%)		Marital status, n (%)	
Single	69 (7.8)	Single	73 (8.2)
Married	616 (69.4)	Married	584 (65.8)
Other status	147 (16.6)	Other status	182 (20.5)
Unknown	55 (6.2)	Unknown	48 (5.5)
Seer stage, n (%)		Seer stage, n (%)	
In situ	66 (7.4)	In situ	N/A
Localized	323 (36.4)	Localized	N/A
Regional	70 (7.9)	Regional	241 (27.2)
Distant	140 (15.8)	Distant	646 (72.8)
Unknown	288 (32.5)	Unknown	N/A
Interval between diagnoses, months		Follow up from diagnosis of gastric cancer, months	
Mean	74.4	Mean	37.2
Median (IQR)	49 (22–95.5)	Median (IQR)	23 (8.3–57.8)

IQR interquartile range

radiotherapy, with a ratio of 1:1 and a calliper of 0.2 [10]. Kaplan–Meier method and log-rank test were utilized to compare differences of OS in patients with no prior cancer vs. any prior cancer, before and after PSM. Multivariate Cox proportional hazards models were also built to determine whether prior cancer affects patients' prognosis independently. Descriptive statistic, Pearson Chi-square test, and Cox proportional hazards model were performed using SPSS 24.0 (IBM Corp). The Kaplan–Meier plot and log-rank test were plotted or conducted by using R software version 4.0.0. A 2-sided P value of < 0.05 was considered as statistical significance unless otherwise stated.

Results

A total of 19,772 eligible APC patients were extracted from SEER database, of whom 887 (4.5%) carried a history of prior cancer. As shown in Table 1, the median age at prior cancer diagnoses was 70 years old, and that

of subsequent APC was 77 years old. The median (interquartile range, IQR) time interval between two cancer diagnoses was 49 (22–95.5) months (Table 1). The Table 2 indicated that a history of prior cancer was more common among the elderly (75.6 years vs. 69.3 year), black (84.7% vs. 75.4%), and married (65.8% vs. 59.8%) individuals. After propensity score matching (PSM), all the baseline characteristics between patients with or without prior cancer history were balanced (Table 2). Figure 1 showed that the most common types of prior cancer in APC survivors included urinary bladder (19%), colon and cecum (16%), melanoma of the skin (9%), and non-hodgkin lymphoma (9%).

The Kaplan–Meier plot was utilized to compare the OS between patients who had, or had not prior cancer. As shown in Fig. 2a, the OS of patients with a history of prior cancer was dramatically lower (P < 0.001) than that of patients without a prior cancer history. After PSM, the Kaplan–Meier plot still showed a worse survival

Table 2 Baseline characteristics of patients with advanced prostate cancer in the original/matched data sets (N = 19,772)

Characteristics	Original data set			Matched data set		
	No prior cancer N = 18,885 (%)	With prior cancer N = 887 (%)	P value	No prior cancer N = 887 (%)	With prior cancer N = 887 (%)	P value
Age (years), mean (SD)	69.3 (11.5)	75.6 (10.3)	< 0.001	75.8 (10.7)	75.6 (10.3)	0.661
Year of diagnose(%)			0.001			0.393
2004–2007	10,185 (53.9)	430 (48.5)		448 (50.5)	430 (48.5)	
2008–2010	8700 (46.1)	457 (51.5)		439 (49.5)	457 (51.5)	
Race			0.025			0.088
White	3442 (18.2)	85 (9.6)		101 (11.4)	85 (9.6)	
Black	14,231 (75.4)	751 (84.7)		717 (80.8)	751 (84.7)	
Others/Unknown	1212 (6.4)	51 (5.7)		69 (7.8)	51 (5.7)	
Marital status			< 0.001			0.174
Single	2636 (14.0)	73 (8.2)		94 (10.6)	73 (8.2)	
Married	11,292 (59.8)	584 (65.8)		543 (61.2)	584 (65.8)	
Others status [a]	3742 (19.8)	182 (20.5)		198 (22.3)	182 (20.5)	
Unknown	1215 (6.4)	48 (5.4)		52 (5.9)	48 (5.4)	
Grade			< 0.001			0.608
Grade I	1209 (6.4)	79 (8.9)		70 (7.9)	79 (8.9)	
Grade II	13,411 (71.0)	555 (62.6)		573 (64.6)	555 (62.6)	
Grade III	4265 (22.6)	253 (28.5)		244 (27.5)	253 (28.5)	
Surgery			0.304			0.159
No/unknown	13,951 (73.9)	669 (75.4)		694 (78.2)	669 (75.4)	
Yes	4934 (26.1)	218 (24.6)		193 (21.8)	218 (24.6)	
Chemotherapy			0.468			0.413
No/unknown	17,843 (94.5)	833 (93.9)		835 (94.1)	833 (93.9)	
Yes	1042 (5.5)	54 (6.1)		52 (5.9)	54 (6.1)	
Radiotherapy			0.013			0.639
No/unknown	14,191 (75.1)	699 (78.8)		707 (79.7)	699 (78.8)	
Yes	4694 (24.9)	188 (21.2)		180 (20.3)	188 (21.2)	

[a] Other status including divorced, widowed, separated or domestic partner

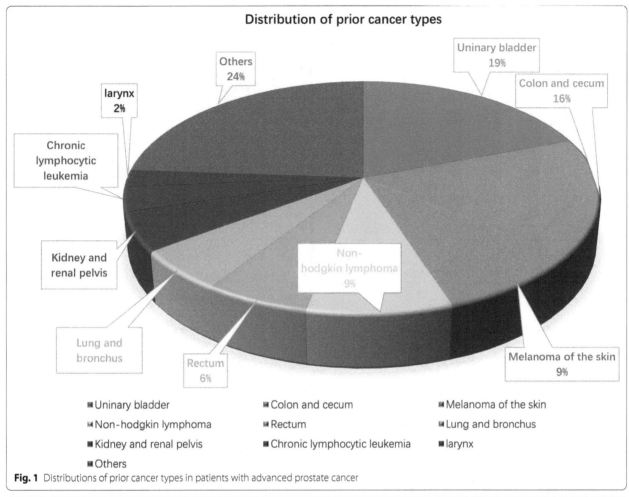

Fig. 1 Distributions of prior cancer types in patients with advanced prostate cancer

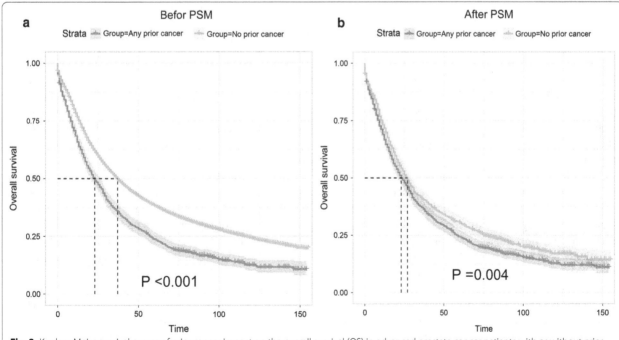

Fig. 2 Kaplan–Meier survival curves of prior cancer impact on the overall survival (OS) in advanced prostate cancer patients with or without prior cancer. **a** The OS analysis before Propensity score matching (PSM); **b** The OS analysis after PSM

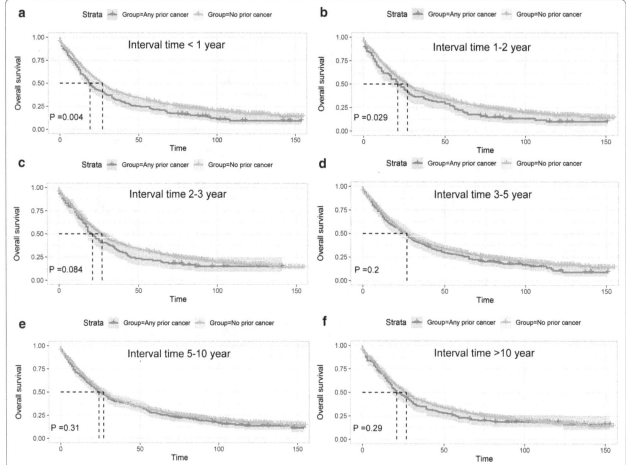

Fig. 3 Kaplan–Meier survival curves of prior cancer impact on the overall survival (OS) stratified by timing of prior cancer in patients with advanced prostate cancer. **a** The OS analysis with time interval less than 1 year; **b** The OS analysis with time interval between 1–2 year; **c** The OS analysis with time interval between 2–3 year; **d** The OS analysis with time interval between 3–5 year; **e** The OS analysis with time interval between 5–10 year; **f** The OS analysis with time interval longer than 10 years

for patients who had a history of prior cancer, presenting a potential adverse effect of a prior cancer history on clinical outcome (P = 0.004) of patients with subsequent advanced prostate cancer (Fig. 2b).

In order to further investigate the survival impact of prior cancer, subgroup analyses were subsequently performed for APC patients stratified by timing (time interval), stage categorization and types of prior cancer. As shown in Fig. 3, we found that patients who had a prior cancer diagnosis with time interval of 2 years or longer showed non-inferior prognosis (P > 0.05) to that of patients without a prior cancer diagnosis. We also found that only prior cancer with advanced stage had significantly adverse impact on OS, while no survival detriment was observed in patients with a prior cancer diagnosed at in situ, localized, or regional stage (Fig. 4). Furthermore, our results also showed that a prior bladder, colon and cecum, lung and bronchus cancer, or CLL

had a dramatically (P < 0.05) adverse effect on survival of patients with subsequent advanced prostate cancer (Fig. 5 and Additional file 1: Fig. S1). However, patients whose prior cancers originating from other sites presented similar OS as compared with that of patients without a prior cancer diagnosis.

After adjusted for age, race, marital status, histologic grade, and treatment modalities, the multivariate Cox regression analysis showed that a prior cancer history was significantly associated with worse OS (HR = 1.13; 95% CI [1.02–1.26]) for patients with advanced prostate cancer (Table 3). Similar to the Kaplan–Meier method, the multivariate Cox analysis for the subgroup analysis further demonstrated that only prior cancer with time interval less than 1 years (HR = 1.35; 95% CI [1.11–1.66]) or within 1–2 years (HR = 1.27; 95% CI [1.02–1.57]), with prior cancer diagnosed at advanced stage (HR = 1.31; 95% CI [1.08–1.58]), or with prior cancer

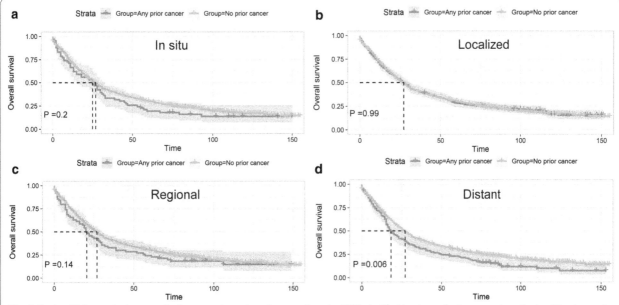

Fig. 4 Kaplan–Meier survival curves of prior cancer impact on the overall survival (OS) stratified by stage of prior cancer in patients with advanced prostate cancer. **a** The OS analysis with prior cancer at *in situ* stage; **b** The OS analysis with prior cancer at localized stage; **c** The OS analysis with prior cancer at regional stage; (D) The OS analysis with prior cancer diagnosed at advanced stage

of bladder (HR = 1.39; 95% CI [1.16–1.66]), colon and cecum (HR = 1.23; 95% CI [1.02–1.48]), lung and bronchus cancer (HR = 1.54; 95% CI [1.15–2.08]) or CLL (HR = 1.47; 95% CI [1.01–2.15]) significantly affected the prognosis of patients with advanced prostate cancer. Nevertheless, patients with other different timing, with other stage categorization or with other types of prior cancer had non-inferior survival to that of patients without a prior cancer diagnosis. Our result also showed that patients with a history of prior cancer presented non-inferior or even slightly superior prostate cancer-specific survival to patients without a prior cancer history. Detailed data can be seen in Table 3.

Discussion

This study focused on survival impact of a prior cancer history on APC patients. Approximately 4.5% of patients with advanced prostate cancer had a prior cancer history. Those patients showed a worse prognosis in comparison with patients without a prior cancer diagnosis. Nevertheless, subgroup analyses indicated that a history of prior cancer didn't adversely affect patients' survival, except for patients with prior cancer diagnosed within 2 year, or those with prior cancer diagnosed at advanced stage, or those with specific types of prior cancer, including bladder, colon and cecum, lung and bronchus cancer, or CLL .

Over the last few decades, the population of cancer survivors has been steadily increasing in the United States because of the aging of the population and the great advances in early detection and cancer treatment [11–13]. This population had a high risk of developing second primary cancer [14, 15]. Previous study reported that about one-tenth of younger adults and one-fourth of the elderly cancer patients had a prior cancer history [16].

Similar to other types of cancer, prostate cancer is frequently diagnosed as a second malignancy. In our study, we focused on assessing the survival impact of a prior cancer history on APC patients who are often candidates for clinical trials. We found that approximately 4.5% of patients had exactly one non-prostate prior cancer before the diagnosis of APC. This proportion was similar to advanced breast cancer but lower than advanced lung cancer [6, 17]. Besides, similar to studies reported by Bluethmann et al. [16] and Murphy et al. [18], our study suggested that the elderly patients were more likely to have a history of prior cancer than the younger patients. The median time interval between advanced prostate cancer and prior cancers was approximately four years, which was longer than some cancers [3, 8]. The urinary bladder, colon and cecum, melanoma of the skin, and Non-hodgkin lymphoma exhibited as the most common types of prior cancer in the APC patients, of which the distribution differs from other cancers, such as nasopharyngeal cancer [3], lung cancer [19] and breast cancer [8].

The cancer trials exerts as a promising way for improving survivorship of advanced cancer patients. However,

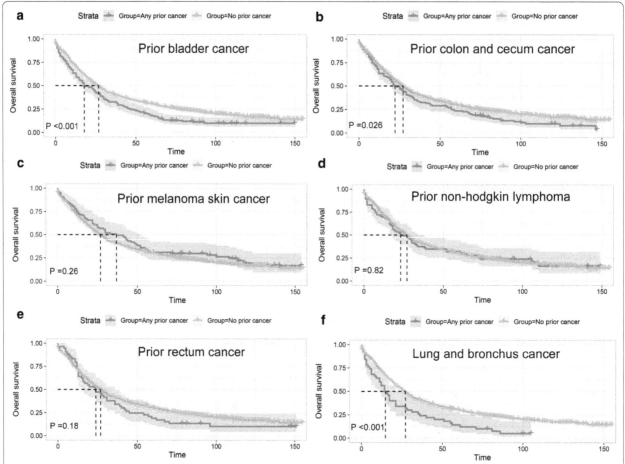

Fig. 5 Kaplan–Meier survival curves of prior cancer impact on the overall survival (OS) stratified by different types of prior cancer in patients with advanced prostate cancer. **a** The impact of prior bladder cancer on OS; **b** The impact of prior colon and cecum cancer on OS; **c** The impact of prior melanoma skin cancer on OS; **d** The impact of prior non-hodgkin lymphoma on OS; **e** The impact of prior rectum cancer on OS; **f** The impact of prior lung and bronchus cancer on OS

fewer than 5% of patients can be enrolled in cancer trials due to the overly restrictive exclusion criteria [20], and a history of prior cancer was the commonly used one in most trials. This could mainly due to the widely accepted belief that a prior cancer can adversely affect patients' survival, though no authoritative data have proved it. The stringent criteria may weed out a large number of patients who had urgent need, which could limit generalizability and lead to premature trial termination [4, 21]. Therefore, liberalizing the exclusion criteria, especially for a history of prior cancer, has been proposed by several working groups [5, 22]. Furthermore, the Food and Drug Administration (FDA) has introduced a draft guidance implying that patients who had a prior cancer history could generally be enrolled in clinical trials [23].

Our data indicated that the overall survival of APC patients with a history of prior cancer was significantly poorer than that of patients without a prior cancer history before and after PSM method. This result was consistent to the pan-cancer study by Zhou et al. [24]. However, subsequent subgroup analyses revealed that a prior cancer history could impair the survival of patients only when the interval time was less than two year. This time-frame finding was different from the study by Lin et al. that demonstrated no survival detriment in patients with advanced breast cancer who had prior cancer outside the timeframe of 4 years [17].

Our study also demonstrated that a prior cancer diagnosed at in situ, localized, or regional stage didn't adversely affect the OS of APC patients. Moreover, subgroup analysis further showed that an inferior OS was only observed in APC survivors who had prior cancer originating from bladder, colon and cecum, or lung and bronchus, or prior CLL. In addition, these aforementioned results were further confirmed by the multivariable Cox analysis after adjusting for various clinicopathological variables. Hence, our data implied that a large number of APC patients who had a history of

Table 3 Multivariable Cox analysis for advanced prostate patients with prior cancer (vs. no prior cancer)

Characteristic	Overall survival		Prostate cancer-specific survival	
	HR (95 % CI)	P	HR (95 % CI)	P
All patients	1.13 (1.02–1.26)	0.017	0.93 (0.81–1.06)	0.248
Part I: Prior cancer timing (vs. no prior cancer)				
≤ 1 year	1.35 (1.11–1.66)	0.003	0.80 (0.60–1.08)	0.152
1–2 year	1.27 (1.02–1.57)	0.033	0.97 (0.72–1.29)	0.818
2–3 year	1.18 (0.93–1.49)	0.176	0.78 (0.56–1.09)	0.150
3–5 year	1.14 (0.94–1.37)	0.180	0.97 (0.77–1.23)	0.792
5–10 year	1.05 (0.89–1.24)	0.535	0.93 (0.76–1.15)	0.512
>10 year	1.11 (0.92–1.33)	0.270	1.09 (0.88–1.35)	0.432
Part II: Prior cancer stage (vs. no prior cancer)				
In situ	1.13 (0.87–1.47)	0.365	0.90 (0.64–1.27)	0.539
Localized	1.05 (0.91–1.21)	0.537	0.87 (0.73–1.05)	0.139
Regional	1.27 (0.97–1.68)	0.083	0.91 (0.70–1.19)	0.488
Distant	1.31 (1.08–1.58)	0.007	0.77 (0.51–1.16)	0.206
Part III: Prior cancer type (vs. no prior cancer)				
Urinary bladder	1.39 (1.16–1.66)	<0.001	0.98 (0.77–1.26)	0.880
Colon and cecum	1.23 (1.02–1.48)	0.034	0.67 (0.67–1.11)	0.243
Melanoma of the skin	1.02 (0.70–1.19)	0.502	0.93 (0.68–1.26)	0.618
Non-hodgkin lymphoma	1.16 (0.89–1.52)	0.277	1.22 (0.89–1.65)	0.213
Rectum	1.10 (0.81–1.48)	0.546	0.78 (0.52–1.19)	0.250
Lung and bronchus	1.54 (1.15–2.08)	0.004	0.90 (0.58–1.42)	0.658
Kidney and renal pelvis	0.79 (0.57–1.09)	0.154	0.70 (0.47–1.06)	0.096
Chronic lymphocytic leukemia	1.47 (1.01–2.15)	0.046	1.10 (0.66–1.85)	0.707
larynx	1.06 (0.64–1.76)	0.819	0.94 (0.50–1.78)	0.850
Others	1.05 (0.89–1.24)	0.576	0.92(0.77–1.14)	0.447

HR hazard ratio, *CI* confidence interval

The multivariate analysis was adjusted for age, race, marital status, histologic grade, and treatment modalities (surgery, chemotherapy, and radiation)

prior cancer may be eligible candidates for relevant cancer trials.

There are also several limitations in our study. First, other information such as efficacy and toxicity of treatment on prior cancer could not be considered due to lack of relevant data. Second, selection bias is inherent because of the intrinsic weaknesses of retrospective study. Therefore, further study is warranted to confirm the generality of our findings.

Conclusion

In conclusion, a large number of APC patients have a prior cancer history. Only prior cancer diagnosed within two year, at advanced stage, or some specific prior cancer adversely affect APC patients' survival. Therefore, for APC cancer patients with prior cancer history, broader inclusion criterion should be adopted

to increase the accrual rate for the relevant clinical cancer trials.

Supplementary Information

Additional file 1: Fig. S1. Kaplan-Meier survival curves of prior cancer impact on the overall survival (OS) stratified by different types of prior cancer in patients with advanced prostate cancer. (A) The impact of prior kidney cancer on OS; (B) The impact of prior chronic lymphocytic leukemia on OS; (C) The impact of prior larynx cancer on OS; (D) The impact of prior others cancer on OS.

Abbreviations

APC: Advanced prostate cancer; SEER: Surveillance, Epidemiology, and End Results; OS: Overall survival; CSS: Cancer-specific survival; PSM: Propensity score matching; HR: Adjusted hazard ratio; IQR: Interquartile range; CLL: Chronic lymphocytic leukemia.

Acknowledgements

The authors acknowledged the efforts of the Surveillance, Epidemiology, and End Results (SEER) Program tumor registries in the creation of the SEER database.

Authors' contributions

YW, TC contributed to study conception and design. YW, XC, DQ contributed to data acquisition. YW, WW, YZ contributed to analysis and interpretation data. JH, JZ, QW contributed to drafting the manuscript. QW, TC were involved in revising the manuscript. All authors have read and approved the manuscript.

Author details

[1] Department of Urology, Baoshan Branch, Shuguang Hospital Affiliated to Shanghai University of Traditional Chinese Medicine, Shanghai 201900, People's Republic of China. [2] Department of Urology, Tongji Hospital, Tongji University School of Medicine, Shanghai 200065, People's Republic of China. [3] Department of Urology, Shanghai Forth People's Hospital Affiliated to Tongji University School of Medicine, Shanghai 200434, People's Republic of China. [4] Department of Urology, Tongji Hospital, Tongji University School of Medicine, Shanghai 200065, People's Republic of China.

References

1. Siegel RL, Miller KD, Jemal A. Cancer statistics, 2018. Cancer J Clin. 2018;68(1):7–30.
2. Saad F, Shore N, Zhang T, Sharma S, Cho HK, Jacobs IA. Emerging therapeutic targets for patients with advanced prostate cancer. Cancer Treat Rev. 2019;76:1–9.
3. Wang YQ, Lv JW, Tang LL, Du XJ, Chen L, Li WF, Liu X, Guo Y, Lin AH, Mao YP, et al. Effect of prior cancer on trial eligibility and treatment outcomes in nasopharyngeal carcinoma: Implications for clinical trial accrual. Oral Oncol. 2019;90:23–9.
4. Filion M, Forget G, Brochu O, Provencher L, Desbiens C, Doyle C, Poirier B, DuRocher M, Camden S, Lemieux J. Eligibility criteria in randomized phase II and III adjuvant and neoadjuvant breast cancer trials: not a significant barrier to enrollment. Clin Trials. 2012;9(5):652–9.
5. Gerber DE, Laccetti AL, Xuan L, Halm EA, Pruitt SL. Impact of prior cancer on eligibility for lung cancer clinical trials. J Natl Cancer Inst. 2014;106(11):302.
6. Laccetti AL, Pruitt SL, Xuan L, Halm EA, Gerber DE. Effect of prior cancer on outcomes in advanced lung cancer: implications for clinical trial eligibility and accrual. J Natl Cancer Inst. 2015;107(4):dvj002.
7. Pierce SR, Stine JE, Gehrig PA, Havrilesky LJ, Secord AA, Nakayama J, Snavely AC, Moore DT, Kim KH. Prior breast cancer and tamoxifen exposure does not influence outcomes in women with uterine papillary serous carcinoma. Gynecol Oncol. 2017;144(3):531–5.
8. Ji F, Yang CQ, Li XL, Zhang LL, Yang M, Li JQ, Gao HF, Zhu T, Cheng MY, Li WP, et al. Risk of breast cancer-related death in women with a prior cancer. Aging. 2020;12(7):5894–906.
9. Cronin KA, Ries LA, Edwards BK. The Surveillance, Epidemiology, and End Results (SEER) Program of the National Cancer Institute. Cancer. 2014;120(Suppl **23**):3755–7.
10. Austin PC. An introduction to propensity score methods for reducing the effects of confounding in observational studies. Multivar Behav Res. 2011;46(3):399–424.
11. de Moor JS, Mariotto AB, Parry C, Alfano CM, Padgett L, Kent EE, Forsythe L, Scoppa S, Hachey M, Rowland JH. Cancer survivors in the United States: prevalence across the survivorship trajectory and implications for care. Cancer Epidemiol Biomark Prev. 2013;22(4):561–70.
12. Miller KD, Siegel RL, Lin CC, Mariotto AB, Kramer JL, Rowland JH, Stein KD, Alteri R, Jemal A. Cancer treatment and survivorship statistics, 2016. Cancer J Clin. 2016;66(4):271–89.
13. Oh CM, Won YJ, Jung KW, Kong HJ, Cho H, Lee JK, Lee DH, Lee KH. Cancer Statistics in Korea: incidence, mortality, survival, and prevalence in 2013. Cancer Res Treat. 2016;48(2):436–50.
14. Travis LB, Demark Wahnefried W, Allan JM, Wood ME, Ng AK. Aetiology, genetics and prevention of secondary neoplasms in adult cancer survivors. Nat Rev Clin Oncol. 2013;10(5):289–301.
15. Wood ME, Vogel V, Ng A, Foxhall L, Goodwin P, Travis LB. Second malignant neoplasms: assessment and strategies for risk reduction. J Clin Oncol. 2012;30(30):3734–45.
16. Murphy CC, Gerber DE, Pruitt SL. Prevalence of prior cancer among persons newly diagnosed with cancer: an initial report from the surveillance, epidemiology, and end results program. JAMA Oncol. 2018;4(6):832–6.
17. Lin C, Wu J, Ding S, Goh C, Andriani L, Shen K, Zhu L. Impact of prior cancer history on the clinical outcomes in advanced breast cancer: a propensity score-adjusted, population-based study. Cancer Res Treat. 2020;52(2):552–62.
18. Bluethmann SM, Mariotto AB, Rowland JH. Anticipating the "Silver Tsunami": prevalence trajectories and comorbidity burden among older cancer survivors in the United States. Cancer Epidemiol Biomark Prev. 2016;25(7):1029–36.
19. Laccetti LA, Pruitt LS, Lei, Xuan AE, Halm ED, Gerber. Effect of prior cancer on outcomes in advanced lung cancer: implications for clinical trial eligibility and accrual.J Natl Cancer Inst 2015.
20. Kim ES, Bruinooge SS, Roberts S, Ison G, Lin NU, Gore L, Uldrick TS, Lichtman SM, Roach N, Beaver JA, et al. Broadening eligibility criteria to make clinical trials more representative: American Society of Clinical Oncology and Friends of Cancer Research Joint Research Statement. J Clin Oncol. 2017;35(33):3737–44.
21. Lemieux J, Goodwin PJ, Pritchard KI, Gelmon KA, Bordeleau LJ, Duchesne T, Camden S, Speers CH. Identification of cancer care and protocol characteristics associated with recruitment in breast cancer clinical trials. J Clin Oncol. 2008;26(27):4458–65.
22. Gerber DE, Pruitt SL, Halm EA. Should criteria for inclusion in cancer clinical trials be expanded? J Comp Effect Res. 2015;4(4):289–91.
23. Administration TFaD. Cancer Clinical Trial Eligibility Criteria: Patients with Organ Dysfunction or Prior or Concurrent Malignancies. Washington, DC: The Food and Drug Administration c2019 [cited 2019 Mar 7]. https://www.fda.gov/Drugs/GuidanceComplianceRegulatoryInformation/Guidances/default.htm.
24. Zhou H, Huang Y, Qiu Z, Zhao H, Fang W, Yang Y, Zhao Y, Hou X, Ma Y, Hong S, et al. Impact of prior cancer history on the overall survival of patients newly diagnosed with cancer: a pan-cancer analysis of the SEER database. Int J Cancer. 2018;143(7):1569–77.

7

Comprehensive analysis of tumour mutational burden and its clinical significance in prostate cancer

Lijuan Wang, Shucheng Pan, Binbin Zhu, Zhenliang Yu and Wei Wang*⬤

Abstract

Background: The tumorigenesis of prostate cancer involves genetic mutations. Tumour mutational burden (TMB) is an emerging biomarker for predicting the efficacy of immunotherapy.

Results: Single-nucleotide polymorphisms were the most common variant type, and C>T transversion was the most commonly presented type of single-nucleotide variant. The high-TMB group had lower overall survival (OS) than the low-TMB group. TMB was associated with age, T stage and N stage. Functional enrichment analysis of differentially expressed genes (DEGs) showed that they are involved in pathways related to the terms spindle, chromosomal region, nuclear division, chromosome segregation, cell cycle, oocyte meiosis and other terms associated with DNA mutation and cell proliferation. Six hub genes, PLK1, KIF2C, MELK, EXO1, CEP55 and CDK1, were identified. All the genes were associated with disease-free survival, and CEP55 and CDK1 were associated with OS.

Conclusions: The present study provides a comprehensive analysis of the significance of TMB and DEGs and infiltrating immune cells related to TMB, which provides helpful information for exploring the significance of TMB in prostate cancer.

Keywords: Prostate cancer, Tumour mutational burden, Gene, Clinical

Background

Prostate cancer ranks as the second most commonly diagnosed malignancy in males [1]. In terms of treatment, challenges still exist, especially for castration-resistant prostate cancer (CRPC). CRPC with metastasis is reported to have a poor prognosis, with a median survival time of less than 2 years [2]. In recent years, immune checkpoint inhibitors blocking programmed cell death 1 and its ligand (PD-1/PD-L1) and cytotoxic T-lymphocyte antigen-4 (CTLA-4) have shown promising preliminary results in various kinds of tumours. Two clinical trials of ipilimumab in metastatic CRPC have shown improved progression-free survival [3, 4]. Nevertheless, the

utilization of immunotherapy is still limited by low efficacy. Some response predictive biomarkers are under investigation, including tumour mutational burden (TMB).

TMB involves the number of non-synonymous somatic mutations per megabase pair (Mbp) of sequenced DNA. Mutations of tumours affect the mutational load, which in turn determines the chance of presenting immunogenically relevant neoantigens [5]. High-TMB tumours tend to harbour more neoantigens than low-TMB tumours, which make the high-TMB tumours more immunogenic, resulting in an improved T cell response and subsequent enhancement of antitumour immunity. Given the function of TMB in immunity, clinical studies focused on melanoma and non-small-cell lung cancer have demonstrated that the TMB is associated with the immunotherapy treatment response [6, 7]. Therefore, TMB is believed

*Correspondence: wangw2005@zju.edu.cn
The First Affiliated Hospital, Zhejiang University School of Medicine, Hangzhou 310003, Zhejiang Province, China

to be one of the candidates for predicting the efficacy of immunotherapy.

Next-generation sequencing (NGS) profiling of patients has enabled advancements, and The Cancer Genome Atlas (TCGA) offers convenient access to relevant information. In this study, the gene expression and mutation profiles of prostate cancer samples were extracted from TCGA, and the data were used to investigate the clinical significance of TMB and its related differentially expressed genes (DEGs) and immune cell infiltration signatures.

Methods

Data collection and processing

Transcriptome data in the HTSeq-FPKM format from 524 samples, including 499 prostate and 25 adjacent normal tissue samples, were acquired from the TCGA databank (https://portal.gdc.cancer.gov/). The data were in masked somatic mutation files, and these data were analysed and visualized using the R software package maftools.

Estimation of TMB and its associations with clinical factors

TMB was defined as the sum of mutations in coding regions per megabase and was calculated as the total number of mutations/the length of exons. The length of exons was estimated to be 38 Mb in previous research [8]. First, Perl scripts were written to obtain the estimated TMB data, which were amalgamated with interrelated survival profiles for each patient. Then, we set the median TMB value as the cutoff, according to which samples were classified into a group with high TMB and a group with low TMB. We utilized the survival R package to analyse the overall survival (OS) differences between the two groups. The differences in TMB between groups categorized based on clinical features (age, T stage and N stage) were analysed using the limma R package.

Identification of DEGs and DEG pathway analysis

First, we performed DEG analysis with |log$_2$ fold change > 1| and false discovery rate (FDR) < 0.05 as cutoffs. We employed the limma package in the R package to analyse the differences and used pheatmap in the R package to generate a heatmap. Subsequently, the gene symbols were transferred into the ID of Entrez using the org.Hs.eg.db package of the R package. Moreover, we employed the ggplot2, enrichplot, and clusterProfiler of R packages to perform Gene Ontology (GO) and Kyoto Encyclopedia of Genes and Genomes (KEGG) analyses of the DEGs. We used GSEA software (https://www.gsea-msigdb.org/gsea/index.jsp) to perform GSEA. We used c2.cp.kegg.v7.0.symbols.gmt as the databank of gene sets. In addition, the TMB level was set as the phenotype

labels. The pathways were considered to be statistically enriched according to a cutoff of FDR < 0.25.

Protein–protein interaction (PPI) network and classification of core genes

We constructed a PPI network of DEGs using STRIING (https://string-db.org/). Evidence-based interactions were generated with a minimum required interaction score > 0.4 [9]. Then, the PPI network was visualized by utilizing Cytoscape 3.8.0 software [10]. Using the Cyto-Hubba plugin, we obtained five protein groups, including the top 30 proteins, with five analytic algorithms, including MCC, MNC, Degree, EPC and EcCentricity, as previously reported [11]. In addition, we acquired the overlapping proteins of the five groups and identified pivotal proteins with more interactions than others as potential hub proteins. These intersections were visualized by a Venn diagram, which was generated online (http://bioinformatics.psb.ugent.be/webtools/Venn/). GEPIA (http://gepia.cancer-pku.cn/) was used to investigate the prognostic significance of the hub proteins.

CIBERSORT

CIBERSORT is an algorithm for characterizing the immune cell composition of certain tissues according to their gene expression profiles [12]. We used CIBERSORT in the R package to analyse 22 types of immune cells. The comparison of the levels of immune cells between the group with low TMB and the group with high TMB was conducted using the Wilcoxon rank-sum test, and the results were presented in a violin diagram generated with the vioplot package of the R package.

Statistical analysis

We used the Kaplan–Meier method to generate the survival curve. The comparisons of OS between different groups categorized according to TMB, age, T stage and N stage was performed using the log-rank test. We used the Shapiro–Wilk test to determine whether the groups categorized according to TMB, age, T stage and N stage had normal distributions. Through the Shapiro–Wilk test, we found that all the groups were not normally distributed, and thus, nonparametric tests were required. The Wilcoxon rank-sum test was used to compare groups classified by age and N stage. The Kruskal–Wallis test was used to compare groups classified by T stage. We used R software (version 3.6.1) to perform the Kaplan–Meier analysis, log-rank test, Wilcoxon rank-sum test and Kruskal–Wallis test. We used SPSS (version 25.0) to perform the Shapiro–Wilk test. The criterion for statistical significance was a P value < 0.05.

Results

Mutations in prostate cancer

We obtained mutation data from TCGA, which were analysed and visualized with the maftools package. Missense mutations were the most common type of variant (Fig. 1a). The frequency of single-nucleotide polymorphisms (SNPs) was greater than that of other variant types (Fig. 1b). C>T transversions represented the largest proportion of single-nucleotide variants (SNVs) in prostate cancer (Fig. 1c). TTN, TP53, SPOP, KMT2D, SYNE1, MUC16, FOXA1, KMT2C, SPTA1 and ATM were the top ten genes with high mutation frequencies.

Associations of TMB with prognostic and clinical factors

Based on the median TMB, we stratified the patients with prostate cancer into a group with high TMB and a group with low TMB. The prognostic analysis revealed that the group with low TMB had increased OS compared with the group with high TMB (Fig. 2a, $P = 0.026$). There was a relationship between age, T stage, N stage and TMB level (Fig. 2b–d). The median age of the patients was 61 years. It was demonstrated that patients older than 61 years had a higher TMB than those who were 61 years or younger(Fig. 2b, $P < 0.001$). In addition, the higher the T stage was, the higher the TMB (Fig. 2c, $P < 0.001$). Similar results were seen for N stage, with the N1 stage group having a higher TMB than the group with other N stages (Fig. 2d, $P < 0.001$).

Comparison of DEGs and functional enrichment analysis

A total of 257 DEGs were identified, and the top 20 DEGs were displayed in the heatmap (Fig. 3a). Functional enrichment analysis of the DEGs was conducted. GO enrichment analysis, including three major categories, was utilized (Fig. 3b). In the biological process (BP) category, the terms nuclear division, organelle fission and chromosome segregation were enriched. The cellular component (CC) category terms included spindle, chromosomal region, kinetochore, midbody and microtubule. The molecular function (MF) category terms involved receptor-ligand activity, growth factor activity and hormone activity. Moreover, we identified pathways related to the terms microRNA in cancer, cell cycle, oocyte meiosis and ECM-receptor interaction in the KEGG enrichment analysis (Fig. 3c). There were 37 pathways enriched in the GSEA, and the top 10 pathways were displayed in a diagram (Fig. 3d). These pathways were related to DNA-level cell proliferation, including mechanisms such as pyrimidine metabolism, DNA replication, DNA degradation, and aminoacyl tRNA biosynthesis, and the findings were in accordance with the above results.

PPI network of DEGs and selected hub genes

A PPI network of 189 nodes and 1789 edges was generated by STRING, and online tool for analysing proteins, and the results were visualized by Cytoscape (Fig. 4a). Five algorithms, MCC, MNC, Degree, EPC and EcCentricity, were utilized, and the overlapping proteins in the results generated from each algorithm were identified with Venn diagrams (Fig. 4b). PLK1, KIF2C, MELK, EXO1, CEP55 and CDK1 were identified as hub genes through this method. High expression of PLK1 and KIF2C was related to poor overall survival, with a P value < 0.05. High expression of PLK1, KIF2C, MELK, EXO1, CEP55 and CDK1 was related to poor disease-free survival, with a P value < 0.05.

Comparison of differential immune cell signatures

A violin diagram was generated to visualize the differences in the proportions of 22 infiltrating immune cells between the group with low TMB and the group with high TMB (Fig. 5). The group with high TMB had higher levels of CD8 T cells and activated CD4 memory cells than the low TMB group ($P < 0.05$). However, there were no other statistically significant findings or trends for the other infiltrating immune cells.

Discussion

Immunotherapies have shown preliminary results in prostate cancer. TMB is considered an emerging biomarker for response evaluation. Therefore, it is meaningful to investigate the relationship between TMB and prostate cancer. This study provides an overview of mutations, the clinical significance of TMB, and DEGs and infiltrating immune cells related to TMB in prostate cancer.

Among the top 10 mutated genes, TP53, SPOP, FOXA1 and ATM showed pivotal functions in the initiation and development of malignant prostate cancer. As a tumour suppressor, TP53 has a high mutation frequency among various kinds of tumours, and the mutant form is equipped with antiproliferative functions and is related to the metastasis and progression of prostate cancer [13, 14]. Mutations in SPOP are considered the most common recurrent point mutations in prostate cancer [15]. SPOP is crucial for the preservation of nuclear genome stability and is essential for the degradation of multiple proteins [16, 17]. FOXA1 is necessary for androgen receptor-mediated activation of prostate genes [18]. Furthermore, the expression of FOXA1 is related to tumorigenesis and the progression of prostate cancer [19]. ATM is considered one of the

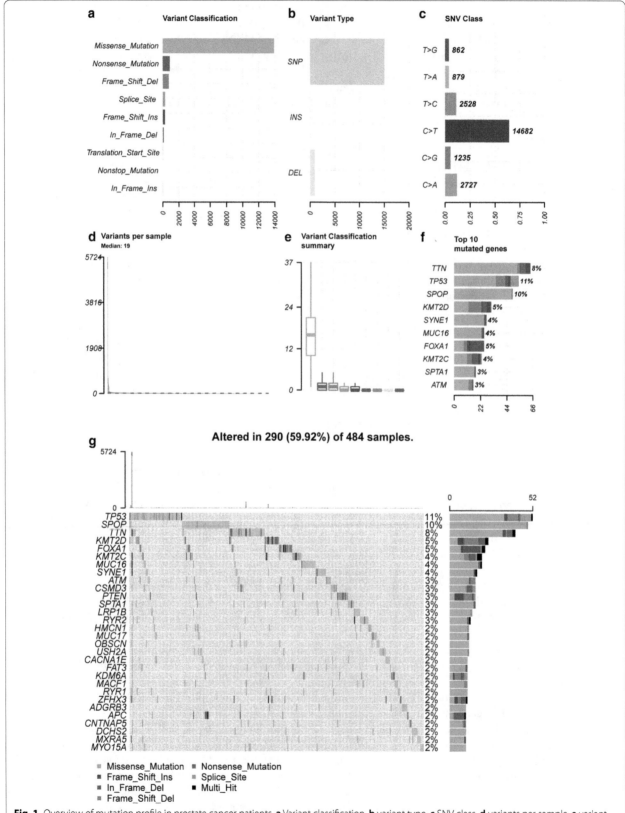

Fig. 1 Overview of mutation profile in prostate cancer patients. **a** Variant classification, **b** variant type, **c** SNV class, **d** variants per sample, **e** variant classification summary, **f** top 10 mutated gene, **g** waterfall diagram of top 30 mutated genes

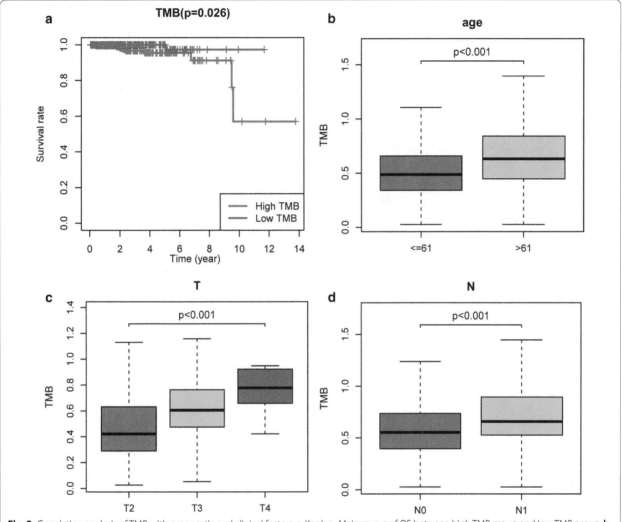

Fig. 2 Correlation analysis of TMB with prognostic and clinical factors. **a** Kaplan–Meier curve of OS between high TMB group and low TMB group, **b** the difference of TMB level between groups classified by age, **c** the difference of TMB level between groups classified by T stage, **d** the difference of TMB level between groups classified by N stage

DNA damage repair genes, and its activation can be seen in the earlier stages of prostate tumorigenesis [20].

The clinical significance of TMB in prostate cancer was assessed. Similar to a previous prostate and renal cancer study, our study found that the group of patients with prostate cancer with high TMB had lower OS than the group of patients with prostate cancer with low TMB[1][21]. Furthermore, we observed higher TMB levels in patients older than 61 years than in those who were 61 years or younger and in the higher T stage and N1 stage groups. According to reports from the TCGA database, the prognostic role of TMB is unclear. In a study of bladder cancer, the high TMB group exhibited increased OS compared with the low TMB group [22]. Two reasons probably account for the results of our research.

One reason is that not all patients with a high TMB have an increased treatment response, as not every generated neoantigen has immunogenicity [23]. That is, high TMB does not always initiate an antitumour response. Another reason is that the high TMB group in this study was older and had a more advanced stage than the low TMB group.

GO and KEGG analyses revealed that the DEGs between the group with high TMB and the group with low TMB were related to the terms spindle, chromosomal region, kinetochore, nuclear division, chromosome segregation, cell cycle, oocyte meiosis, receptor-ligand activity, growth factor activity and ECM-receptor interaction, all of which are associated with DNA mutation and cell proliferation. Furthermore, the results of GSEA also supported this observation, showing enrichment of

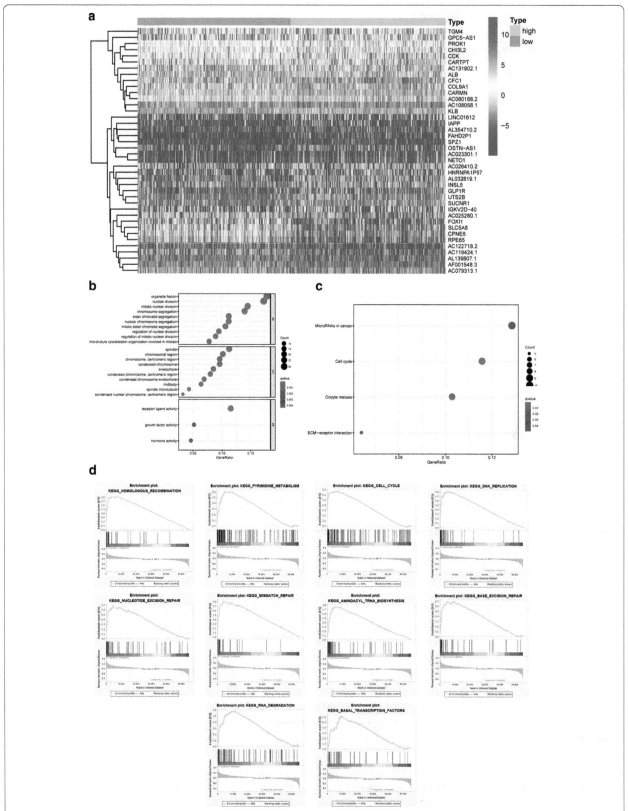

Fig. 3 DEGs and its corresponding enrichment analysis. **a** Heatmap of the top 20 DEGs, **b** GO enrichment of the DEGs, **c** KEGG enrichment of the DEGs, **d** top 10 pathways of the GSEA enrichment

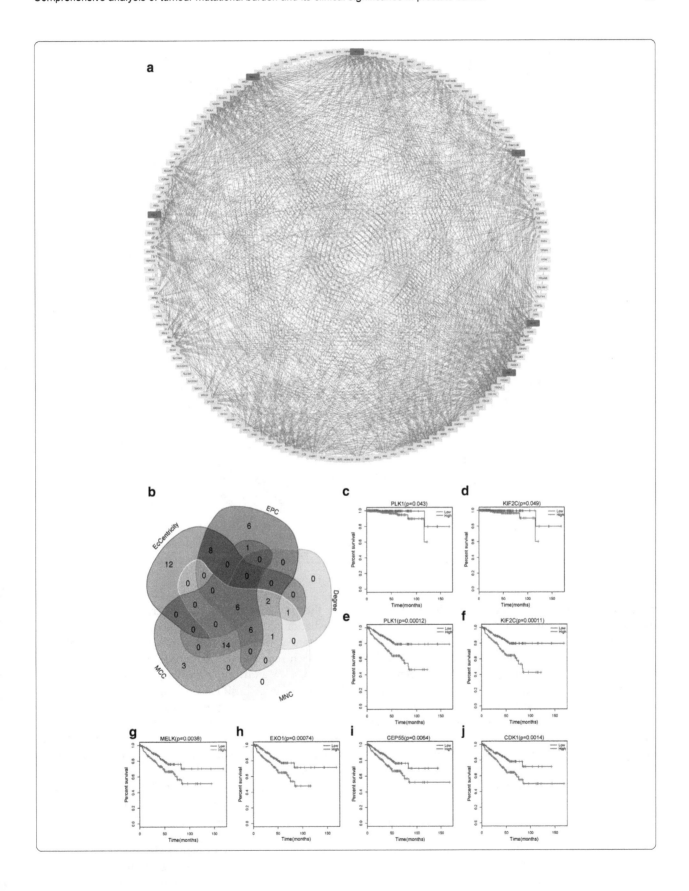

(See figure on previous page.)
Fig. 4 PPI network and hub genes with their correlation to survival. **a** PPI network of DEGs generated by Cytoscape with hub genes showing red color, **b** Venn dots of intersections from five methodology involved MCC, MNC, Degree, EPC and EcCentricity, **c–j** Logrank analysis of hubgenes. The relation of PLK1 (**c**) and KIF2C (**d**) with overall survival in prostate cancer patients. The relation of PLK (**e**), KIF2C (**f**), MELK (**g**), EXO1 (**h**), CEP55 (**i**) and CDK1 (**j**) with disease free survival in prostate cancer patients

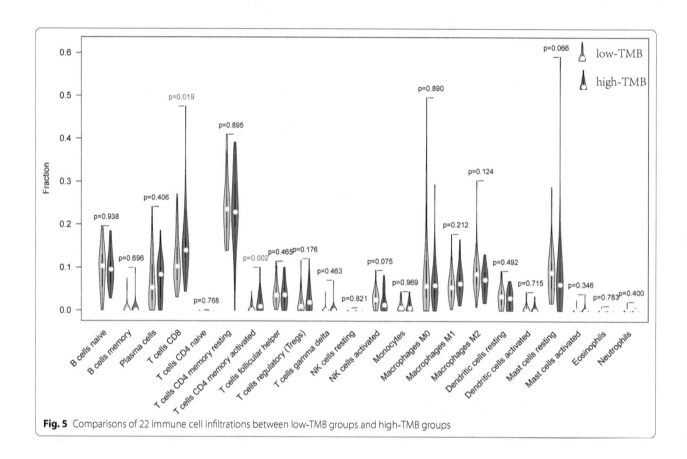

Fig. 5 Comparisons of 22 immune cell infiltrations between low-TMB groups and high-TMB groups

pathways related to pyrimidine metabolism, DNA replication, DNA degradation and aminoacyl tRNA biosynthesis. None of the analyses showed associations with pathways related to immune mediation or response. This phenomenon is likely because the immunogenicity of prostate cancer cases with low TMB is poorer than that of lung cancer and melanoma [24]. Because of this poor immunogenicity, the numbers of neoantigens generated by prostate cancer patients may be less than those generated by high-TMB cancer patients. The subsequent immune response in patients with low TMB is probably also weaker than that of high-TMB cancer patients.

Through CytoHubba analysis of the PPI network, we identified six hub genes: PLK1, KIF2C, MELK, EXO1, CEP55 and CDK1. All the genes were correlated with DFS, and CEP55 and CDK1 were associated with OS. PLK1 and MELK have been suggested to be potential targets in prostate cancer. As PLK1 plays a critical role

in the proliferation of cells, centrosome abnormalities, mediation of the cell cycle and apoptosis, it is considered a potential treatment target in prostate cancer [25]. It has been reported that targeting PLK1 can enhance the response to androgen signalling inhibitors or olaparib in CRPC [26, 27]. MELK is upregulated in prostate cancer and related to aggressiveness. Furthermore, in vitro silencing of MELK can weaken the proliferation of prostate cancer cells, and in vivo tests also proved that an inhibitor of MELK could repress the growth of prostate cancer.

Different kinds of immune cells play a pivotal role in the tumour microenvironment and are also determinants of immunotherapy efficacy. Therefore, our study explored differences in the levels of immune cells between the group with high TMB and the group with low TMB. The analysis indicated that the group with high TMB had a significantly higher proportion of CD8

T cells and activated CD4 memory cells than the group with low TMB. These findings were similar to those in previous reports of bladder cancer [22]. Generally, a high TMB can produce more neoantigens, eliciting a subsequent immune response. CD8 T cells are one of the determinants of antigen-specific responses. Therefore, the high TMB group with higher levels of CD8 T cells is likely to experience superior immunotherapy efficacy. However, a recent study demonstrated that metastatic CRPC with low TMB but a high density of CD8 T cells could also benefit from immune checkpoint inhibitors [28]. Our findings suggesting that TMB has an interaction with immune infiltration are only preliminary, and further validation in clinical cohorts and investigations to explore the underlying mechanisms of the correlations are needed.

The study has some limitations that should be considered. Firstly, all the data were retrospectively collected which had bias. Secondly, the results of our study were preliminary exploration and should be further tested through in vitro or in vivo experiments. Thirdly, our study lacked sub-group analysis including CRPC patients and non-CRPC patients.

Conclusion

In conclusion, we performed a comprehensive and systematic analysis of TMB in prostate cancer and analysed its clinical significance. Furthermore, we also identified enriched pathways of DEGs, hub genes with prognostic roles and infiltrating immune cells related to TMB. Our results elucidate the association between TMB and infiltrating immune cells in prostate malignancy and will likely be useful for future investigations of TMB in prostate cancer.

Supplementary Information

Additional file 1. Table S1. Setting items of the transcriptome data. **Table S2.** Setting items of the clinical data. **Table S3.** Setting items of the mutation data.

Abbreviations

TMB: Tumour mutational burden; SNPs: Single nucleotide polymorphisms; SNV: Single-nucleotide variant; OS: Overall survival; DFS: Disease free survival; CRPC: Castration-resistant prostate cancer; PD-1/PD-L1: Programmed cell death 1 and its ligand; CTLA-4: Cytotoxic T-lymphocyte antigen-4; Mbp: Megabase pair; NGS: Next-generation sequencing; TCGA: The Cancer Genome Atlas; GO: Gene Ontology; KEGG: Kyoto Encyclopedia of Genes and Genomes; PPI: Protein–protein interaction; BP: Biological process; CC: Cellular component; MF: Molecular function.

Acknowledgments

Not applicable.

Authors' contributions

LJW performed data analysis work and wrote the manuscript. SCP, BBZ and ZLY edited the manuscript. WW designed the study. All authors read and approved the final manuscript.

References

1. Center MM, Jemal A, Lortet-Tieulent J, et al. International variation in prostate cancer incidence and mortality rates. Eur Urol. 2012;61(6):1079–92.
2. Zhu Y, Ye D. Chinese Expert Consensus on the Diagnosis and Treatment of Castration-Resistant Prostate Cancer (2019 Update). Cancer Manag Res. 2020;12:2127–40.
3. Kwon ED, Drake CG, Scher HI, et al. Ipilimumab versus placebo after radiotherapy in patients with metastatic castration-resistant prostate cancer that had progressed after docetaxel chemotherapy (CA184-043): a multicentre, randomised, double-blind, phase 3 trial. Lancet Oncol. 2014;15(7):700–12.
4. Beer TM, Kwon ED, Drake CG, et al. Randomized, double-blind, phase III trial of ipilimumab versus placebo in asymptomatic or minimally symptomatic patients with metastatic chemotherapy-naive castration-resistant prostate cancer. J Clin Oncol. 2017;35(1):40–7.
5. Riaz N, Morris L, Havel JJ, Makarov V, Desrichard A, Chan TA. The role of neoantigens in response to immune checkpoint blockade. Int Immunol. 2016;28(8):411–9.
6. Snyder A, Makarov V, Merghoub T, et al. Genetic basis for clinical response to CTLA-4 blockade in melanoma. N Engl J Med. 2014;371(23):2189–99.
7. Rizvi NA, Hellmann MD, Snyder A, et al. Cancer immunology. Mutational landscape determines sensitivity to PD-1 blockade in non-small cell lung cancer. Science. 2015;348(6230):124–8.
8. Chalmers ZR, Connelly CF, Fabrizio D, et al. Analysis of 100,000 human cancer genomes reveals the landscape of tumor mutational burden. Genome Med. 2017;9(1):34.
9. Szklarczyk D, Morris JH, Cook H, et al. The STRING database in 2017: quality-controlled protein-protein association networks, made broadly accessible. Nucleic Acids Res. 2017;45(D1):D362–8.
10. Shannon P, Markiel A, Ozier O, et al. Cytoscape: a software environment for integrated models of biomolecular interaction networks. Genome Res. 2003;13(11):2498–504.
11. Liu Z, Meng J, Li X, et al. Identification of Hub genes and key pathways associated with two subtypes of diffuse large B-cell lymphoma based on gene expression profiling via integrated bioinformatics. Biomed Res Int. 2018;2018:3574534.
12. Newman AM, Liu CL, Green MR, et al. Robust enumeration of cell subsets from tissue expression profiles. Nat Methods. 2015;12(5):453–7.
13. Kandoth C, McLellan MD, Vandin F, et al. Mutational landscape and significance across 12 major cancer types. Nature. 2013;502(7471):333–9.
14. Petitjean A, Achatz MI, Borresen-Dale AL, Hainaut P, Olivier M. TP53 mutations in human cancers: functional selection and impact on cancer prognosis and outcomes. Oncogene. 2007;26(15):2157–65.
15. Barbieri CE, Baca SC, Lawrence MS, et al. Exome sequencing identifies recurrent SPOP, FOXA1 and MED12 mutations in prostate cancer. Nat Genet. 2012;44(6):685–9.
16. Geng C, He B, Xu L, et al. Prostate cancer-associated mutations in speckle-type POZ protein (SPOP) regulate steroid receptor coactivator 3 protein turnover. Proc Natl Acad Sci USA. 2013;110(17):6997–7002.
17. Boysen G, Barbieri CE, Prandi D, et al. SPOP mutation leads to genomic instability in prostate cancer. Elife. 2015;4:e09207.
18. Gao N, Zhang J, Rao MA, et al. The role of hepatocyte nuclear factor-3 alpha (Forkhead Box A1) and androgen receptor in transcriptional regulation of prostatic genes. Mol Endocrinol. 2003;17(8):1484–507.
19. Alvarez-Cubero MJ, Martinez-Gonzalez LJ, Robles-Fernandez I, et al. Somatic mutations in prostate cancer: closer to personalized medicine. Mol Diagn Ther. 2017;21(2):167–78.
20. Fan C, Quan R, Feng X, et al. ATM activation is accompanied with earlier stages of prostate tumorigenesis. Biochim Biophys Acta. 2006;1763(10):1090–7.
21. Zhang C, Li Z, Qi F, Hu X, Luo J. Exploration of the relationships between tumor mutation burden with immune infiltrates in clear cell renal cell carcinoma. Ann Transl Med. 2019;7(22):648.

22. Zhang C, Shen L, Qi F, Wang J, Luo J. Multi-omics analysis of tumor mutation burden combined with immune infiltrates in bladder urothelial carcinoma. J Cell Physiol. 2020;235(4):3849–63.

23. Chabanon RM, Pedrero M, Lefebvre C, Marabelle A, Soria JC, Postel-Vinay S. Mutational landscape and sensitivity to immune checkpoint blockers. Clin Cancer Res. 2016;22(17):4309–21.

24. De Velasco MA, Uemura H. Prostate cancer immunotherapy: where are we and where are we going? Curr Opin Urol. 2018;28(1):15–24.

25. Ahmad N. Polo-like kinase (Plk) 1: a novel target for the treatment of prostate cancer. FASEB J. 2004;18(1):5–7.

26. Zhang Z, Hou X, Shao C, et al. Plk1 inhibition enhances the efficacy of androgen signaling blockade in castration-resistant prostate cancer. Cancer Res. 2014;74(22):6635–47.

27. Li J, Wang R, Kong Y, et al. Targeting Plk1 to enhance efficacy of olaparib in castration-resistant prostate cancer. Mol Cancer Ther. 2017;16(3):469–79.

28. Subudhi SK, Vence L, Zhao H, et al. Neoantigen responses, immune correlates, and favorable outcomes after ipilimumab treatment of patients with prostate cancer. Sci Transl Med. 2020;12(537):eaaz3577.

8

Holmium laser enucleation of the prostate with Virtual Basket mode: Faster and better control on bleeding

Giorgio Bozzini[1,2]* ⬤, Matteo Maltagliati[1,3], Umberto Besana[1], Lorenzo Berti[1,3], Albert Calori[1], Maria Chiara Sighinolfi[3], Salvatore Micali[2,3], Jean Baptiste Roche[4], Ali Gozen[5], Alexander Mueller[6], Dimitry Pushkar[7], Evangelos Liatsikos[8], Marco Boldini[9], Carlo Buizza[1] and Bernardo Rocco[2,3]

Abstract

Background: To compare clinical intra and early postoperative outcomes between conventional Holmium laser enucleation of the prostate (HoLEP) and Holmium laser enucleation of the prostate using the Virtual Basket tool (VB-HoLEP) to treat benign prostatic hyperplasia (BPH).

Methods: This prospective randomized study enrolled consecutive patients with BPH, who were assigned to undergo either HoLEP (n = 100), or VB-HoLEP (n = 100). All patients were evaluated preoperatively and postoperatively, with particular attention to catheterization time, operative time, blood loss, irrigation volume and hospital stay. We also evaluated the patients at 3 and 6 months after surgery and assessed maximum flow rate (Qmax), postvoid residual urine volume (PVR), the International Prostate Symptom Score (IPSS) and the Quality of Life score (QOLS).

Results: No significant differences in preoperative parameters between patients in each study arm were found. Compared to HoLEP, VB-HoLEP resulted in less hemoglobin decrease (2.54 vs. 1.12 g/dl, $P = 0.03$) and reduced operative time (57.33 ± 29.71 vs. 42.99 ± 18.51 min, $P = 0.04$). HoLEP and VB-HoLEP detrmined similar catheterization time (2.2 vs. 1.9 days, $P = 0.45$), irrigation volume (33.3 vs. 31.7 l, $P = 0.69$), and hospital stay (2.8 vs. 2.7 days, $P = 0.21$). During the 6-month follow-up no significant differences in IPSS, Qmax, PVR, and QOLS were demonstrated.

Conclusions: HoLEP and VB-HoLEP are both efficient and safe procedures for relieving lower urinary tract symptoms. VB-HoLEP was statistically superior to HoLEP in blood loss and operative time. However, procedures did not differ significantly in catheterization time, hospital stay, and irrigation volume. No significant differences were demonstrated in QOLS, IPSS, Qmax and PVR throughout the 6-month follow-up.

Trial Registration: Current Controlled Trials ISRCTN72879639; date of registration: June 25th, 2015. Retrospectively registred.

Keywords: Benign prostatic hyperplasia, Holmium laser, Laser therapy, Prostate

Background

Benign prostatic hyperplasia (BPH), with consequent lower urinary tract symptoms (LUTS), is one of the most common diseases in aging men. Many surgical treatments are available to handle BPH refractory to pharmacological therapy [1]. Transurethral resection of the prostate (TURP) remains the gold standard surgical

*Correspondence: gioboz@yahoo.it
[1] Department of Urology, ASST Valle Olona, Via Arnaldo da Brescia, 21052 Busto Arsizio, VA, Italy
Full list of author information is available at the end of the article

treatment for prostates with a total volume between 30 and 80 ml. Open prostatectomy (OP), instead, is used for enlarged glands (> 80 ml) [2]. Today, laser enucleation of the prostate is gradually replacing these old techniques due to the advantage of decreased bleeding complications and increased safety. Laser procedures are indicated for the treatment of prostates > 80 ml and they can be considered as alternatives to TURP for prostates with a total volume between 30 and 80 ml [1, 3].

BPH laser surgery comprises many different technologies and techniques [4]. HoLEP was introduced 20 years ago by Fraundorfer and Gilling [5] and, since then, several studies have demonstrated that it determines a reduction in hospital stay, catheterization time, and intraoperative and postoperative bleeding [6]. During the procedure, the surgeons detach the adenoma from the prostate surgical capsule with a blunt dissection, using the holmium laser and the tip of the resectoscope. The laser also allows to perform an accurate hemostasis. With regard to energy and frequency settings, 1.8–2.5 J and 20–50 Hz are normally used, delivering a total power of 80–120 W.

Thanks to its pulsed activity, the Ho:YAG laser is also ideal for stone lithotripsy. However, the energy impact against the stone can cause its migration from the ureter to the renal cavities, or from one calyx to another. Stone migration increases operative time, patient morbidity and healthcare cost. Antiretropulsion devices have been created to prevent stone migration. The "Virtual Basket™" technology is a result of the laser's pulse modulation, usually employed for holmium laser lithotripsy: the laser emits part of the energy to create an initial bubble and the remaining energy is discharged once the bubble is formed, so that it can pass through the previously created vapor channel.

We applied the Virtual Basket™ mode to HoLEP (VB-HoLEP), in order to compare clinical, intra and early postoperative outcomes between conventional HoLEP and VB-HoLEP for the treatment of benign prostatic hyperplasia (BPH).

Methods

This prospective randomized study enrolled consecutive patients with BPH who received an indication to HoLEP according to EAU GuideLines [1]. Ethical committee approval was obtained (No. 2019/267 ATSIns) and a subsequent consent form was signed by each patient that entered the study (Clinical trial registration: ISRCTN72879639). A simple 1:1 randomization was used to assign each patient to either HoLEP, or VB-HoLEP. Exclusion criteria were: age under 18, or over 90, presence of acute infection (fever more than 38°C, total leucocyte count more than 15,000/dl or preoperative positive urinary colture), coexisting urethral, or prostate

disease and presence of bladder stones. Furthermore, all the recruited patients who refused to give their consent to the study were excluded. Coagulation during the procedure was performed by only using the laser and not with a monopolar, or bipolar resector.

Both groups were treated using the Cyber Ho 100 laser platform (Quanta System, Samarate, Lombardia, Italy) set to 1.8 J at 45 Hz for cutting, with 550 μm reusable laser fibres. The Virtual Basket mode was enabled on the left pedal (used for cutting) in the second group only. The same settings in both groups were also used for coagulation (0.6 J at 35 Hz). The adopted technique was the traditional 3 lobes technique.

A Storz resectoscope with a 12 degrees optic, a Kuntz element (Karl Storz Tuttlingen Germany) and a guide (to allow the 550 μm fiber to pass) were used for all the procedures.

After completing the enucleation, the dissected tissue was morcellated with the DrillCut morcellator (Karl Storz, Tuttlingen, Germany).

All of the patients were evaluated postoperatively with regards to blood loss, catheterization time, irrigation volume, hospital stay and operative time. At 3 and 6 months after surgery, patients were also evaluated with the International Prostate Symptom Score (IPSS), the Quality of Life Score (QOLS), maximum urinary flow rate (Qmax) and postvoid residual urine volume (PVR).

Statistical analysis

Simple Block Randomization was obtained using the "Adaptative Randomization" software (University of Texas) to reach a good number balance between the two groups. To reach a good allocation concealment we used a centralized service to rule all the partecipanting centers. To avoid any outcome bias blinding of the participants was ensured for the duration of hospitalization (they actually did not know which surgical technique was used for their enucleation) and data were never analyzed by one of the operating surgeons.

A statistical analysis was carried out to assess patients' data and outcomes. All of the reported P-values were obtained with the two-sided exact method at the conventional 5% significance level. Data were analyzed with the April 2016 by R software v.3.2.3 (R Foundation for Statistical Computing, Vienna, Austria), according to previously published guidelines for the reporting of statistics. We calculated the sample size with a confidence level of 95% and a confidence interval of 5%.

Results

From June 2019 to January 2020, 278 patients received the indication to be treated with a HoLEP procedure for BPH and met the inclusion criteria of the study. 21

of them refused to sign the consent, leaving 125 patients assigned to the HoLEP group and 132 to the VB-HoLEP one. Three months after surgery 112 and 120 patients were controlled and 100 patients for each arm were able to attend the 6-month scheduled control. CONSORT flow chart Fig. 1.

Patients' preoperative data are presented in Table 1. Early postoperative outcomes are summarized in Table 2. No significant differences in preoperative parameters between the two study arms were found. Compared to HoLEP, VB-HoLEP resulted in reduced hemoglobin decrease (2.54 vs. 1.12 g/dl, $P = 0.03$) and operative time (57.33 ± 29.71 vs. 42.99 ± 18.51 min, $P = 0.04$). Patients in the HoLEP and VB-HoLEP groups presented similar catheterization time (2.2 vs. 1.9 days, $P = 0.45$), irrigation volume (33.3 vs. 31.7 l, $P = 0.69$), and hospital stay (2.8 vs. 2.7 days, $P = 0.21$). During the 6-month follow-up no significant differences in IPSS, Qmax, PVR and QOLS were found (Table 3).

Complications in the twogroups are presented in Table 2.

Discussion

HoLEP is a surgical option for the management of BPH and an alternative treatment to TURP, or open prostatectomy, according to EAU Guidelines. One of the main advantages of HoLEP is that it reduces intraoperative and

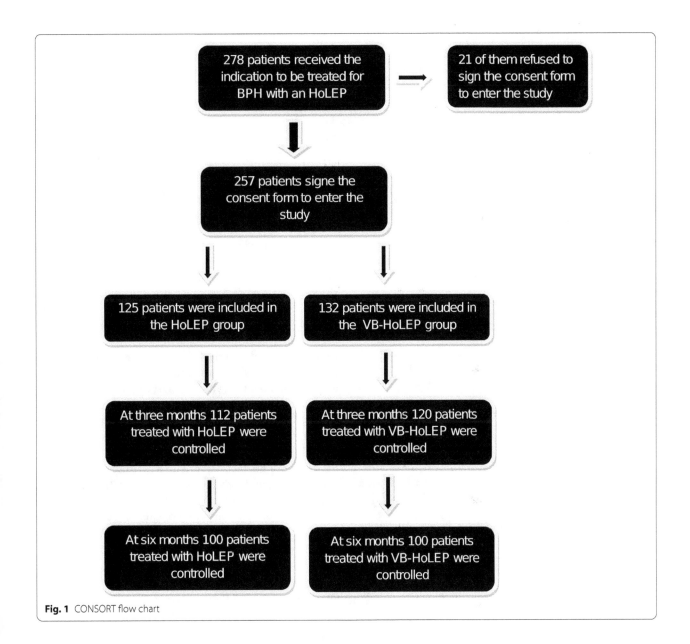

Fig. 1 CONSORT flow chart

Table 1 Patient's data

	Group A Holep	Group B VB Holep	P
No.	100	100	>0.05
Age yrs (mean±SD)	72.1±11.6	70.9±12.8	>0.05
Preoperative prostatic volume ml. (mean±SD)	74.2±36.2	77.1±29.4	>0.05
PSA ng/ml (mean±SD)	2.7±4.12	2.8±3.89	>0.05
Preoperative Hb g/dl (mean±SD)	13.4±2.45	13.9±2.23	>0.05
IPSS (mean±SD)	19.9±7.01	18.1±6.69	>0.05
Q max ml/sec (mean±SD)	6.9±5.54	7.1±6.12	>0.05
Post void volume ml (mean±SD)	118.8±161.95	124.1±148.92	>0.05

Table 2 Intra and early post operative outcomes and postoperative complications

	Group A	Group B	P
Operative time, min (mean±SD)	57.33±29.71	42.99±18.51	=0.04
Haemoglobin decrease, g/dl (mean±SD)	2.54±1.23	1.12±1.78	=0.03
Catheterization time, days (mean±SD)	2.2±3.55	1.9±2.81	=0.45
Continuous irrigation volume, liters (mean±SD)	33.3±24.78	31.7±25.22	=0.69
Enucleated/resected prostatic volume, g (mean±SD)	47.75±18.54	51.03±14.84	=0.321
Hospital stay, days (mean±SD)	2.8±3.19	2.7±2.89	=0.21
Complication	(No. patients, %)	(No. patients, %)	
Blood transfusion	1 (1)	0 (0)	
Post void retention	2 (2)	7 (7)	
Stress Incontinence	9 (9)	2 (2)	
Urge Incontinence	7 (7)	4 (4)	
Urethral Strictures	2 (2)	1 (1)	
Bladder injury	1 (1)	1 (1)	

Table 3 Postoperative functional outcomes (after 3 and 6 months)

	Group A	Group B	P
3 months			
Qmax ml/s (mean±SD)	20.76±9.78	22.42±11.09	>0.05
IPSS (mean±SD)	6.12±3.75	5.87±5.18	>0.05
PostVoid residual, ml (mean±SD)	45.3±25.16	42.3±22.71	>0.05
QOLS (mean±SD)	44.2±13.22	42.9±11.86	>0.05
6 months			
Qmax ml/s (mean±SD)	19.43±12.56	23.04±8.54	>0.05
IPSS (mean±SD)	7.34±5.43	5.45±3.24	>0.05
Post void residual, ml (mean±SD)	31.9±20.35	38.7±21.62	>0.05
QOLS (mean±SD)	45.6±11.59	41.8±11.77	>0.05

postoperative bleeding, leading to a lower transfusion rate, shorter hospitalization and catheterization [7].

This enucleating technique is performed with the Ho:YAG laser, which emits a pulsed laser beam, with a wavelength of about 2.1 μm, obtaining tissue vaporization, coagulation and necrosis limited to a depth of 0.3–0.4 mm [8]. The Ho:YAG laser is also used for stone lithotripsy, during which, the impact of the energy against the stone can cause its migration from the ureter to the renal cavities or from one calyx to another. To prevent this phenomenon, anti-retropulsion devices have been engineered, like the "Virtual Basket" mode, which is a result of the laser's pulse modulation: the laser creates an initial bubble with the first part of its energy and discharges the remaining energy once the bubble is formed, so that it can pass through the formed vapor channel. In this study, we report our results on the application of the Virtual Basket mode to HoLEP (VB-HoLEP) compared to the conventional technique, with a 6-month follow-up.

Vizziello et al. firstly reported their in vitro experience regarding the use of the Virtual Basket in stone phantom lithotripsy [9]. The authors concluded that this mode was associated with significantly fewer events of stone migration and better target stability during the procedure. Another study [10] investigated this emission mode in the treatment of ureteral and renal stones. In particular, it was reported that when compared to the regular mode, the Virtual Basket technology was associated with significantly lower retropulsion, fragmentation time and total procedural time, with no significant differences in total emitted energy.

Based on these studies, this mode may grant a smoother effect not only on stones but also on soft tissues, resulting in less trauma and bleeding.

Because of its double pulse pattern, we hypothesized that the use of the Virtual Basket during HoLEP may result in a first energy portion creating an initial separation of the prostatic tissues and the remaining energy being discharged through the incision, expanding it further and clotting bleeding vessels. As the laser's second pulse travels through the vapor tunnel created by the first pulse, a lower attenuation of the second pulse should occur, resulting in a stronger effect on the tissue (sealing and/or incision). This system, with the emission of two energy pulses fired with a small time gap between one another, seems to allow faster coagulation, reducing the risk of bleeding and, therefore, operative time. Indeed, as reported in our results, compared to HoLEP, the VB-HoLEP was faster (57.33 ± 29.71 vs. 42.99 ± 18.51 min, $P = 0.04$) and resulted in less hemoglobin decrease (2.54 vs. 1.12 g/dl, $P = 0.003$). Despite being inferior, compared to older surgical techniques, bleeding risk with HoLEP still remains. Some studies report a risk of severe hemorrhage in 5.2% of patients and a risk of bladder tamponade that required cystoscopy and evacuation of blood clots in 2.3% [11]. In some Centers, to reduce the risk of bleeding in the early post-operative period, surgeons use a bipolar resector to obtain prostatic loggia coagulation. This lengthens the operating time, increasing the risk of anesthesiologic complications. The use of the Virtual Basket could improve coagulation with the laser, allowing to avoid the use of the bipolar resector and reduce morcellation time, thanks to a good endoscopic vision, without residual bleeding.

Moreover, HoLEP has proven to be safe and effective in anticoagulated patients. The hemostatic efficacy of the Ho:YAG laser makes HoLEP more effective and safer than other BPH treatments in patients taking anticoagulant agents. Specifically, the low penetration depth of the holmium laser limits eschar formation, which can contribute to delayed bleeding seen after other BPH procedures [12]. The use of VB-HoLEP, thanks to its observed better coagulation capability, could further reduce the risk of bleeding in patients under anticoagulation therapy [13].

The comparison between HoLEP and VB-HoLEP during the 6-month follow-up did not demonstrate significant differences in Qmax, IPSS, PVR, and QOLS.

Urinary incontinence (UI) is one of the most worrying postoperative complications. Postoperative UI occurs in about 20% of patients and most of them recover within the first year. Long operative time is the first risk factor: the longer the resectoscope remains in the urethra, the higher the possibility of sphincter damage. Some studies stated that high prostate volume, a conspicuous reduction in postoperative PSA and diabetes mellitus are significant risk factors for stress UI [14]. Various authors have suggested that postoperative incontinence could be related to either thermal injury to the pericapsular structures, resulting in urge incontinence, or linked to the presence of a urinary tract infection, or BPH-related detrusor instability [15]. Another risk factor for UI is the presence of a large prostatic fossa, created after the removal of adenoma, which leads to urine entrapment and leakage with stress maneuvers [16]. VB-HoLEP could reduce the risk of UI thanks to a better cut on the tissue, resulting in reduced traction and stress on the urethra and external sphincter.

The long learning curve is the major negative factor that hinders widespread use of this procedure to date [17]. The inexperience of the surgeon elevates the risk of bleeding and UI after HoLEP because of long operative time, frequent intraoperative complications and inadequate enucleation.

As the use of VB-HoLEP proved to reduce operative time in our study, the risk of UI may be reduced with this technique. Moreover, as the use of the Virtual Basket reduced bleeding, improving the quality of the endoscopic vision, the use of VB-HoLEP may help to reduce the learning curve. These aspects may be verified in future multicentric studies.

Together with the long learning curve associated with the enucleation technique, the cost associated with the purchase of high power laser platforms has probably represented another factor hindering the spread of laser enucleation. However, the possibility to use the VB technology, with reusable fibers and on medium power platforms might help to foster the adoption of HoLEP in upcoming years. Indeed, the non-inferiority of low-power HoLEP with respect to high power HoLEP has been investigated [18, 19]. For instance, Elshal et al. compared 50 W and 100 W HoLEP techniques, reaching comparable improvement in IPSS, Qmax and median PSA reduction, with similar perioperative and late postoperative complications [18].

There is growing interest for new pulse modulation technologies which can potentially enhance lithotripsy effectiveness and which have been recently launched on the market [9, 20, 21]. However, so far the potential advantages of these modulations have been mainly explored for stone application, whereas little has been reported regarding the effect of these pulse modulations on soft tissue treatments. One exception consists in the study performed by Large et al., who shared their experience with the Moses™ technology for HoLEP [22]; Large et al. reported that the use of this modality resulted in increased OR efficiency and hemostasis, regardless of prostate size, when compared to standard HoLEP. Both his study and ours suggest that advanced pulse modulation of the Ho:YAG laser results in increased hemostatic effect. Nevertheless, there are differences between these two technologies. First, the second pulse of Virtual Basket is emitted when the vapor bubble, originated by the first pulse, is at the maximum expansion; instead, the second pulse of the Moses is emitted during the collapse of the bubble originated by the first pulse. Moreover, another difference is in the fiber compatibility with these pulse modulations: Virtual Basket, unlike the Moses, is pulse modulation which is compatible with any standard fiber, without the need of a "special" fiber in order to enable this pulse modulation.

To our knowledge, this is the first study describing the use of the Virtual Basket mode for HoLEP and one of a small group of papers reporting the use of advanced Ho:YAG pulse modulation for soft tissue applications, such as the Moses™ technology, which has been used since 2017. Further investigations by other centers are needed in order to corroborate the findings of our study.

Limitations of this study are linked to the fact that all the procedures were notperformed by only one skilled surgeon. Another limitation is that hemostasis effectiveness was judged only by measuring hemoglobin drop. Potentially, recording of the time spent on hemostasis (for example the time with the right pedal pushed) may have represented an additional comparison term to corroborate our outcomes regarding hemostatic properties. Furthermore, only a single emission setting was tested in this study for both groups.

Conclusions

Compared to conventional HoLEP, VB-HoLEP determines faster operative time and results in less hemoglobin decrease, due to better coagulation, but there are no differences with regard to catheterization time, irrigation volume, hospital stay, Qmax, IPSS, PVR and QOLS at 3 and 6 months. Based on these results VB-HoLEP may be better than conventional HoLEP, but from our experience in the field of laser enucleation of prostate, it may not overcome the efficacy, safety and early and late outcomes of thulium laser enucleation of the prostate (ThuLEP) [23].

Abbreviations

BPH: Benign prostate hyperplasia; HoLEP: Holmium laser enucleation of the prostate; IPSS: International Prostate Symptom Score; LUTS: Lower urinary tract symptoms; OP: Open prostatectomy; PVR: Postvoid residual urine volume; Qmax: Maximum flow rate; VB: Virtual Basket; VB-HoLEP: Holmium laser enucleation of the prostate with Virtual Basket mode.

Acknowledgements

Our abstracts "Thulium laser enucleation (ThULEP) versus Holmium laser enucleation of the prostate (HoIEP): A two institution trial to compare intra and early postoperative outcomes" (EAU 2019) and "Thulium laser enucleation (thULEP) versus Holmium laser enucleation of the prostate: a two institution trial to compare intra and early postoperative outcomes" (WCET19) were published.

Authors' contributions

All authors have contributed to the information or material submitted for publication, and that all authors have read and approved the manuscript. GB and DP has made the study design and the critical review; MM, LB, UB and AC have been involved in data interpretation, performed the statistical analysis and drafting the manuscript; MCS has been involved in data collection; AG, CB, MS and JBR have reviewed the references; AM and MB have been involved in tables drawn; BR, SM and EL have reviewed the manuscript.

Author details

[1] Department of Urology, ASST Valle Olona, Via Arnaldo da Brescia, 21052 Busto Arsizio, VA, Italy. [2] ESUT, European Section for UroTechnology, Arnhem, Italy. [3] Department of Urology, Ospedale Policlinico e Nuovo Ospedale Civile S. Agostino Estense, University of Modena and Reggio Emilia, Modena, Italy. [4] Department of Urology, Clinique Saint Augustin, Bordeaux, France. [5] Department of Urology, SLK Kliniken, Heilbron, Germany. [6] Department of Urology, Spital Limmattal, Schlieren, Switzerland. [7] Department of Urology, Moscow State University, Moscow, Russia. [8] Department of Urology, University of Patras, Patras, Greece. [9] Department of Urology, Clinica Sant'Anna, Lugano, Switzerland.

References

1. Gravas S, et al. EAU guidelines of management of non-neurogenic male lower urinary tract symptoms (LUTS), incl. Benign Prostatic Obstruction (BPO), EAU Guidelines; 2019.
2. Leonardo C, Lombardo R, Cindolo L. What is the standard surgical approach to large volume BPE? Systematic review of existing randomized clinical trials. Minerva Urol Nefrol. 2020;72(1):22–9.
3. Herrmann Thomas RW, Bach T. Thulium laser enucleation of the prostate (ThuLEP): transurethral anatomical prostatectomy with laser support. Introduction of a novel technique for the treatment of benign prostatic obstruction. World J Urol. 2010;28:45–51.
4. Nguyen DD, Misraï V, Bach T. Operative time comparison of aquablation, greenlight PVP, ThuLEP, GreenLEP, and HoLEP. World J Urol. 2020;38:3227–33.
5. Fraundorfer MR, Gilling PJ. Holmium:YAG laser enucleation of the prostate combined with mechanical morcellation: preliminary results. Eur Urol. 1998;33(1):69–72.
6. Cornu JN, Ahyai S, Bachmann A, et al. Asystematic review and meta-analysis of functional outcomes and complicationsfollowing transurethral procedures for lower urinary tract symptoms resultingfrom benign prostatic obstruction: an update. Eur Urol. 2015;67(6):1066–96.
7. Tooher R, Sutherland P, Costello A, et al. A systematic review of holmium laser prostatectomy for benign prostatic hyperplasia. J Urol. 2004;171(5):1773–81.
8. Gilling PJ, Cass CB, Malcolm AR, et al. Combination holmium and Nd:YAG laser ablation of the prostate: initial clinical experience. J Endourol. 1995;9(2):151–3.
9. Vizziello D, Acquati P, Clementi M, et al. Virtual Basket technology-impact on high frequency lithotripsy in a urological simulator. J Endourol. 2018;32:A277.
10. Bozzini G, Besana U, Maltagliati M, et al. "VirtualBasket" ureteroscopic Holmium laser lithotripsy: intraoperative and early postoperative outcomes. J Urol. 2020;203:e464.
11. Davydov DS, Tsarichenko DG, Bezrukov E, et al. Complications of the holmium laser enucleation of prostate for benign prostatic hyperplasia. Urologia. 2018;1:42–7.
12. Elzayat E, Habib E, Elhilali M. Holmium laser enucleation of the prostate in patients on anticoagulant therapy or with bleeding disorders. J Urol. 2006;175:1428–32.

13. Sun J, Shi A, Tong Z, et al. Safety and feasibility study of holmium laser enucleation of the prostate (HOLEP) on patients receiving dual antiplate let therapy (DAPT). World J Urol. 2018;36(2):271–6.

14. Elmansy HM, Kotb A, Elhilali MM. Is there a way to predict stress urinary incontinence after holmium laser enucleation of the prostate? J Urol. 2011;186:1977–81.

15. Montorsi F, Naspro R, Salonia A, et al. Holmium laser enucleation versus transurethral resection of the prostate: results from a 2-center, prospective, randomized trial in patients with obstructive benign prostatic hyperplasia. J Urol. 2004;172(5 Pt 1):1926–9.

16. Shah HN, Mahajan AP, Hegde SS, et al. Peri-operative complications of holmium laser enucleation of the prostate: experience in the first 280 patients, and a review of literature. BJU Int. 2007;100:94–101.

17. Kampantais S, Dimopoulos P, Tasleem A, et al. Assessing the learning curve of holmium laser enucleation of prostate (HoLEP). A systematic review. Urology. 2018;120:9–22.

18. Elshal AM, El-Nahas AR, Ghazy M, et al. Low-powervs. high-power holmium laser enucleation of the prostate: critical assessmentthrough randomized trial. Urology. 2018;121:58–65.

19. Becker B, Gross AJ, Netsch C. Safety and efficacy using a low-powered holmium laser for enucleation of the prostate (HoLEP): 12-month results from a prospective low-power HoLEP series. World J Urol. 2018;36(3):441–7.

20. Mullerad M, Aguinaga JRA, Aro T, et al. Initial clinical experience with a modulated holmium laser pulse-moses technology: Does it enhance laser lithotripsy efficacy? Rambam Maimonides Med J. 2017;8(4):e0038.

21. Terry RS, Whelan PS, Lipkin ME. New devices for kidney stone management. Curr Opin Urol. 2020;30(2):144–8.

22. Large T, Nottingham C, Stoughton C, et al. Comparative study of holmium laser enucleation of the prostate with MOSES enabled pulsed laser modulation. Urology. 2020;136:196–201.

23. Bozzini G, Seveso M, Melegari S, et al. Thulium laser enucleation (ThuLEP) versus transurethral resection of the prostate in saline (TURis): a randomized prospective trial to compare intra and early postoperative outcomes. Actas Urol Esp. 2017;41(5):309–15.

9

Sensitizing the cytotoxic action of Docetaxel induced by Pentoxifylline in a PC3 prostate cancer cell line

Martha E. Cancino-Marentes[1], Georgina Hernández-Flores[2], Pablo Cesar Ortiz-Lazareno[2], María Martha Villaseñor-García[2], Eduardo Orozco-Alonso[2], Erick Sierra-Díaz[3], Raúl Antonio Solís-Martínez[2], Claudia Carolina Cruz-Gálvez[1] and Alejandro Bravo-Cuellar[2,4]*

Abstract

Background: Prostate cancer is one of the most frequently diagnosed types of cancers worldwide. In its initial period, the tumor is hormone-sensitive, but in advanced states, it evolves into a metastatic castration-resistant tumor. In this state, chemotherapy with taxanes such as Docetaxel (DTX) comprises the first line of treatment. However, the response is poor due to chemoresistance and toxicity. On the other hand, Pentoxifylline (PTX) is an unspecific inhibitor of phosphodiesterases; experimental, and clinically it has been described as sensitizing tumor cells to chemotherapy, increasing apoptosis and decreasing senescence. We study whether the PTX sensitizes prostate cancer cells to DTX for greater effectiveness.

Methods: PC3 human prostate cancer cells were treated in vitro at different doses and times with PTX, DTX, or their combination. Viability was determined by the WST-1 assay by spectrophotometry, cell cycle progression, apoptosis, generic caspase activation and senescence by flow cytometry, DNA fragmentation and caspases-3, -8, and -9 activity by ELISA.

Results: We found that PTX in PC3 human prostate cancer cells induces significant apoptosis per se and increases that generated by DTX, while at the same time it reduces the senescence caused by the chemotherapy and increases caspases-3,-8, and -9 activity in PTX + DTX-treated cells. Both treatments blocked the PC3 cell in the G1 phase.

Conclusions: Our results show that PTX sensitizes prostate tumor cells to apoptosis induced by DTX. Taken together, the results support the concept of chemotherapy with rational molecular bases.

Keywords: Pentoxifylline, Docetaxel, Prostate cancer, Apoptosis, Senescence

Background

Prostate cancer (PCa) is the second most common cancer worldwide in males, and an estimated 1.28 million new cases and 358,989 deaths were reported in 2018 [1]. This cancer is among the main leading causes of cancer deaths in developed countries, with 278,539 deaths registered in 2018; however, in the United States, 31,620 deaths were estimated for 2019 [1, 2]. PCa is a clinically heterogeneous disease during which some patients may have an aggressive state of the disease with high progression and metastasis. In contrast, others have a low rate of disease progression [3]. This disease is essentially a cancer of older men. It is characterized by patterns of abnormal glandular growth in which poorly differentiated tumors are observed with a high mortality rate, while well-differentiated tumors have a favorable clinical

*Correspondence: abravocster@gmail.com
[2] División de Inmunología, Centro de Investigación Biomédica de Occidente del IMSS, Sierra Mojada 800, Col. Independencia, CP 44340 Guadalajara, Jalisco, México
Full list of author information is available at the end of the article

outcome [4–7]. During the initial period of PCa, tumor growth is androgen-dependent; therefore, surgical castration and or Androgen-Deprivation Therapy (ADT) is the mainstay of treatment in metastatic Hormone-Sensitive Prostate Cancer (mHSPC) [8, 9]. Frequently the use of such treatments results in a temporary regression of the disease; however, after a time comprising 2–3 years, the tumor progresses despite continuous hormonal manipulation. This type of cancer is known as metastatic Castration-Resistant Prostate Cancer (mCRPC), [10, 11]. Cytotoxic chemotherapy remains the only treatment option in mCRPC, providing modest survival and palliative benefits [12, 13]. Taxanes represent the most active chemotherapeutic drugs that prolong survival in mHSPC and that are used as standard first-line chemotherapy and mCRPC, as second-line chemotherapy [13, 14]. Docetaxel (DTX) is one of the most important taxanes for the treatment of PCa [15]. It has been employed as treatment for 15 years, on occasion, in addition to another chemotherapeutic drug. Nonetheless, mostly as the most important treatment. DTX acts at the level of the centrosome in the mitotic spindle, thus preventing cell division [16]. However, not all patients respond to treatment with DTX due to its toxicity and a heterogenous taxane resistance, which is related to multidrug-resistant genes, *TMPRSS2–ERG* fusion genes, kinesins, cytokines, to the components of other signalling pathways [11], and a recently discovered factor: the overexpression of microRNA-323 [10, 14]. Thus, efforts have been made to improve the effectiveness of such therapeutic schemes. For its part, Pentoxifylline (PTX) (1-[5-oxohexyl]-3, 7-dimethylxanthine) is a synthetic derivative of the methylxanthines, initially developed as a hemorheological agent for circulatory problems and considered as a non-selective adenosine antagonist [17]. Currently, its clinical usefulness is due to its anti-inflammatory, antioxidant, and immunomodulatory properties [18, 19]. The anti-inflammatory action of PTX lies in its blocking of proinflammatory cytokine production (IL-1, IL-6, and TNF-α) by increasing cyclic Adenosine Monophosphate c (cAMP) limiting the formation of ATP [20]. In previous studies, a decreased activity in the Transcription Factor kB (NF-κB) was described as an antitumoral manner, through the inhibition of IκB phosphorylation [21].

In this respect, our work group previously found, clinically and experimentally, the sensitization to PTX-mediated chemotherapy of different drugs, such as Adriamycin (ADM), Cisplatin, and Perillyl Alcohol in cervical cancer cells and in other tumors, increasing apoptosis and decreasing cell senescence [22–26]. There are also reports of sensitization to radiotherapy in prostate cancer lines in which PTX induces a cell cycle arrest in the G2 phase [27]. The aim of the present study was to determine the effects of PTX in combination with DTX in an in vitro model with the PC3 cell line from a castrate-resistant prostate cancer.

Materials and methods
Drugs
Docetaxel (DTX) was obtained from Pisa Farmacéutica, México, stored at 4 °C for fewer than 4 days, and adjusted to the desired concentration with F-12K culture medium immediately before use. Pentoxifylline (PTX), (Sigma, St. Louis, MO, USA) was dissolved in sterile saline solution at a concentration of 0.5 M and maintained at − 4 °C for fewer than 4 days.

Cell line
We worked with the PC3 cell line (ATCC CRL 1435; Manassas, VA, USA). This cell line is epithelial, derived from bone metastasis of an independent androgen grade-IV prostate adenocarcinoma of a 62-year-old caucasian patient and was authenticated using the Multiplex Cell Authentication system by Multiplexion GmbH (Friedrichshafen, Germany) report 2386 and tested for mycoplasma contamination using the Universal Mycoplasma Detection Kit (ATCC, Manassas, VA, USA), and the cells were negative throughout the study.

Cell culture
PC3 cells (1×10^6 cells) were cultured at 37 °C in an atmosphere containing 5% CO_2 and 95% air, in 150-cm^2 culture flasks for adherent cells (Corning CLS430825) suspended in 18 mL of F-12K Medium (Kaighn's Modification of Ham's F-12 Medium) from GIBCO (Invitrogen Co.) with the addition of 10% Bovine Fetal Serum (BFS) (GIBCO), 1% 100X L-glutamine solution (GIBCO), and antibiotics/antimycotics (Penicillin–Streptomycin-Neomycin). This supplemented culture medium will be designated F-12KS and was replaced every 48 h. Prior to the experiments, PC-3 cells were detached with Accutase (GIBCO™) [28]; then, the cells were washed 3 times in PBS 4 °C, pH 7.4, and live cells were then resuspended at the desired concentration in F-12KS culture medium. Depending on the experiment, live PC3 cells determined by Trypan Blue exclusion (>95%) were seeded at concentrations of 1×10^4 to 1×10^6 cells in 6-, 48-, or 96-well plates and cultured for 24 h before the application of treatments. The ideal concentrations of the treatments were determined by means of a dose–response curve and kinetics at 24, 48, and 72 h (Fig. 1).

In vitro treatments
The groups utilized were as follows: an Untreated Control Group (UCG) as negative control; an 8 mM PTX group; a 25 nM DTX group, and a group for 8 mM PTX + 25 nM

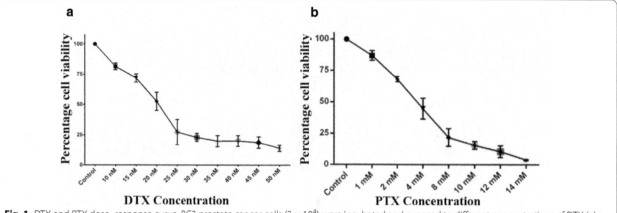

Fig. 1 DTX and PTX dose–response curve. PC3 prostate cancer cells (3×10^4) were incubated and exposed to different concentrations of DTX (**a**) or PTX (**b**). Viability was evaluated by the WST-1 assay. The results represent the mean $\pm$ SD of the normalized percentages of the three independent experiments carried out in triplicate

DTX. In all experiments, PC3 cells treated with PTX were administered 1 h before DTX, in that there is evidence that better results can be obtained in this manner [21, 22]. In the same way peripheral blood monocluear cells from healt voluntary were obtained and treated with PTX (4 and 8 mM) during 24 h to investigate toxicity of PTX in normal cells.

Cell viability assay

The effects of both drugs on the cells were determined by the WST-1 4-(3-(4-Iodophenyl)2-(4-nitrophenyl)2H-5-tetrazolium)-1,3-benzene disulfonate) assay. This study is based on the reduction of tetrazolium salts into formazan; the rate of WST-1 cleavage by mitochondrial dehydrogenases correlates with the number of viable cells. Exponentially grown cells were harvested and seeded in 96-well plates (1×10^4 cells/well) and allowed to attach to wells overnight. After 24 h, the medium was replaced with fresh medium and then the cells were treated according to the treatment scheduled at 24 h, 48 h and 72 h. After the incubation, 10 µL/well of WST-1/ECS reagent (Quick Cell Proliferation Colorimetric Assay Kit WST-1; BioVision, Inc. Milpitas, CA, USA) was added to each well and the PC3 cells were incubated for another 2 h. Absorbance was measured in a microtiter plate reader (Synergy™ HT Multi-Mode Microplate Reader; Biotek, Winooski, VT, USA) at 450 nm. The percentage of viability was calculated utilizing the following formula: viability $= (1 - $ [absorbance of experimental well $-$ absorbance of blank)/(absorbance of untreated control well $-$ absorbance of blank) $\times 100\%$. Data are reported as the percentage of cell viability in comparison to that of its respective UCG considered as 100% [29]. The IC_{50} of the DXT or PTX treatment in PC3 cells was determined from survival curves generated for each

experiment. Data are reported in percentage $\pm$ Standard Deviation (SD) of cell survival as compared with the UCG considered as 100% [30].

Assessment of apoptosis

Apoptosis was evaluated by flow cytometry after treatment with 8 mM PTX, 25 nM DTX, and PTX (8 mM) $+$ DTX (25 nM) employing the Annexin-V-Fluos staining kit (Roche, Basel, Switzerland) according to the manufacturer's instructions. For this, 1×10^6 PC3 live cells from each of the different experimental conditions were treated. Etoposide at a concentration of 1 µg/mL was used as positive control and UCG as a negative control. The cells were harvested using Accutase as described previously and were washed 3 times with PBS. After that, the cells were then resuspended in 200 µL of incubation buffer, which contained 3 µL of Annexin V-Fluorescein Isothiocyanate (FITC) and 5 µL Propidium Iodide (PI) (1 µg/mL stock solution). These were mixed gently and incubated at 20 °C for 10 min in the dark. Finally, 400 µL of incubation buffer was added to the suspension, which was analyzed by flow cytometry. At least 20,000 events were acquired with Attune (Applied Biosystem), and the analysis was performed using. FlowJo ver. 7.6.5 software (Tree Star, Inc., Ashland, OR, USA). Annexin V-FITC-negative and PI-negative cells were considered live cells. Cells positive for Annexin V-FITC but negative for PI were regarded as being in early apoptosis. Cells positive for both Annexin V-FITC and PI were taken as undergoing late apoptosis. Cells positive for PI and negative for Annexin V-FITC were considered necrotic. The data will be represented as the mean $\pm$ SD of the percentage of cells and represent the addition of early and late apoptosis.

ELISA apoptosis assay

For the determination of the apoptosis assay by histone-associated fragmented DNA, 2×10^4 PC3 live cells were seeded per well (200 µL volume) in a 96-well plate and were treated under the same conditions described above for 24 h at 37 °C, 95% air, and 5% CO_2. The cell plates were centrifuged at 1200 rpm for 10 min at 4 °C. Supernatants were decanted and the cells were lysed for 30 min in 200 µL of lysis buffer, centrifuged at $200 \times g$ for 10 min. Twenty µL of lysate of each sample was transferred onto the Streptavidin-coated microplate plus 80 µL immunoreagent per well. The samples were incubated for 30 min and were protected from light at between 15 and 25 °C. The cells were centrifuged at 1200 rpm for 10 min at 4 °C, and 20 µL of the supernatant from each well was taken and placed into the ELISA 96-well kit plate. Eighty µL of immunoreactive was added to each well (Incubation Buffer 72 µl, Anti-Histone 4 µl, Anti-DNA 4 µL), the plates were covered with an adhesive cover, and these were incubated in a shaker at 300 rpm for 2 h at between 15 and 25 °C. The plates with the supernatants were removed. Each plate well was washed 3 times with 300 µL of incubation buffer; 100 µL of ABTS solution was added to each well. The plates were incubated in a shaker at 250 rpm for 20 min; 100 µL of ABTS stop solution was added to each well. The absorbance of each sample was determined using a microplate reader (Sinregy HT Multi-Mode Microplate Reader, Biotek at 450 nm). In the DNA fragmentation test, the rate of apoptosis is reflected by the Enhanced factor (fold change) of mono- and oligonucleosomes accumulated in the cytoplasm, both of which were calculated and normalized versus UCG.

Caspases activity assay by flow cytometry

The generic caspase activity (Caspases-1, -3, -4, -5, -6, -7, -8, and -9) was determined by flow cytometry using the Generic Caspase Activity Assay kit (Abcam, Cambridge, UK). The activation of caspase is an indicator for cell apoptosis, TF2-VAD-FMK is a fluorescent reporter that binds to active caspases in apoptotic cells. Briefly, PC3 cells were seeded at a density of 1×10^6 cells in 6-well plates and treated for 24 h with the different drugs as described previously. After this, the cells were harvested and collected by centrifugation, suspended in 500 µL of F-12KS. Then, 1 µL of 500X TF2-VAD-FMK was added and incubated at room temperature for 1 h. Finally, the cells were washed with PBS at 4 °C pH 7.4 and resuspended in 500 µL of assay buffer for immediate determination. The samples were processed using Attune™ Applied Biosystem flow cytometry equipment. For each sample, at least 20,000 events were analyzed with the FlowJo ver. 7.6.5 software (Tree Star, Inc; Ashland, OR,

USA). Data are presented as a percentage of caspase-positive cells.

ELISA assay to determine caspases activity-3, -8, and -9

The activity of caspases-3, -8, and -9 was measured using the Caspases Colorimetric Assay kit (Abcam) following the manufacturer's protocol. PC3 cells (5×10^6) were cultured and treated for 24 h under the conditions previously described. Afterward, the cells were washed with PBS at 4 °C, pH 7.4, 50 µL of cell lysis buffer was added and incubated on ice for 10 min, homogenized was centrifuged at $10,000 \times g$ for 1 min. The protein concentration was determined by Bradford assay (Bio-Rad, CA, USA), and 100 µg of protein was used for each test. Subsequently, the absorbance at 405 nm was determined in a microplate reader (Synergy HT Multi-Mode Microplate Reader Biotek). Results are represented as a percentage of caspase activity and compared with the respective percentage in UCG cells, considered as 100%.

β-galactosidase-associated senescence

Cell senescence was evaluated by flow cytometry using the C12FDG kit (5-Dodecanoylaminofluorescein Di-β-D-Galactopyranoside; Invitrogen), which acts as a substrate for β-galactosidase. Briefly, PC3 cells were seeded at a density of 1×10^6 cells in 6-well plates and treated for 24 h with the different drugs. Afterward, we added 100 nM of bafilomycin A1 for 1 h at 37 °C afterwards the cells were washed, harvested, collected by centrifugation, and incubated with 10 µM C12FDG (Invitrogen) according to the manufacturer's instructions. Acquisition of the samples was carried out in Attune (Life Technologies, Carlsbad, CA, USA) flow cytometry equipment. For each sample, at least 20,000 events were analyzed with Attune cytometer and the data were analyzed with the FlowJo ver7.6.5. Software (Tree Star, Inc). Data are expressed by the percentage of positive senescent cells compared with the respective percentage in UCG cells (considered as 100%). In Additional file 1: Figure S1 is shown the gating strategy for apoptosis, generic caspase activity, and senescence analyzed by flow cytometry.

Determination of the cell cycle by flow cytometry

For the cell-cycle analysis, the PC3 cells were initially synchronized. In brief, cells were cultured in F-12K culture medium containing 5% FBS for 12 h. Subsequently, the cells were washed with PBS and were incubated in serum-free medium for 18 h. Finally, the cells were split and were released into cell cycle by the addition of 10% FBS in F-12K culture medium. A total of 1×10^6 PC3 cells were treated with each drug alone or with both drugs for 24 h. The BD Cycletest Plus DNA reagent kit was utilized according to the manufacturer's instructions

(BD Biosciences, San Jose, CA, USA). DNA QC Particles (BD, Biosciences) equipment was employed to verify the instrument performance and quality control of the equipment used for cell cycle analysis (Attune cytometer; Applied Biosystems). The samples were analyzed by flow cytometry (Attune; Life Technologies, Carlsbad, CA, USA). For each sample, at least 20,000 events were analyzed with the Attune Cytometric Software PC v2.1(Life Technologies). The percentage of cells represents the cell cycle distribution in the G1, S, and G2 phase; this was assessed by using the obtained data and processed with FlowJo ver. 7.6.5 software (Tree Star, Inc., Ashland, OR, USA) [31].

Statistical analysis

Each experiment was carried out in triplicate and repeated on at least three occasions. The results are expressed as the mean ± Standard Deviation (SD) of the values obtained. The difference between groups was determined by the non-parametric Mann–Whitney U test considering a significant difference of $p < 0.05$. In some experiments, the Δ% was calculated, which represents the percentage of increase or decrease in relation to UCG.

Results

Determination of IC_{50} of PTX and DTX in PC3 cells of prostate cancer

The IC_{50} of PTX and DTX were determined in PC3 cell cultures treated for 24 h. After receiving the results, we observed that both drugs produced a decrease in the viability effect in a dose-dependent manner. The IC_{50} is reached at a concentration of 20 nM DTX (Fig. 1a). Thus, a concentration of 4 mM of PTX was sufficient to reach IC_{50} (Fig. 1b). However, we were also able to observe the antitumor activity of this drug, which decreases 25% of the cell viability at a concentration of 2 mM.

Effect of PTX alone or in combination with DTX on the cell viability of PC3 cells

The viability of PC3 cells incubated with different doses of PTX + DTX, using concentrations close to the IC_{50}, was determined by WST-1 assay. Table 1 shows the results of the percentage of viability achieved after the administration of treatments at 24, 48, and 72 h. It presents an evident decrease in viability by combining DTX and PTX, compared versus the UCG. We also observed similar results with both doses of PTX 4 and 8 mM ($p < 0.05$). With this kinetic and dose–response evaluation, we concluded that the ideal concentrations of treatment for our future experiments will be DTX at 25 nM and PTX at 8 mM, alone or combined, for each respective experimental group. Surprisingly, also in Table 1, it can be observed that PTX, mainly at 4 and 8 mM, by itself reaches levels of cytotoxicity comparable to those obtained with the combination of both drugs in particular to 48 and 72 h. In contrast to prostate tumor cells, the viability of normal peripheral blood mononuclear cells practically was not affected by the PTX (3 ± 0.9 and 5 ± 1.3% decreases in viability for the doses of 4 and 8 mM respectively).

Effect of PTX in apoptosis induction by DTX in the PC3 line cell

Initially, apoptosis induction was studied by Annexin V/Propidium Iodide (IP) assay (Fig. 2a). After 24 h of treatment, we found a statistical difference between treated groups compared versus the UCG; however, it is noteworthy that the percentage of apoptosis was considerably higher in the groups treated with PTX + DTX or with PTX even in comparison with the DTX group ($p < 0.005$). At 48 h, we found the same behaviour with higher values: the PTX and PTX + DTX groups exhibited apoptosis of 57.6% and 72.1%, respectively, compared with 30% of apoptosis in DTX and UCG ($p < 0.005$). Furthermore, apoptosis was determined by apoptotic DNA fragmentation using a sandwich ELISA assay. Figure 2b depicts the results, noting a significant increase of apoptosis in the

Table 1 Viability of PC3 cells treated with PTX alone or in combination with DTX

GROUP/HOURS	PTX			DTX		PTX + DTX	
	2 mM	4 mM	8 mM	15 nM	25 nM	4 mM/25 nM	8 mM/25 nM
24	70.0 ± 3.6	34.7 ± 8.2[+]	26.3 ± 2.6[+]	87.3 ± 2.1	45.8 ± 2.5	24.7 ± 2.5[+]	22.3 ± 3.2[+]
48	61.7 ± 4.2	29.4 ± 3.3[+]	19.7 ± 3.1[+]	69.5 ± 2.1	42.3 ± 7.4	23.7 ± 2.5[+]	21.3 ± 4.2[+]
72	59.1 ± 2.2	20.7 ± 1.5[+]	17.3 ± 3.5[+]	62.3 ± 3.2	25.7 ± 2.1	19.2 ± 2.3[+]	17.3 ± 1.5[+]

PTX decreases viability, alone or in combination with DTX, in PC3 cells after 24, 48, and 72 h of treatment. A total of 3×10^4 PC3 cells were seeded and were initially treated (24 h prior) with different concentrations of PTX and DTX, alone or combined. Later, cell viability was evaluated by WST-1 assays. The results represent the mean ± SD of the values obtained of three experiments carried out in triplicate. Untreated control cells were considered as 100%. + Mann–Whitney U test, $p < 0.05$ versus DTX-treated groups

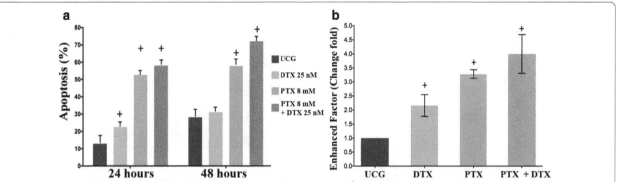

Fig. 2 Apoptosis of PC3 cells treated with DTX, PTX, or their combination. The 1×10^6 live cells were seeded and exposed to DTX 25 nM, PTX 8 mM, or PTX 8 mM + DTX 25 nM. **a** Apoptosis was evaluated by Flow Cytometry using Annexin V/PI assay. **b** Apoptosis was evaluated by ELISA, the results were normalized in relation to UCG, and represent the mean ± SD of three independent assays. Statistical analysis in both Figures: Mann–Whitney U test, $p < 0.05$ in all PTX-treated groups versus UCG and DTX groups

PTX + DTX group ($\Delta\% = 298\%$ above that of the UCG). Similarly, the DTX ($\Delta\% = 115\%$) and PTX ($\Delta\% = 225\%$) groups also demonstrated increased apoptotic activity compared with the UCG group ($p < 0.05$ all PTX-treated groups vs. UCG and DTX groups). Taken together, the results concluded with the sensibilization in DTX by PTX, increasing apoptosis in PC3 tumor cells. Thus, PTX reveals antitumor activity per se, a novel effect of this drug.

PTX alone or in combination with DTX induces caspase activity in PC3 cells

The role of caspases in apoptosis was analyzed. First, we determined the general caspase activity (Fig. 3a), and afterward, we studied in particular caspase-8 (extrinsic pathway), caspase-9 (intrinsic pathway), and caspase-3 (common pathway) activity (Fig. 3b). The treated groups produced greater general caspase activity at a level that was statistically significant compared to that of the UCG group ($p < 0.05$) being higher and comparable between

themselves in PTX and PTX + DTX-treated groups ($p < 0.005$ vs., the DTX group). However, we can observe that DTX does not receive sufficient caspase activation in the intrinsic and extrinsic pathways to find statistically significant results compared with the UCG ($p > 0.05$). On the other hand, the PTX group demonstrated a preference for caspase-9 activation ($p < 0.05$ vs., all groups), PTX + DTX also achieves higher labels of caspase-9 activation, near those found in the PTX group ($p < 0.05$ vs. DTX and UCG). Meanwhile, in PTX-treated groups, both pathways are activated, finding a notable increase of caspase-8 activation that is statistically significant as compared with the UCG and DTX groups ($p < 0.05$). The PTX + DTX group exhibited a similar activation of caspase-3 to that of the PTX group, but higher than the caspase-3 activation in the UCG- and DTX-treated groups ($p < 0.05$), with these results, taken together, indicating that PTX plays an important role in the induction of apoptosis.

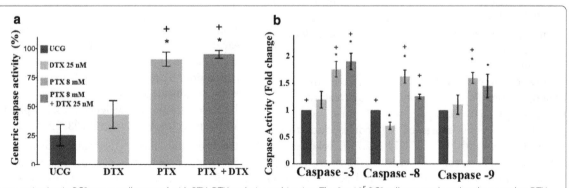

Fig. 3 Caspase activation in PC3 tumor cells treated with PTX, DTX or their combination. The 2×10^5 PC3 cells were cultured and exposed to DTX 25 nM, PTX 8 mM, or PTX 8 mM + DTX 25 nM for 24 h. **a** General caspase activity was determined by flow cytometry. **b** Caspases-3, -8, and -9 activity was determined by sandwich ELISA assay. The results were normalized in relation to UCG, and represent the mean ± SD of the three experiments carried out in triplicate. Statistical analysis: Mann–Whitney U test *($p < 0.05$) versus UCG, + ($p < 0.05$) versus DTX 25 nM

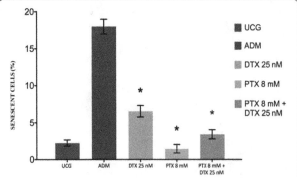

Fig. 4 Senescent PC3 cells treated with DTX, PTX or their combination. The 1×10^6 PC3 cells were cultured and treated with DTX 25 nM, PTX 8 mM, or PTX 8 mM + DTX 25 nM for 48 h. Cell senescence was determined by the levels of the β-galactosidase enzyme by flow cytometry. UCG = Untreated Control Group, ADM = Adriamycin (ADM) use as a positive control. The results represent the mean ± SD of the three replicated experiments. Statistical analysis: Mann–Whitney U test *($p < 0.05$) versus UCG, + ($p < 0.05$) versus DTX 25 nM

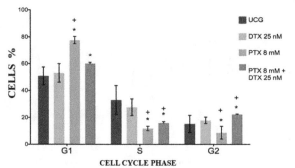

Fig. 5 Cell cycle phases arrested in PC3 cells treated with PTX and/or DTX. The 1×10^6 PC3 cells were cultured and treated with DTX 25 nM, PTX 8 mM, or PTX 8 mM + DTX 25 nM for 24 h. The cell cycle was determined by flow cytometry. The results represent the mean ± SD of the three replicated experiments. Statistical analysis: Mann–Whitney U test *($p < 0.05$) versus UCG, + ($p < 0.05$) versus DTX 25 nM

Role of PTX in the induction of the senescence of PC3 cells treated with DTX

The levels of the β-galactosidase enzyme were determined to measure senescence. Built on the premise that chemotherapy induces senescence, there is major logical senescence in the DTX group, as reported in Fig. 4, which shows a significant increase compared with the control group (Δ% = 192%). For its part, the senescence values of the PTX group demonstrated lower values than UCG (Δ% = − 35%), but are statistically and significantly lower compared with the DTX group, since it represents a Δ% = − 77% ($p < 0.05$). The PTX + DTX group exhibited a smaller percentage of senescence than DTX, but slightly higher than the PTX-treated group.

Cell cycle phases arrested in PC3 cells treated with PTX and/or DTX

The main objective of this experiment was to determine how PTX + DTX could modify the cell cycle in all experimental groups. In Additional file 2: Figure S2 is shown a representative example of cell cycle analysis using FlowJo software.

Flow cytometry analyzed this through the DNA obtained from PC3 cells after 24 h of treatment. Figure 5 shows that, during in the G1 phase, we found that the higher percentage of cells corresponds to the group treated with PTX (77.7% ± 2.7%), followed by the PTX + DTX group (60% ± 1.0%), both with a significant difference ($p < 0.05$) compared with the UCG group (50.8% ± 6.7%) and the DTX group (53.0 ± 7.8%), which is strictly comparable with UCG. Furthermore, PTX alone or combined with DTX showed no arresting

activity during the S phase and activity lower than the close percentages of the UCG and DTX groups (UCG- and DTX vs. PTX-treated groups $p < 0.05$). Finally, the lower percentage of cells in phase G2 corresponding to the group of PC3 cells treated exclusively with PTX 8.7 ± 2.1% ($p < 0.05$ vs. the other groups), and the other groups revealed very close percentages to about 20%. On the other hand, we found an arresting cell cycle during the G2 phase by PTX + DTX, a statistically significant increase compared with the control and the DTX group ($p < 0.05$), but with values very close to those the other groups.

Discussion

In the present work, it is shown that PTX can sensitize PC3 prostate cancer cells to the toxicity of the DTX, and it is essential to note that the PTX also demonstrates antitumor activity per se. The importance of the latter is that metastatic prostate cancer has a poor prognosis, and DTX is the first line of treatment for this tumor [8, 15].

Both drugs, either isolated or in combination, show a clear dose- and time-dependent effect on the survival of the PC3 tumor cells, indicating the treatments' specificity-of-action. The doses of PTX are in agreement with previous clinical and experimental observations with other tumor cells, such as leukemias, lymphoma, cervical cancer, and retinoblastoma [22, 23, 29, 32, 33].

On the other hand, it is well known that the most critical effect of chemotherapy against tumor cells is the induction of apoptosis [34]. In the present work, we observed that PTX could sensitize prostate tumor cells to the toxic effects of DTX, increasing apoptosis significantly in terms of the apoptosis induced by DTX.

In addition, with regard to this point, it is noteworthy that the label of antitumor activity exhibited by PTX per se is near those showed revealed in the PTX + DTX-treated cells; this is also in agreement with previous observations with respect to other tumor cell lines and supports the idea of the possible utilization of PTX as a direct antitumor drug [23], but additional studies are necessary to confirm this possibility.

The fact that strictly similar observations have been reported with ADM, Cisplatin, and Perillyl Alcohol permits us to think that PTX have a common target in different tumor cells with the same effects, sensitizing tumor cells to chemotherapy and showing per se an antitumor effect [22, 23].

The apoptosis observed in the PTX-treated groups, as depicted in Fig. 3, is dependent on caspases involving both extrinsic and intrinsic apoptotic pathways. The most important of these is the mitochondrial pathway, and the higher labels of caspase activity principally in the intrinsic pathway in PTX-treated groups can explain the persistence of the most top labels of apoptosis observed and afford security to our observations. In addition, the differences observed with caspases suggest a specific mechanism of action of each treatment, the main effect of DTX is die the cells and PTX have other effects, this may explain the difference of caspase activity between different groups.

The senescence initially was considered as a defence mechanism of the cells against the malignization of the cells. However, this is now in doubt, because cells in senescence are live and secrete factors that favor a tumor microenvironment that facilitates their growth and expansion and an inhibitor of the immune response [28]. In the present work, we observed that PTX does not induce senescence and that it diminishes the senescence produced by DTX. Therefore, the use of PTX is an advantage because a defence mechanism of the tumor cells against chemotherapy is the induction of senescence, as we can observe in the DTX group (Fig. 5) and is inhibited by the PTX.

We observed, in all groups, that the higher percentage of cells were in the G1 phase; however, this was more intensely observed in PTX and PTX + DTX groups. Concerning phase G2, lower results were observed with the PTX and PTX + DTX groups and, as expected, the lower percentages found in phase S was practically without a difference between groups. The importance of these observations is that it is well-known that, in the G0 and G1 phase cycles, tumor cells are more sensitive to the toxic effects of chemotherapy [35, 36]. Additionally, the finding that PTX-treated groups also showed a lower percentage of these in phase S, strongly suggesting the lower ability of PC3 cells to divide.

It is important to note that there was an agreement with all of the experiments carried out, in that the work helps to support the use of PTX in Oncology. It also has been reported that increased chemotherapy efficiency [18, 23, 32, 37] inhibits side effects of chemo- and radio-therapy [18], which is certain even when used in children with leukemia, and in addition exerted an antitumor impact per se [22, 23]. Another possible advantage of PTX pretreatment is that as the tumour cells are more sensitive to chemotherapy, so requiring lower doses of chemotherapy avoiding or reducing side effects, at this respect it was observed experimentally in lymphoma-bearing mice treated with PTX + ADM survived more than 1 year after receiving only one half of the standard therapeutically active ADM dose compared to single treatment of ADM [29].

In conclusion, PTX sensitizes prostate PC3 cells to DTX toxicity increasing apoptosis. The agreement of the results of this work, as well as the previous reports in the literature, provide additional evidence supporting the concept of chemotherapy with rational molecular bases [29].

Abbreviations

cAMP: Cyclic adenosine monophosphate c; ADT: Androgen-deprivation therapy; DTX: Docetaxel; mHSPC: metastatic Hormone-sensitive prostate cancer; PTX: Pentoxifylline; PCa: Prostate cancer; mCRPC: metastatic Castration resistant prostate cancer; ADM: Adryamicin; UCG: Untreated control group.

Supplementary Information

Additional file 1. Figure S1: Representative analyses of apoptosis, generic caspase activity and senescence in PC3 cells treated or not with PTX, DTX or PTX + DTX.

Additional file 2. Figure S2: Representative cell cycle analyses of PC3 cells treated or not with PTX, DTX or PTX + DTX.

Acknowledgements

We are grateful to Joo Hyun Lee for his critique of the manuscript.

Authors' contributions

ABC responsible for the project, design, data analysis, manuscript writing. MECM design, data analysis. GHF, PCOL, MMVG performed flow cytometry and ELISA studies, analysis of data. EOA, RASM, CCCG, performed apoptosis and survival studies, ESD performed the statistical analysis. All authors helped to draft the manuscript and approved this final version.

Author details

[1] Doctorado en Farmacología, Centro Universitario de Ciencias de la Salud, Universidad de Guadalajara, Guadalajara, Jalisco, México. [2] División de Inmunología, Centro de Investigación Biomédica de Occidente del IMSS, Sierra Mojada 800, Col. Independencia, CP 44340 Guadalajara, Jalisco, México. [3] Servicio de Urología, Hospital de Especialidades, CMNO-IMSS, Guadalajara, Jalisco, México. [4] Centro Universitario de los Altos, Universidad de Guadalajara, Tepatitlán de Morelos, Jalisco, México.

References

1. Bray F, Ferlay J, Soerjomataram I, Siegel RL, Torre LA, Jemal A. Global cancer statistics 2018: GLOBOCAN estimates of incidence and mortality worldwide for 36 cancers in 185 countries. CA Cancer J Clin. 2018;68(6):394–424.
2. Siegel RL, Miller KD, Jemal A. Cancer statistics, 2019. CA Cancer J Clin. 2019;69(1):7–34.
3. Testa U, Castelli G, Pelosi E. Cellular and molecular mechanisms underlying prostate cancer development: therapeutic implications. Medicines (Basel). 2019;6(3):1–139.
4. Gleason DF. Histologic grading of prostate cancer: a perspective. Hum Pathol. 1992;23(3):273–9.
5. Johansson JE, Adami HO, Andersson SO, Bergström R, Holmberg L, Krusemo UB. High 10-year survival rate in patients with early, untreated prostatic cancer. JAMA. 1992;267(16):2191–6.
6. Johansson JE, Adami HO, Andersson SO, Bergström R, Krusemo UB, Kraaz W. Natural history of localised prostatic cancer. A population-based study in 223 untreated patients. Lancet. 1989;1(8642):799–803.
7. Lu-Yao GL, Yao SL. Population-based study of long-term survival in patients with clinically localised prostate cancer. Lancet. 1997;349(9056):906–10.
8. Nevedomskaya E, Baumgart SJ, Haendler B. Recent advances in prostate cancer treatment and drug discovery. Int J Mol Sci. 2018;19(5):1–25.
9. Gomella LG, Petrylak DP, Shayegan B. Current management of advanced and castration resistant prostate cancer. Can J Urol. 2014;21(2 Suppl 1):1–6.
10. Karantanos T, Corn PG, Thompson TC. Prostate cancer progression after androgen deprivation therapy: mechanisms of castrate resistance and novel therapeutic approaches. Oncogene. 2013;32(49):5501–11.
11. Mahon KL, Henshall SM, Sutherland RL, Horvath LG. Pathways of chemotherapy resistance in castration-resistant prostate cancer. Endocr Relat Cancer. 2011;18(4):R103–23.
12. de Morrée E, van Soest R, Aghai A, de Ridder C, de Bruijn P, Ghobadi Moghaddam-Helmantel I, et al. Understanding taxanes in prostate cancer; importance of intratumoral drug accumulation. Prostate. 2016;76(10):927–36.
13. Huebner NA, Shariat SF, Resch I, Gust K, Kramer G. The role of taxane-based chemotherapy in the treatment of prostate cancer. Curr Opin Urol. 2020;30(4):527–33.
14. Joerger M. Treatment regimens of classical and newer taxanes. Cancer Chemother Pharmacol. 2016;77(2):221–33.
15. Nader R, El Amm J, Aragon-Ching JB. Role of chemotherapy in prostate cancer. Asian J Androl. 2018;20(3):221–9.
16. Antonarakis ES, Armstrong AJ. Evolving standards in the treatment of docetaxel-refractory castration-resistant prostate cancer. Prostate Cancer Prostatic Dis. 2011;14(3):192–205.
17. Aviado DM, Dettelbach HR. Pharmacology of pentoxifylline, a hemorheologic agent for the treatment of intermittent claudication. Angiology. 1984;35(7):407–17.
18. Golunski G, Woziwodzka A, Piosik J. Potential use of pentoxifylline in cancer therapy. Curr Pharm Biotechnol. 2018;19(3):206–16.
19. Jain M, Ratheesh A, Gude RP. Pentoxifylline inhibits integrin-mediated adherence of 12(S)-HETE and TNFalpha-activated B16F10 cells to fibronectin and endothelial cells. Chemotherapy. 2010;56(1):82–8.
20. Speer EM, Dowling DJ, Ozog LS, Xu J, Yang J, Kennady G, et al. Pentoxifylline inhibits TLR- and inflammasome-mediated in vitro inflammatory cytokine production in human blood with greater efficacy and potency in newborns. Pediatr Res. 2017;81(5):806–16.
21. Hernandez-Flores G, Ortiz-Lazareno PC, Lerma-Diaz JM, Dominguez-Rodriguez JR, Jave-Suarez LF, Aguilar-Lemarroy Adel C, et al. Pentoxifylline sensitizes human cervical tumor cells to cisplatin-induced apoptosis by suppressing NF-kappa B and decreased cell senescence. BMC Cancer. 2011;11:483.
22. Bravo-Cuellar A, Ortiz-Lazareno PC, Lerma-Diaz JM, Dominguez-Rodriguez JR, Jave-Suarez LF, Aguilar-Lemarroy A, et al. Sensitization of cervix cancer cells to Adriamycin by Pentoxifylline induces an increase in apoptosis and decrease senescence. Mol Cancer. 2010;9:114.
23. Cruz-Galvez CC, Ortiz-Lazareno PC, Pedraza-Brindis EJ, Villasenor-Garcia MM, Reyes-Uribe E, Bravo-Hernandez A, et al. Pentoxifylline enhances the apoptotic effect of carboplatin in Y79 retinoblastoma cells. In Vivo. 2019;33(2):401–12.
24. Gómez-Contreras PC, Hernández-Flores G, Ortiz-Lazareno PC, Del Toro-Arreola S, Delgado-Rizo V, Lerma-Díaz JM, et al. In vitro induction of apoptosis in U937 cells by perillyl alcohol with sensitization by pentoxifylline: increased BCL-2 and BAX protein expression. Chemotherapy. 2006;52(6):308–15.
25. Gonzalez-Ramella O, Ortiz-Lazareno PC, Jiménez-López X, Gallegos-Castorena S, Hernández-Flores G, Medina-Barajas F, et al. Pentoxifylline during steroid window phase at induction to remission increases apoptosis in childhood with acute lymphoblastic leukemia. Clin Transl Oncol. 2016;18(4):369–74.
26. Angel MJLSR, Paulina RV, Angel MJP, Georgina HF, Alejandro BC. Management of hepatocarcinoma with celecoxib and pentoxifylline: report of three cases. J Clin Exp Pharmacol. 2018;8(5):1–6.
27. Serafin AM, Binder AB, Böhm L. Chemosensitivity of prostatic tumour cell lines under conditions of G2 block abrogation. Urol Res. 2001;29(3):221–7.
28. Solís-Martínez R, Cancino-Marentes M, Hernández-Flores G, Ortiz-Lazareno P, Mandujano-Álvarez G, Cruz-Gálvez C, et al. Regulation of immunophenotype modulation of monocytes-macrophages from M1 into M2 by prostate cancer cell-culture supernatant via transcription factor STAT3. Immunol Lett. 2018;196:140–8.
29. Lerma-Díaz JM, Hernández-Flores G, Domínguez-Rodríguez JR, Ortíz-Lazareno PC, Gómez-Contreras P, Cervantes-Munguía R, et al. In vivo and in vitro sensitization of leukemic cells to adriamycin-induced apoptosis by pentoxifylline. Involvement of caspase cascades and IkappaBalpha phosphorylation. Immunol Lett. 2006;103(2):149–58.
30. Bravo-Cuellar A, Hernández-Flores G, Lerma-Díaz JM, Domínguez-Rodríguez JR, Jave-Suárez LF, De Célis-Carrillo R, et al. Pentoxifylline and the proteasome inhibitor MG132 induce apoptosis in human leukemia U937 cells through a decrease in the expression of Bcl-2 and Bcl-XL and phosphorylation of p65. J Biomed Sci. 2013;20(1):13.
31. Gomez-Contreras PC, Hernandez-Flores G, Ortiz-Lazareno PC, Del Toro-Arreola S, Delgado-Rizo V, Lerma-Diaz JM, et al. In vitro induction of apoptosis in U937 cells by perillyl alcohol with sensitization by pentoxifylline: increased BCL-2 and BAX protein expression. Chemotherapy. 2006;52(6):308–15.
32. Meza-Arroyo J, Bravo-Cuellar A, Jave-Suárez LF, Hernández-Flores G, Ortiz-Lazareno P, Aguilar-Lemarroy A, et al. Pentoxifylline added to steroid window treatment phase modified apoptotic gene expression in pediatric patients with acute lymphoblastic leukemia. J Pediatr Hematol Oncol. 2018;40(5):360–7.
33. Rishi L, Gahlot S, Kathania M, Majumdar S. Pentoxifylline induces apoptosis in vitro in cutaneous T cell lymphoma (HuT-78) and enhances FasL mediated killing by upregulating Fas expression. Biochem Pharmacol. 2009;77(1):30–45.
34. Bravo-Cuellar A, Gómez-Contreras PC, Lerma-Díaz JM, Hernández-Flores G, Domínguez-Rodríguez JR, Ortíz-Lazareno P, et al. In vivo modification of adriamycin-induced apoptosis in L-5178Y lymphoma cell-bearing mice by (+)-alpha-tocopherol and superoxide dismutase. Cancer Lett. 2005;229(1):59–65.
35. Jin Z, Dicker DT, El-Deiry WS. Enhanced sensitivity of G1 arrested human cancer cells suggests a novel therapeutic strategy using a combination of simvastatin and TRAIL. Cell Cycle. 2002;1(1):82–9.
36. Bai J, Li Y, Zhang G. Cell cycle regulation and anticancer drug discovery. Cancer Biol Med. 2017;14(4):348–62.
37. Mosalam EM, Zidan AA, Mehanna ET, Mesbah NM, Abo-Elmatty DM. Thymoquinone and pentoxifylline enhance the chemotherapeutic effect of cisplatin by targeting Notch signaling pathway in mice. Life Sci. 2020;244:117299.

10

MicroRNA-4429 suppresses proliferation of prostate cancer cells by targeting distal-less homeobox 1 and inactivating the Wnt/β-catenin pathway

Jinguo Wang, Sheng Xie, Jun Liu, Tao Li, Wanrong Wang and Ziping Xie[*]

Abstract

Background: Emerging evidence suggests that microRNAs (miRNAs) play multiple roles in human cancers through regulating mRNAs and distinct pathways. This paper focused on the functions of miR-4429 in prostate cancer (PCa) progression and the molecules involved.

Methods: Expression of miR-4429 in PCa tissues and cells was determined. Upregulation of miR-4429 was introduced in PCa cells to examine its role in the malignant behaviors of cells. The putative target mRNA of miR-4429 involved in PCa progression was predicted from a bioinformatic system and validated through luciferase assays. Overexpression of distal-less homeobox 1 (DLX1) was further induced in cells to validate its implication in miR-4429-mediated events. The activity of Wnt/β-catenin pathway was determined.

Results: miR-4429 was poorly expressed in PCa tissues and cells. Artificial upregulation of miR-4429 significantly reduced proliferation, growth, invasion, migration and resistance to death of cancer cells and inactivated the Wnt/β-catenin pathway. DLX1 mRNA was found as a target of miR-4429. Upregulation of DLX1 restored the malignant behaviors of PCa cells which were initially suppressed by miR-4429, and it activated the Wnt/β-catenin pathway.

Conclusion: Our study highlights that miR-4429 inhibits the growth of PCa cells by down-regulating DLX1 and inactivating the Wnt/β-catenin pathway. This finding may offer novel insights into PCa treatment.

Keywords: Prostate cancer, MicroRNA-4429, Wnt/β-catenin pathway, DLX1, Biological behavior

Background

Prostate cancer (PCa) is the second most common malignant tumor and the sixth leading cause of cancer-associated death among males around the world [1]. Recently, the incidence of PCa has been elevating steadily in China with the economy improvement [2]. Established risk factors for PCa comprise black race, advancing age, family history and certain genetic polymorphisms [3, 4]. Currently, digital rectal examination, prostate-specific antigen testing and prostate needle biopsies are applied in the diagnosis and monitoring of PCa progression [5]. It is essential to identify more biomarkers for PCa prediction and treatment, which requires a better recognition of the molecular pathogenesis of the disease.

MicroRNAs (miRNA) are a major type of small noncoding RNAs that can negatively modulate gene expression via binding to the 3′untranslated region (3′UTR) of target mRNAs [6]. The miRNAs play versatile roles in many key cellular processes, such as carcinogenesis,

*Correspondence: xieziping12121@163.com
Department of Andrology, Renmin Hospital, Hubei University of Medicine, No. 39 Chaoyang Middle Road, Maojian District, Shiyan 442000, Hubei, People's Republic of China

proliferation and metastasis [7]. Aberrant expression of miRNAs, either upregulation or downregulation, has been frequently found in PCa tissues versus normal tissues [5]. miR-4429 was discovered to have a suppressive effect on several types of malignancies such as thyroid cancer [8] and cervical cancer [9]. However, there is little evidence concerning its role in the tumorigenesis of PCa. Distal-less homeobox 1 (DLX1) was firstly found in Drosophila melanogaster and found to mediate development of nerves and embryo [10]. DLX1 downregulation has been demonstrated to lead to PCa cell growth arrest, revealing that DLX1 might serve as an oncogene [11]. Wnt signaling is a pivotal pathway controlling adult tissue homeostasis and β-catenin is an essential effector of this signaling [12]. The Wnt/β-catenin pathway exerts key functions in a variety of cellular processes such as cell fate determination, cell growth and polarity, and stem cell maintenance [13]. This pathway has been reported to induce invasive behaviors of PCa cells [14]. In this study, DLX1 was confirmed as a target of miR-4429. We hypothesized that miR-4429 could inhibit PCa progression through regulating DLX1 and the Wnt/β-catenin pathway, with gain- and loss-of function studies of these molecules performed to validate this hypothesis.

Methods
Ethical approval
This study was ratified by the Ethics Committee of Renmin Hospital, Hubei University of Medicine and performed in line with the *Declaration of Helsinki*. Signed informed consent form was obtained from each eligible participant.

Collection of clinical samples
Biopsy specimens of primary PCa tissues and the adjacent normal prostate tissues were collected from 35 patients with PCa in People's Hospital Affiliated to Hubei University of Medicine from February 2017 to November 2019. The patients aged from 42 to 68 years at a median age of 57 years. The tissues were stored at -80 °C until further use. The inclusion criteria were: 1. Patients were diagnosed with PCa by prostate puncture, digital rectal examination, computerized tomography or magnetic resonance imaging, or prostate specific antigen test; 2. Patients aged between 40 and 70 years; 3. Gleason score was not less than 6. Patients with a history of hormone therapy, radiotherapy, chemotherapy or surgery, or those with other malignancies were excluded.

Cell culture
PCa cell lines PC-3, LNCAP, and DU145 and a human normal prostate epithelial cell line RWPE-1 were procured from the American Standard Bacterial Bank

(ATCC, Rockville, Maryland, USA). Cells were cultured in RPMI-1640 medium (Gibco, Gaithersburg, MD, USA) supplemented with 10% fetal bovine serum (FBS) in a 37°C incubator with 5% CO_2.

Reverse transcription quantitative polymerase chain reaction (RT-qPCR)
Total RNA in cells and tissues was extracted using a TRIzol kit (TAKARA, Shiga, Japan). A SYBR Green qPCR Mix Kit (Thermo Fisher Scientific, Waltham, MA, USA) was used for quantitative PCR after the addition of templates and primers. The gene expression was detected on the ABI real-time PCR platform (Thermo Fisher Scientific). Primers were purchased from Invitrogen (Shanghai, China). Internal references were U6 (for miRNA) and glyceraldehyde phosphate dehydrogenase (GAPDH) (for mRNA). The primer sequences are as follows: miR-4429 (GenBank ACCESSION: NR_039627.1): forward primer: 5'-GGCCAGGCAGTCTGAGTTG-3'; reverse primer: 5'-GGGAGAAAAGCTGGGCTGAG-3'. DLX1 (GenBank ACCESSION: NM_178120): forward primer: 5'-GCGGCCTCTTTGGGACTCACA-3'; reverse primer: 5'-GGCCAACGCACTACCCTCCAGA-3'. GAPDH (GenBank ACCESSION: NM_001289746.2): forward primer: 5'-GAGTCCACTGGCGTCTTCAC-3'; reverse primer: 5'-ATCTTGAGGCTGTTGTCATACTTCT-3'. U6 (GenBank ACCESSION: NR_004394.1): forward primer: 5'-CTCGCTTCGGCAGCACA-3'; reverse primer: 5'-AACGCTTCACGAATTTGCGT-3'. Axin2 (GenBank ACCESSION: NM_004655.4): forward primer: 5'-CAGATCCGAGAGGATGAAGAGA-3'; reverse primer: 5'-AGTATCGT CTGCGGGTCTTC-3'. CD44 (GenBank ACCESSION: NM_000610.4): forward primer: 5'-ACCCTCCCCTCATTCACCAT-3'; reverse primer: 5'-GTTGTACTACTAGGAGTTGCCTGGATT-3'. Relative gene expression was examined by the $2^{-\Delta\Delta Ct}$ method.

Cell apoptosis detection
Exponentially growing cells were seeded in 6-well plates, and the cells were rinsed twice with pre-chilled phosphate-buffered saline (PBS) and stained using a PI/Annexin-V kit at room temperature without light exposure for 15 min. Then, the cells were appended with 300 μL 1 × binding buffer and suspended, and transferred into a 5-mL flow tube. A flow cytometer (Thermo Fisher Scientific) was adopted to detect the number of apoptotic cells within one hour.

Cell transfection
DU145 and PC-3 cells in good growth conditions were sorted in 6-well plates (4×10^5 cells/mL) and incubated in DMEM with 10% FBS for 24 h of pre-transfection. Next, the cells were introduced with miR-4429 mimic/inhibitor

and the corresponding miR-4429 mimic/inhibitor control, pcDNA-DLX1, or empty pcDNA (all procured from Thermo Fisher Scientific). Transfection was conducted using Lipofectamine 2000 reagent (Thermo Fisher Scientific) according to the manufacturer's protocols. Forty-eight hours later, cells were harvested for subsequent experiments, and miR-4429 expression was detected by RT-qPCR to evaluate the transfection efficiency.

Determination of cell proliferation

A cell counting kit-8 (CCK-8) assay was performed to evaluate cell proliferation. In brief, cells were treated with 10 µL/well CCK-8 solution (Beyotime Biotechnology, Shanghai, China) and cultured at 37 °C for 2 h. The optical density at 450 nm was measured with a microplate reader (BioTek Instruments).

Colony formation assay

Cells were detached in trypsin, seeded onto 6-well plates (200 cells/well), and then incubated in DMEM with 10% FBS for 2 w. The medium was renewed every three days. Next, cells were fixed in methanol for 15 min and then stained with crystal violet (1%) for 30 min. The images (containing more than 50 cells/colonies) were captured using a light microscope (magnification: $100 \times$; Olympus Optical Co., Ltd, Tokyo, Japan) and the number of cell colonies was counted.

Cell invasion assay

The Transwell apical chamber was pre-coated with Matrigel (BD Biosciences, Franklin Lakes, NJ, USA) under sterile conditions. Then, each apical chamber was loaded with 30 µL of serum-free RPMI 1640 medium, and then placed in a CO_2 incubator for later use. Each basolateral chamber was loaded with 200 µL cell suspension and 500 µL RPMI 1640 medium containing 10% FBS. The chambers were incubated in a 37°C incubator with 5% CO_2 for 24 h. After that, the non-invaded cells were wiped with a cotton swab, and cells invaded to the lower membranes were fixed in 4% paraformaldehyde and stained by crystal violet for 10 min. The count of invading cells was evaluated under a light microscope.

Luciferase activity assay

The binding sequence between miR-4429 and DLX1 mRNA was first predicted on a bioinformatic system Starbase (http://starbase.sysu.edu.cn/). To validate the binding relationship between miR-4429 and DLX1 mRNA, DLX1 3′UTR containing the putative binding site with miR-4429 was designed and inserted into pmirGLO reporter vectors (LMAIBio Co., Ltd., Shanghai, China) to construct wild-type luciferase vectors. A mutant type vector was designed by mutating the binding sequence

between miR-4429 and DLX1 mRNA. Well-constructed reporter vectors were co-transfected with miR-4429 mimic or mimic control into PCa cells. Forty-eight hours later, the cells were harvested and lysed, and luciferase activity in cells was determined on a dual luciferase reporting system (Promega Corp., Madison, Wisconsin, USA) according to the manufacturer's protocol.

Western blot analysis

Cells were lysed in Western and IP cell lysis buffer (Beyotime) to extract total protein, and the protein concentration was determined using a bicinchoninic acid kit (No. P0009, Beyotime). Next, the proteins were separated by polyacrylamide gel (5% spacer gel and 12% separation gel), transferred on polyvinylidene fluoride membranes and treated with 5% bovine serum albumin to block the non-specific binding. After that, the membranes were co-incubated with the primary antibodies at 4°C overnight and then with the secondary antibody at 37°C for 2 h. Next, the protein bands were developed using enhanced chemiluminescence reagent (WBKLS0100, Millipore, Billerica, MA, USA). Relative gray value analysis was performed on all immunoblotted bands, and the ratio of the gray value of the target band to the internal reference band was considered as the relative expression of the protein. Primary antibodies included DLX1 (UniProt Entry ID: P56177) (1:2000, ab126054), β-catenin (UniProt Entry ID: P35222) (1: 7500, ab32572) and GAPDH (1: 2500, ab9485) and secondary antibody was (1:50,000, ab205718) (Abcam, NY, USA).

Statistical analysis

Data were processed using the SPSS 21.0 (IBM Corp. Armonk, NY, USA) statistical software. Results were shown as mean $\pm$ standard deviation (SD) from three independent experiments. The two-group comparison was analyzed by the t test. Comparisons among three or more groups were implemented using one-way analysis of variance (ANOVA) or two-way ANOVA. Pairwise comparison after ANOVA was implemented using Tukey's multiple comparisons test. P less than 0.05 was considered statistically significant.

Results

miR-4429 is poorly expressed in PCa cells and tissues

First, the miR-4429 expression in PCa tissues and cells was detected. Compared to the adjacent normal tissues, the expression of miR-4429 was significantly reduced in PCa tissues (Fig. 1a). Compared to that in human normal prostate epithelial cell line RWPE-1, the expression of

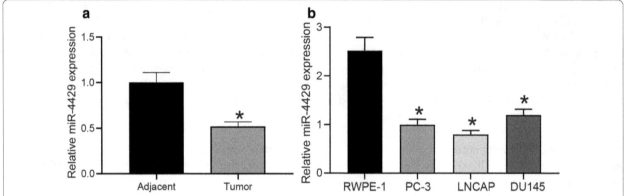

Fig. 1 miR-4429 is lowly expressed in PCa cells and tissues. **a** miR-4429 expression in 35 pairs of PCa tissues and the adjacent normal tissues determined by RT-qPCR (paired *t* test, *P* = 0.0023). **b** miR-4429 expression in PCa cell lines (PC-3, LNCAP and DU145) and human normal prostate epithelial cell line RWPE-1 determined by RT-qPCR (one-way ANOVA, *P* < 0.0001). Data were expressed as mean ± SD from three independent experiments. *P < 0.05 was considered to show statistical significance

miR-4429 was also declined in the PCa cell lines (PC-3, LNCAP and DU145) (Fig. 1b).

miR-4429 mimic suppresses the biological activity of PCa cells

Next, to explore the function of miR-4429 in the activity of PCa cells, miR-4429 mimic, miR-4429 inhibitor and the corresponding negative controls (NCs) were administrated into DU145 and PC-3 cells. RT-qPCR analysis showed that miR-4429 expression in cells was significantly elevated by miR-4429 mimic but reduced by miR-4429 inhibitor (Fig. 2a). Then, the CCK-8 and colony formation assays suggested that miR-4429 mimic restricted proliferation and colony formation ability of the PCa cells, while miR-4429 inhibitor led to inverse results (Fig. 2b, c). As for apoptosis and invasion, it was found that the invasion and migration abilities of cells were reduced by miR-4429 mimic but enhanced by miR-4429 inhibitor (Fig. 2d, e). It can be concluded that miR-4429 mimic can repress the biological activity of PCa cells.

DLX1 is a target mRNA of miR-4429

A luciferase assay was implemented to validate the targeting relationship between miR-4429 and DLX1. According to the data from the bioinformatics system StarBase, DLX1 mRNA was suggested as a potential target of tumor-associated miR-4429. DLX1 3′-UTR contains a putative binding site with miR-4429 (Fig. 3a). We then explored the expression profiles of DLX1 in PCa according to the data available from the Gene Expression Profiling Interactive Analysis (GEPIA) dataset (http://gepia.cancer-pku.cn/detail.php?clicktag= degenes###). It was suggested that DLX1 was highly expressed in PCa samples, while its expression showed no significant relevance to the overall survival rate of patients (Fig. 3b). This might be attributed to the individual differences between patients (Fig. 3c).

The binding relationship between miR-4429 and DLX1 mRNA was validated through a luciferase assay. It was found that the luciferase activity of the wild-type DLX1 3′-UTR luciferase vector was significantly reduced by miR-4429 mimic, while the activity of mutant-type luciferase vector was not significantly changed (Fig. 3d). In addition, the RT-qPCR and western blot assay results suggested that the expression of DLX1 in PCa cells was significantly reduced by miR-4429 mimic but elevated by miR-4429 inhibitor (Fig. 3e, f). Taken together, these results indicate that DLX1 is a target mRNA of miR-4429 in PCa cells.

miR-4429 mimic inhibits Wnt/β-catenin while DLX1 activates this pathway

Since the Wnt/β-catenin pathway is implicated in many human malignancies, we investigated whether the Wnt/β-catenin pathway activation was involved in the events mediated by miR-4429. Importantly, it was found that miR-4429 mimic suppressed the protein level of β-catenin in PCa cells (Fig. 4a). In addition, artificial upregulation of DLX1 was introduced in the PCa cells. In this setting, the protein level of β-catenin in cells was restored (Fig. 4b).

DLX1 overexpression suppresses the antitumor effect of miR-4429 in PCa cells

To explore the involvement of DLX1 inhibition in the miR-4429-mediated events, pcDNA DLX1 was further

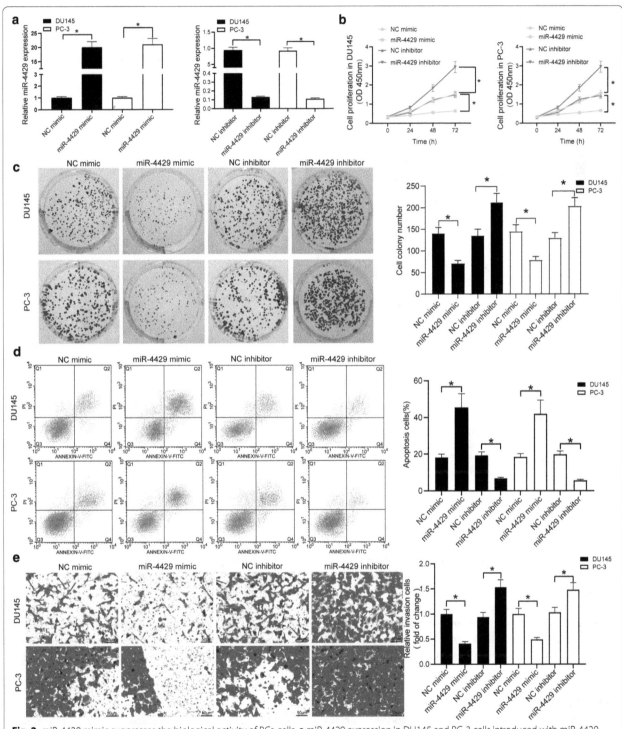

Fig. 2 miR-4429 mimic suppresses the biological activity of PCa cells. **a** miR-4429 expression in DU145 and PC-3 cells introduced with miR-4429 mimic/miR-4429 inhibitor determined by RT-qPCR (unpaired *t* test, *P* < 0.0001). **b** PCa cell proliferation in DU145 and PC-3 cells introduced with miR-4429 mimic/miR-4429 inhibitor determined by CCK-8 assay (two-way ANOVA, *P* < 0.0001). **c** Number of colonies in DU145 and PC-3 cells introduced with miR-4429 mimic/miR-4429 inhibitor determined by colony formation assay (one-way ANOVA, *P* < 0.0001). **d** Apoptosis in DU145 and PC-3 cells introduced with miR-4429 mimic/miR-4429 inhibitor determined by flow cytometry (one-way ANOVA, *P* < 0.0001). **e** Invasion ability in DU145 and PC-3 cells introduced with miR-4429 mimic/miR-4429 inhibitor determined by Transwell assay (one-way ANOVA, *P* < 0.0001). Data were expressed as mean ± SD from three independent experiments. **P* < 0.05 was considered to show statistical significance

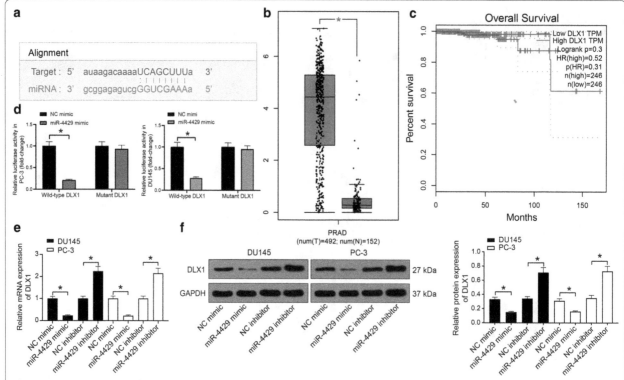

Fig. 3 DLX1 is a target gene of miR-4429 in PCa cells. **a** Putative binding site between miR-4429 and the DLX1 3′-UTR. **b–c** PCa expression (**b**) and its relevance to the overall survival of patients (**c**) predicted according to the data on the GEPIA database (**d**). Binding relationship between miR-4429 and DLX1 3′-UTR evaluated via a dual luciferase reporter gene analysis. DLX1 3′-UTR luciferase vector and miR-4429 mimic or NC mimic were co-transfected into DU145 and PC-3 cells and incubated for 48 h before measuring luciferase activity (one-way ANOVA, $P < 0.0001$). **e** miR-4429 mimic/inhibitor or NC mimic/inhibitor transfected into DU145 and PC-3 cells for 48 h, and DLX1 mRNA expression was measured by RT-qPCR (one-way ANOVA, $P < 0.0001$). **f** miR-4429 mimic/inhibitor or NC mimic/inhibitor transfected into DU145 and PC-3 cells for 48 h, and DLX1 protein expression was measured by western blot analysis (one-way ANOVA, $P < 0.0001$) (see original western blots in Additional file 1: Figure S1). Data were expressed as mean ± SD from three independent experiments. *$P < 0.05$ was considered to show statistical significance

transfected into DU145 and PC-3 cells after miR-4429 mimic administration. As shown in Fig. 5a, it was found that pcDNA DLX1 partially blocked the inhibitory effect of miR-4429 mimic on DLX1 expression. The proliferation, invasion and colony formation abilities of cells and the expression of PCa-biomarker Axin2 and CD44 in cells initially inhibited by miR-4429 mimic were recovered after further DLX1 overexpression. Accordingly, DLX1 reduced the apoptosis rate in the PCa cells (Fig. 5b–f).

Discussion

In recent years, novel promising PCa-specific targets have been recognized in many researches, while only a few of them have reached clinical practice [15]. It is well-known that both overtreatment and overdiagnosis would be decreased if PCa-specific targets could distinguish inactive from aggressive tumors. Therefore, developing novel biomarkers may help a lot in PCa management. In this article, we confirmed that miR-4429 plays a

tumor-suppressive role in PCa via mediating DLX1 and Wnt/β-catenin pathway (Fig. 6).

The miR-4429 has been identified as a tumor suppressor in several kinds of tumors while its role in PCa has not been concerned. Here, the initial finding of this research was that miR-4429 was poorly expressed in both PCa tissue samples and cell lines compared to the normal tissues or cells. Next, artificial up-regulation of miR-4429 significantly reduced proliferation, invasion, colony formation, and resistance to apoptosis of cells. These results were partially in concert with the tumor-suppressing roles of miR-4429 in several previous studies. For instance, miR-4429 was found as a sponge for long non-coding RNA LINC00313 and was expressed at a low lever in thyroid cancer, and its upregulation reduced proliferation and the migratory and colony-forming abilities of thyroid cancer cells [8]. Likewise, miR-4429 has been reported to be reduced in cervical cancer cells versus normal cell lines and it enhanced the sensitivity of cells to irradiation [9]. Furthermore, miR-4429 has been reported as a tumor

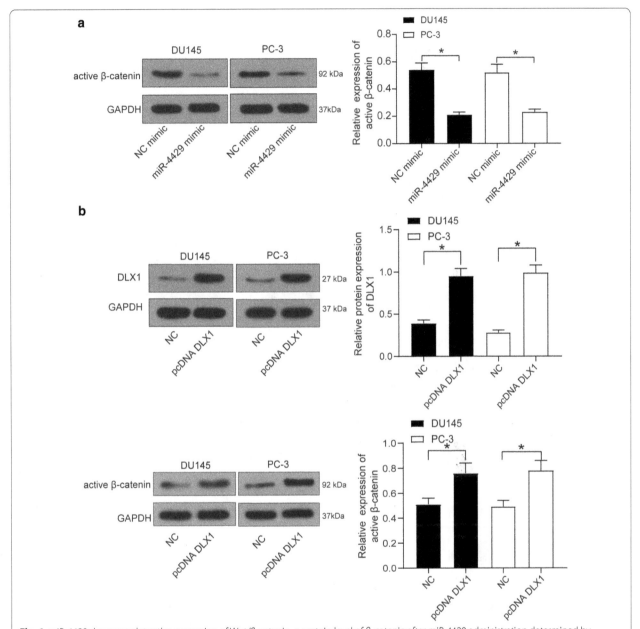

Fig. 4 miR-4429 down-regulates the expression of Wnt/β-catenin. **a** protein level of β-catenin after miR-4429 administration determined by western blot analysis (one-way ANOVA, $P < 0.0001$) (see original western blots in Additional file 1: Figure S2); **b** protein level of β-catenin after pcDNA-DLX1 administration determined by western blot analysis (one-way ANOVA, $P = 0.0009$) (see original western blots in Additional file 1: Figure S3). Data were expressed as mean ± SD from three independent experiments. *$P < 0.05$ was considered to show statistical significance

suppressor in clear cell renal cell carcinoma (ccRCC), and its downregulation was associated with poor prognosis of ccRCC patients while its upregulation inhibited growth of ccRCC cells [16]. Likewise, silencing of miR-4429 was also found to increase the viability of glioblastoma multiforme cells [17].

Data from the StarBase system suggested that miR-4429 owns a binding relationship with DLX1 mRNA, and the direct binding was confirmed by a luciferase assay. Although the correlation between DLX1 and miR-4922 has never been documented before, the involvements of target mRNAs have been well-established in the antioncogenic role of miR-4922, such as CDK6 downregulation in the above-mentioned ccRCC inhibition [16]. Another study has elucidated that miR-4429 prevented the onset of gastric cancer via targeting METTL3 [18].

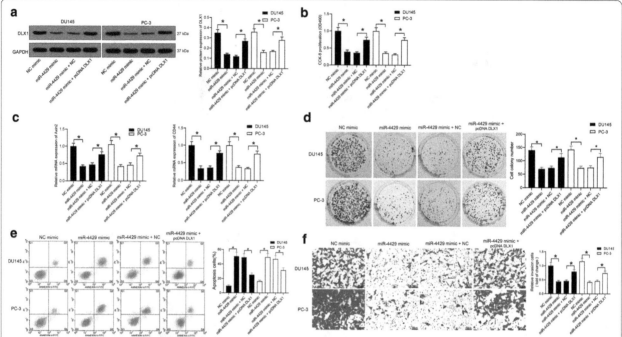

Fig. 5 DLX1 blocks the antitumor function of miR-4429 in PCa cells. **a** DLX1 protein level in DU145 and PC-3 cells introduced with miR-4429 mimic and pcDNA DLX1 determined by western blot analysis (one-way ANOVA, $P < 0.0001$) (see original western blots in Additional file 1: Figure S5). **b** Proliferation of DU145 and PC-3 cells introduced with miR-4429 mimic and pcDNA DLX1 determined by CCK-8 assay (one-way ANOVA, $P < 0.0001$). **c** Expression of Axin2 and CD44 in DU145 and PC-3 cells introduced with miR-4429 mimic and PcDNA DLX1 determined by RT-qPCR (one-way ANOVA, $P < 0.0001$). **d** Number of colonies of DU145 and PC-3 cells introduced with miR-4429 mimic and PcDNA DLX1 determined by colony formation assay (one-way ANOVA, $P < 0.0001$). **e** Apoptosis in DU145 and PC-3 cells introduced with miR-4429 mimic and PcDNA DLX1 determined by flow cytometry (one-way ANOVA, $P < 0.0001$). **f** Invasion ability in DU145 and PC-3 cells introduced with miR-4429 mimic and PcDNA DLX1 determined by Transwell assay (one-way ANOVA, $P < 0.0001$). Data were expressed as mean ± SD from three independent experiments. *$P < 0.05$ was considered to show statistical significance

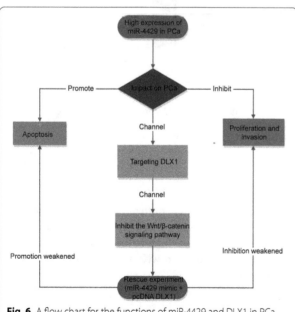

Fig. 6 A flow chart for the functions of miR-4429 and DLX1 in PCa cells

As for DLX1, it has been suggested as an important target of FOXM1 to enhance the aggressiveness of ovarian cancer [19]. More relevantly, DLX1 expression has been found to be elevated in PCa tissues, indicating a possible association between DLX1 and PCa progression, [20]. In concert with this, DLX1 has been suggested as a potent biomarker for high-grade PCa detection [15]. A study by Liang et al. suggested that DLX1 was elevated in PCa clinical samples, and DLX1 promoted growth of PCa cells through activating the β-catenin/TCF pathway [21]. Here, our study found that overexpression of DLX1 partially blocked the inhibitory effect of miR-4429 on the PCa cells. In addition, miR-4429 suppressed was found to inactivate the Wnt/β-catenin pathway, while the activity of this pathway was restored after DLX1 upregulation. Aberrant activation of the Wnt/β-catenin is closely associated with onset and progression of multiple human cancers, leaving this signaling as a potential target for cancer therapy [22, 23]. There is no exception for PCa [14, 24]. As reported, distinct miRNAs could directly mediate the Wnt/β-catenin pathway in many malignancies [25, 26]. Wnt signaling aberrant activation is able

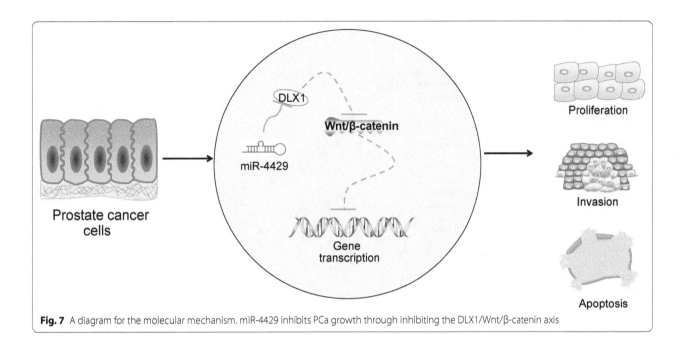

Fig. 7 A diagram for the molecular mechanism. miR-4429 inhibits PCa growth through inhibiting the DLX1/Wnt/β-catenin axis

to induce nuclear β-catenin accumulation, contributing to transcriptional activation of proto-oncogenes that are associated with cell progression [27]. Furthermore, Wnt/β-catenin pathway has been revealed to induce tumor cell malignancy in hormone-refractory PCa cells in a ligand-independent manner [28]. In addition to the finding that miR-4429 inactivated this pathway, overexpression of DLX1 was found to increase the protein level of β-catenin, indicating that down-regulation of Wnt/β-catenin was implicated in the miR-4429/DLX1-mediated events.

Conclusion

To sum up, our study reports that miR-4429 is lowly expressed in PCa tissues and cells compared to the normal healthy ones. Overexpression of miR-4429 can inhibit PCa growth through regulation of DLX1/Wnt/β-catenin axis (Fig. 7). These finding suggest that low expression of miR-4429 may serve as an indicator for PCa prediction and diagnosis, and miR-4429 may serve as a potential tool for PCa cancer intervention. We also hope that more researches in this field be performed to provide more insights and help the development of novel less-invasive treatments for PCa.

Abbreviations

ANOVA: Analysis of variance; BSA: Bovine serum albumin; CCK-8: Cell Counting Kit-8; ccRCC: Clear cell renal cell carcinoma; DLX1: Distal-less 1; FBS: Fetal bovine serum; GAPDH: Glyceraldehyde phosphate dehydrogenase; miRNAs: MicroRNAs; Pca: Prostate cancer; NCs: Negative controls; PBS: Phosphate buffered saline; UTR: Untranslated region.

Supplementary Information

Additional file 1: Figure S1–S4. Full-length western blots for Fig. 3f, Fig. 4a, Fig. 4b and Fig. 5a.

Acknowledgements

Not applicable.

Authors' contributions

JGW is the guarantor of integrity of the entire study and contributed to the concepts and design of this study; SX and JL contributed to the experimental studies; TL and WRW contributed to the data and statistical analysis; ZPX took charge of the manuscript preparation. All authors read and approved the final manuscript.

References

1. Culp MB, Soerjomataram I, Efstathiou JA, Bray F, Jemal A. Recent global patterns in prostate cancer incidence and mortality rates. Eur Urol. 2020;77:38–52.
2. Chen W, Zheng R, Baade PD, Zhang S, Zeng H, Bray F, Jemal A, Yu XQ, He J. Cancer statistics in China. CA Cancer J Clin. 2015;66(2016):115–32.
3. Bostwick DG, Burke HB, Djakiew D, Euling S, Ho SM, Landolph J, Morrison H, Sonawane B, Shifflett T, Waters DJ, Timms B. Human prostate cancer risk factors. Cancer. 2004;101:2371–490.
4. Zhou CK, Check DP, Lortet-Tieulent J, Laversanne M, Jemal A, Ferlay J, Bray F, Cook MB, Devesa SS. Prostate cancer incidence in 43 populations worldwide: an analysis of time trends overall and by age group. Int J Cancer. 2016;138:1388–400.
5. Walter BA, Valera VA, Pinto PA, Merino MJ. Comprehensive microRNA profiling of prostate cancer. J Cancer. 2013;4:350–7.
6. Shukla GC, Singh J, Barik S. MicroRNAs: processing, maturation, target recognition and regulatory functions. Mol Cell Pharmacol. 2011;3:83–92.
7. Schickel R, Boyerinas B, Park SM, Peter ME. MicroRNAs: key players in the immune system, differentiation, tumorigenesis and cell death. Oncogene. 2008;27:5959–74.

8. Wu WJ, Yin H, Hu JJ, Wei XZ. Long noncoding RNA LINC00313 modulates papillary thyroid cancer tumorigenesis via sponging miR-4429. Neoplasma. 2018;65:933–42.

9. Sun H, Fan G, Deng C, Wu L. miR-4429 sensitized cervical cancer cells to irradiation by targeting RAD51. J Cell Physiol. 2020;235:185–93.

10. McDougall C, Korchagina N, Tobin JL, Ferrier DE. Annelid Distal-less/Dlx duplications reveal varied post-duplication fates. BMC Evol Biol. 2011;11:241.

11. Alinezhad S, Vaananen RM, Mattsson J, Li Y, Tallgren T, Tong Ochoa N, Bjartell A, Akerfelt M, Taimen P, Bostrom PJ, Pettersson K, Nees M. Validation of novel biomarkers for prostate cancer progression by the combination of bioinformatics, clinical and functional studies. PLoS ONE. 2016;11:e0155901.

12. Guan H, Liu C, Fang F, Huang Y, Tao T, Ling Z, You Z, Han X, Chen S, Xu B, Chen M. MicroRNA-744 promotes prostate cancer progression through aberrantly activating Wnt/beta-Catenin signaling. Oncotarget. 2017;8:14693–707.

13. Jung SJ, Oh S, Lee GT, Chung J, Min K, Yoon J, Kim W, Ryu DS, Kim IY, Kang DI. Clinical significance of Wnt/beta-Catenin signalling and androgen receptor expression in prostate cancer. World J Mens Health. 2013;31:36–46.

14. Kypta RM, Waxman J. Wnt/beta-Catenin signalling in prostate cancer. Nat Rev Urol. 2012;9:418–28.

15. Van Neste L, Hendriks RJ, Dijkstra S, Trooskens G, Cornel EB, Jannink SA, de Jong H, Hessels D, Smit FP, Melchers WJ, Leyten GH, de Reijke TM, Vergunst H, Kil P, Knipscheer BC, Hulsbergen-van de Kaa CA, Mulders PF, van Oort IM, Van Criekinge W, Schalken JA. Detection of high-grade prostate cancer using a urinary molecular biomarker-based risk score. Eur Urol. 2016;70:740–8.

16. Pan H, Hong Y, Yu B, Li L, Zhang X. miR-4429 inhibits tumor progression and epithelial-mesenchymal transition via targeting CDK6 in Clear cell renal cell carcinoma. Cancer Biother Radiopharm. 2019;34:334–41.

17. Liu X, Chen R, Liu L. SP1-DLEU1-miR-4429 feedback loop promotes cell proliferative and anti-apoptotic abilities in human glioblastoma. Biosci Rep. 2019;39:BSR20190994.

18. He H, Wu W, Sun Z, Chai L. MiR-4429 prevented gastric cancer progression through targeting METTL3 to inhibit m(6)A-caused stabilization of SEC62. Biochem Biophys Res Commun. 2019;517:581–7.

19. Chan DW, Hui WW, Wang JJ, Yung MM, Hui LM, Qin Y, Liang RR, Leung TH, Xu D, Chan KK, Yao KM, Tsang BK, Ngan HY. DLX1 acts as a crucial target of FOXM1 to promote ovarian cancer aggressiveness by enhancing TGF-beta/SMAD4 signaling. Oncogene. 2017;36:1404–16.

20. Sun B, Fan Y, Yang A, Liang L, Cao J. MicroRNA-539 functions as a tumour suppressor in prostate cancer via the TGF-beta/Smad4 signalling pathway by down-regulating DLX1. J Cell Mol Med. 2019;23:5934–48.

21. Liang M, Sun Y, Yang HL, Zhang B, Wen J, Shi BK. DLX1, a binding protein of beta-catenin, promoted the growth and migration of prostate cancer cells. Exp Cell Res. 2018;363:26–32.

22. Li YF, Zhang J, Yu L. Circular RNAs regulate cancer onset and progression via Wnt/beta-Catenin signaling pathway. Yonsei Med J. 2019;60:1117–28.

23. Vallee A, Lecarpentier Y, Vallee JN. Targeting the canonical WNT/beta-Catenin pathway in cancer treatment using non-steroidal anti-inflammatory drugs. Cells. 2019;8:726.

24. Schneider JA, Logan SK. Revisiting the role of Wnt/beta-Catenin signaling in prostate cancer. Mol Cell Endocrinol. 2018;462:3–8.

25. Strillacci A, Valerii MC, Sansone P, Caggiano C, Sgromo A, Vittori L, Fiorentino M, Poggioli G, Rizzello F, Campieri M, Spisni E. Loss of miR-101 expression promotes Wnt/beta-Catenin signalling pathway activation and malignancy in colon cancer cells. J Pathol. 2013;229:379–89.

26. Zheng K, Zhou X, Yu J, Li Q, Wang H, Li M, Shao Z, Zhang F, Luo Y, Shen Z, Chen F, Shi F, Cui C, Zhao D, Lin Z, Zheng W, Zou Z, Huang Z, Zhao L. Epigenetic silencing of miR-490-3p promotes development of an aggressive colorectal cancer phenotype through activation of the Wnt/beta-Catenin signaling pathway. Cancer Lett. 2016;376:178–87.

27. Kawahara K, Morishita T, Nakamura T, Hamada F, Toyoshima K, Akiyama T. Down-regulation of beta-catenin by the colorectal tumor suppressor APC requires association with Axin and beta-catenin. J Biol Chem. 2000;275:8369–74.

28. Schweizer L, Rizzo CA, Spires TE, Platero JS, Wu Q, Lin TA, Gottardis MM, Attar RM. The androgen receptor can signal through Wnt/beta-Catenin in prostate cancer cells as an adaptation mechanism to castration levels of androgens. BMC Cell Biol. 2008;9:4.

11

Favorable intermediate risk prostate cancer with biopsy Gleason score of 6

Jong Jin Oh[1,2†], Hyungwoo Ahn[3†], Sung Il Hwang[3], Hak Jong Lee[3,4], Gheeyoung Choe[5], Sangchul Lee[1], Hakmin Lee[1], Seok-Soo Byun[1,2] and Sung Kyu Hong[1,2*]

Abstract

Background: To identify potential prognostic factors among patients with favorable intermediate risk prostate cancer with a biopsy Gleason score 6.

Methods: From 2003 to 2019, favorable intermediate risk patients who underwent radical prostatectomy were included in this study. All patients were evaluated preoperatively with MRI. Using PI-RADS scores, patients were divided into two groups, and clinic-pathological outcomes were compared. The impact of preoperative factors on significant pathologic Gleason score upgrading ($\geq 4+3$) and biochemical recurrence were assessed via multivariate analysis. Subgroup analysis was performed in patients with PI-RADS ≤ 2.

Results: Among the 239 patients, 116 (48.5%) were MRI-negative (PI-RADS ≤ 3) and 123 (51.5%) were MRI-positive (PI-RADS > 3). Six patients in the MRI-negative group (5.2%) were characterized as requiring significant pathologic Gleason score upgrading compared with 34 patients (27.6%) in the MRI-positive group ($p < 0.001$). PI-RADS score was shown to be a significant predictor of significant pathologic Gleason score upgrading (OR $= 6.246$, $p < 0.001$) and biochemical recurrence (HR $= 2.595$, $p = 0.043$). 10-years biochemical recurrence-free survival was estimated to be 84.4% and 72.6% in the MRI-negative and MRI-positive groups ($p = 0.035$). In the 79 patients with PI-RADS ≤ 2, tumor length in biopsy cores was identified as a significant predictor of pathologic Gleason score (OR $= 11.336$, $p = 0.014$).

Conclusions: Among the patients with favorable intermediate risk prostate cancer with a biopsy Gleason score 6, preoperative MRI was capable of predicting significant pathologic Gleason score upgrading and biochemical recurrence. Especially, the patients with PI-RADS ≤ 2 and low biopsy tumor length could be a potential candidate to active surveillance.

Keywords: Prostate cancer, Intermediate risk group, MRI

Background

Clinically localized prostate cancer can be managed with active surveillance (AS) [1]. Importantly, AS has emerged as a preferred initial management strategy for patients with low-risk (LR) PCa as it helps decrease the overtreatment of clinically indolent disease [2]. The safety and utility of AS in patients with LR PCa was confirmed and its use has rapidly increased worldwide. However, the utility of AS in patients with intermediate risk (IR) PCa remains unclear [3].

In the United States SEER (Surveillance, Epidemiology and End Results)-Medicare program, expectant management of LR PCa cases increased from 22 to 43% between 2004 and 2011; 15% to 18% of IR PCa cases were managed conservatively [4]. According to the National Comprehensive Cancer Network (NCCN) stratification, those classified within the favorable intermediate risk (FIR)

*Correspondence: skhong@snubh.org

†Jong Jin Oh and Hyungwoo Ahn have contributed equally to this work

[2] Department of Urology, Seoul National University College of Medicine, Seoul, Korea

Full list of author information is available at the end of the article

group had better prognoses compared with those within the unfavorable intermediate risk (UFIR) group [5]; other studies revealed similar oncological results compared to LR PCa [6, 7]. Data from one long-term study revealed that a similar percentage of those in the IR group with a biopsy Gleason score of 6 and PSA between 10–20 ng/ml experienced 15-year metastatic-free survival compared to those with LR PCa (94% for both groups) [3]. Therefore, here we evaluated the potential utility of AS in individuals within the IR group, specifically those characterized as FIR.

Biochemical recurrence rates (BCR) following definitive primary treatment for IR PCa vary dramatically, with 5-year rates ranging from 2 to 70% [8–11]. Of note, current criteria for AS have a misclassification rate of between 15–30% [12–15]. Another study revealed that individuals with a bGS of 6 and a PSA between 10 and 20 ng/ml are at higher risk of pathologic Gleason score upgrading (PGU) and upstaging, making them poor candidates for AS [2]. A rate of 50% PGU has been reported in a variety of studies [16–18], suggesting that not all patients with bGS of 6 may be characterized appropriately.

Therefore, in this study, we characterized the outcomes of patients with FIR PCa who have a bGS of 6 and PSA between 10 and 20 ng/ml. Prognosis using MRI according to stratification was analyzed, and potential prognosticators were investigated among patients (and subgroups) with FIR PCa and clear MRI results.

Methods

All data analysis was carried out in accordance with applicable laws and regulations described in the Declaration of Helsinki and approved by institutional review board approval (Seoul National University Bundang Hospital (B-2004–608-104), we reviewed the records of patients who underwent radical prostatectomy (RP) in a single tertiary hospital between November 2003 and April 2019. Among them, patients with FIR PCa, preoperative bGS of 6, PSA between 10 and 20 ng/ml and a percent of positive biopsy cores < 50% were finally enrolled. All patients received ≥ 12 core transrectal prostate biopsy (MR fusion) and preoperative prostate MRI.

Prostate MRI exams were conducted 2–6 weeks after transrectal ultrasound–guided biopsy and before surgery. Prostate MRI up to 2006 was acquired in a biparametric manner including T2-weighted image (T2WI) and diffusion-weighted image (DWI). Since 2007, multiparametric prostate MRI, including dynamic contrast-enhanced (DCE) image, have been obtained. As PI-RADS was released and revised during this period, and to minimize the bias that may occur due to accumulated MRI reading experience over time, an experienced uroradiologist

blinded from relevant information reviewed the preoperative MRI of the included patients for this retrospective study. Final scores for each patient were assigned according to PI-RADS (version 2) standards on a 5-point scale [19, 20]. The probability of clinically significant cancer was defined as follows: 1 (very low), 2 (low), 3 (intermediate), 4 (high), and 5 (very high).

Enrolled patients were stratified into two group according to preoperative MRI findings—the MRI-negative group (PI-RADS < 4) and the MRI-positive group (PI-RADS ≥ 4). Baseline characteristics [ie, age, body mass index (BMI), prostate volume, PSA, percent of positive biopsy core (%), total tumor length in cores, percentage of total tumor of all cores] between the two groups were compared using the student-t and chi-square tests.

RP specimens were assessed as previously reported [21]. Pathological parameters [ie, pGS, PGU, extracapsular extension (ECE), seminal vesicle invasion (SVI), positive surgical margin (PSM), pathologic tumor volume] were compared. We defined significant PGU (SPGU) as pathologic Gleason score ≥ 4 + 3 from bGS 6. All biopsy and RP pathology was newly reviewed by one uro-pathologist. A multivariate analysis was performed to predict SPGU using preoperative parameters and the PI-RADS grouping. Median follow-up duration was 58 months. BCR was defined as postoperative PSA ≥ 0.2 ng/mL taken twice at least 6 weeks apart [22]. Multivariate Cox proportional hazard model was also performed to predict BCR using preoperative parameters. A subgroup analysis was conducted in patients whose preoperative MRI showed no significant lesions and identified other preoperative parameters that could be predictors of PGU.

Results

In all, 239 patients with bGS of 6 and PSA between 10 and 20 ng/ml were enrolled in this study. Among them, 116 (48.5%) were placed into the MRI-negative group and 123 (51.5%) into the MRI-positive group. As shown in Table 1, those in the MRI-positive group had: i) a higher percentage of positive cores (28.51 vs. 20.42%, p = 0.003), ii) longer tumor lengths (0.51 vs. 0.32, mm, p < 0.001) and iii) percentage of total tumors of cores (32.02 vs. 20.76, %, p < 0.001). In the MRI-positive group, 64 (52.0%) and 59 (48.0%) of patients had PI-RADS scores of 4 and 5, respectively.

Pathological outcomes are presented in Table 2. A total of 199 (83.3%) and 40 (16.7%) of patients, respectively demonstrated PGU and SPGU. The percentage of patients demonstrated PGU was significantly higher in the MRI-positive group (96.7%) compared with the MRI-negative group (69.0%) (p < 0.001); similar results were noted for SPGU (≥ 4 + 3) (27.6% vs 5.2% in the MRI-positive and MRI-negative group, respectively) (p < 0.001).

Table 1 Baseline characteristics who intermediate risk prostate cancer patients with biopsy Gleason score 6 and comparisons according to multi-parametric MRI finding

	Total	MR-negative	MR-positive	p value
Number	239	116 (48.5)	123 (51.5)	
Mean Age (years, ± SD)	65.79 ± 6.60	65.37 ± 7.15	66.19 ± 6.03	0.340
Mean BMI (± SD)	24.49 ± 2.64	24.41 ± 2.75	24.56 ± 2.55	0.678
Prostate volume	42.22 ± 18.43	45.27 ± 19.76	39.35 ± 16.65	0.013
PSA	13.51 ± 2.82	13.46 ± 2.86	13.56 ± 2.79	0.801
Median PSA	12.64	12.32	13.00	
Mean PSA density	0.37 ± 0.16	0.36 ± 0.17	0.39 ± 0.15	0.085
DM (%)	25 (10.5)	11 (9.5)	14 (11.4)	0.395
HTN (%)	113 (47.3)	54 (46.6)	59 (48.0)	0.464
Number of biopsy (%)				0.262
12	164 (68.6)	80 (69.0)	84 (68.3)	
≥ 13	75 (31.4)	36 (31.0)	39 (31.7)	
Mean percentage of positive core (%, ± SD)	24.44 ± 19.97	20.42 ± 17.09	28.51 ± 21.85	0.003
Mean tumor length (mm, ± SD)	0.41 ± 0.34	0.32 ± 0.26	0.51 ± 0.39	< 0.001
Mean percentage of total tumor of core (%, ± SD)	26.47 ± 22.50	20.76 ± 18.05	32.02 ± 24.96	< 0.001
PIRADS score (%)				
2	79 (33.1)	79		
3	37 (15.5)	37		
4	64 (26.8)		64	
5	59 (24.7)		59	

BMI; body mass index, PSA; prostate specific antigen, DM; diabetes mellitus, HTN; hypertension, PIRADS; Prostate Imaging Reporting and Data System,

Table 2 Pathological outcomes after radical prostatectomy among favorable intermediate risk prostate cancer patients with biopsy Gleason score 6 and comparison according to multi-parametric MRI finding

	Total	MR-negative	MR-positive	p-value
Number	239	116 (48.5)	123 (51.5)	
Pathologic Gleason score (%)				< 0.001
6	40 (16.7)	36 (31.0)	4 (3.3)	
3 + 4	159 (66.5)	74 (63.8)	85 (69.1)	
4 + 3	38 (15.9)	5 (4.3)	33 (26.8)	
8	2 (0.8)	1 (0.9)	1 (0.8)	
Pathologic Gleason score upgrading (%)	199 (83.3)	80 (69.0)	119 (96.7)	< 0.001
Pathologic significant Gleason score upgrading (≥ 4 + 3) (%)	40 (16.7)	6 (5.2)	34 (27.6)	< 0.001
Extracapsular invasion (%)	50 (20.9)	10 (8.6)	40 (32.5)	< 0.001
Seminal vesicle invasion (%)	9 (3.8)	4 (3.4)	5 (4.1)	0.813
Bladder neck invasion (%)	6 (2.5)	1 (0.9)	5 (4.1)	0.116
Lymph node invasion	0			
Positive surgical margin (%)	53 (22.2)	13 (11.2)	40 (32.5)	< 0.001
Mean pathologic tumor volume (%, ± SD)	0.13 ± 0.14	0.07 ± 0.97	0.18 ± 0.16	< 0.001
Mean pathologic tumor volume (cc, ± SD)	5.16 ± 6.39	3.09 ± 3.96	7.11 ± 7.53	< 0.001

Other parameters (ie, ECE, PSM, pathologic tumor volume) were also higher in the MRI-positive group compared with the MRI-negative group (all p < 0.001).

A multivariate analysis revealed that SPGU, PI-RADS (OR 6.246, 95% CI 2.400–16.255, p < 0.001) and percentage of total tumors of core (OR 1.049, 95% CI

1.014–1.086, p < 0.006) were significant predictors of SPGU (Table 3).

During a median follow-up of 58 months, 31 patients experienced BCR. 10-year BCR-free survival was achieved by 83.2% and 54.8% of those in the MRI-negative and MRI-positive groups, respectively (log rant test p = 0.027, Fig. 1). A mutivariate Cox proportional hazard model revealed that prostate volume (HR = 0.956, 95% CI 0.923–0.991, p = 0.013) and PI-RADS score (HR = 2.595, 95% CI 1.949–7.098, p = 0.043) were significant predictors of BCR (Table 4).

A subgroup analysis of the 79 patients with bGS of 6, PSA between 10-20 ng/ml and PI-RADS < 3, revealed that 48 (60.8%) and 10 (12.7%) required PGU and SPGU, respectively. Among this subgroup, BCR occurred in only 4 patients (5.1%). 10-year BCR-free survival was 84.4%. Multivariate analysis was used to predict PGU in this group and results are presented in Table 5. Tumor length as assessed from biopsy cores was a significant predictor of PGU (OR: 11.336, p = 0.014).

Discussion

In the current study, we investigated potential prognosticators of individuals with FIR PCa, a bGS of 6 and a PSA between 10 and 20 ng/ml. Among the 239 patients included: i) 10-year BCR-free survival was estimated to be 70.9%, ii) PGU and SPGU from bGS 6 were determined to be 83.3% and 16.7%, respectively, iii) and preoperative MRI findings were significantly predictors of PGU and SPGU. These results could help inform the selection of FIR patients who would be most appropriate for AS.

The possibility of using AS for patients in the IR risk group has been previously raised. Accumulating evidence suggests that FIR PCa may be similar biologically to LR

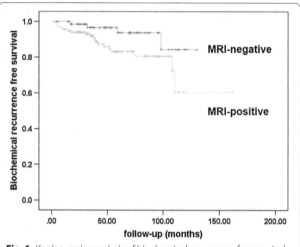

Fig. 1 Kaplan-meier analysis of biochemical recurrence free survival according to MRI negative and positive

PCa. For instance, a previous study revealed that there was no significant difference in BCR between those with FIR and LR PCa [5]. Additionally, this study reported 5-year progression-free survival (PFS) rates of 93% and 87% in LR and FIR risk groups, respectively (p = 0.054). These results are similar to what was observed in this study, namely a 10-year BCR-free survival rate of 70.9% in the FIR group.

Reports suggest that less aggressive IR cancer could be a potential candidate for AS. In particular, patients with Grade Group 1 (bGS 6) IR have been shown to have a low risk of progression to metastasis [23–26]. One large surveillance study (Sunnybrook in Toronto) reported data from a cohort of individuals receiving conservative treatment for IR PCa. Although the

Table 3 Univariate and multivariate logistic regression analysis to predict pathologic significant Gleason score upgrading (≥ 4 + 3)

	Univariate analysis			Multivariate analysis		
	OR	95%CI	p-value	OR	95%CI	p-value
Age	1.000	0.950–1.053	0.998			
Bdoy mass index	1.092	0.958–1.245	0.186			
DM	0.937	0.303–2.892	0.909			
HTN	1.273	0.645–2.515	0.486			
Prostate volume	0.981	0.960–1.003	0.087			
PSA	0.936	0.824–1.063	0.310			
PSA density	2.755	0.352–21.536	0.334			
PIRADS (< 3 vs. ≥ 3)	6.940	2.788–17.275	< 0.001	6.246	2.400–16.255	< 0.001
Number of biopsy (12 vs. ≥ 13)	0.319	0.093–1.099	0.070			
Mean percentage of positive core	1.007	0.990–1.025	0.431			
Mean tumor length	3.667	1.493–9.005	0.005	0.133	0.014–1.285	0.081
Mean percentage of total tumor of core	1.027	1.012–1.041	< 0.001	1.049	1.014–1.086	0.006

Table 4 Univariate and multivariate Cox proportional hazards analysis to predict biochemical recurrence after radical prostatectomy

	Univariate analysis			Multivariate analysis		
	HR	95%CI	p-value	HR	95%CI	p-value
Age	0.967	0.911–1.027	0.274			
Bdoy mass index	1.116	0.962–1.295	0.148			
DM	0.314	0.042–2.327	0.257			
HTN	1.854	0.793–4.335	0.154			
Prostate volume	0.953	0.921–0.986	0.005	0.956	0.923–0.991	0.013
PSA	1.043	0.907–1.199	0.555			
PSA density	14.810	2.307–95.077	0.004			
PIRADS (<3 vs. ≥3)	3.002	1.024–8.800	0.035	2.595	1.949–7.098	0.043
Number of biopsy (12 vs. ≥13)	1.162	0.422–3.202	0.772			
Mean percentage of positive core	1.022	0.005–1.040	0.012	1.345	0.632–2.863	0.442
Mean tumor length	2.114	0.786–5.681	0.138			
Mean percentage of total tumor of core	1.012	0.997–1.027	0.117			

Table 5 Univariate and multivariate logistic regression analysis to predict pathologic Gleason score upgrading among PIRADS ≤ 2 patients

	Univariate analysis			Multivariate analysis		
	OR	95%CI	p-value	OR	95%CI	p-value
Age	1.021	0.958–1.088	0.523			
Bdoy mass index	1.100	0.925–1.307	0.280			
DM	0.804	0.198–3.261	0.760			
HTN	0.981	0.394–2.440	0.967			
Prostate volume	0.984	0.962–1.007	0.173			
PSA	0.991	0.844–1.164	0.915			
PSA density	1.811	0.688–4.764	0.329			
Number of biopsy (12 vs. ≥13)	0.615	0.196–1.933	0.406			
Mean percentage of positive core	3.400	1.010–11.451	0.048	0.962	0.905–1.022	0.206
Mean tumor length	6.500	2.114–19.987	0.001	11.336	1.630–78.845	0.014
Mean percentage of total tumor of core	3.274	1.210–8.861	0.020	1.042	0.976–1.112	0.220

15-year PCa metastatsis rate was 3.7 times higher in the IR risk group compared with the LR group, the presence of Gleason 7 cancer at initial diagnosis accounted for almost all of this increase in risk [3]. Patients with a bGS of 6 and PSA between 10 and 20 ng/ml had an estimated 15-year metastasis-free survival rate of 94%, a rate very similar to patients with LR PCa. This group highlighted that a PSA above 10 did not confer a significantly increased risk of metastasis in those without a cancer with a Gleason score of 4 [27]. Loeb et al. [28] revealed the patients with a bGS of 6 (Grade Group 1), PSA between 10 and 15 mg/ml and a PSA density less than 0.15 ng/ml did not significantly differ in adverse pathology findings when compared to those with LR

PCa. As a result, the authors concluded that patients with bGS 6 IR PCa could be candidates for AS.

It should be noted, however, that other studies with contradictory findings have also been published. Aghazadeh et al. [5] conducted a large study (3,686 patients) which compared prognoses between FIR and LR PCa. The rate of adverse pathological findings in those with FIR was significantly higher when compared with those with lower risk PCa and significantly lower when compared with those with unfavorable intermediate risk PCa (27.4% vs 14.8% and 48.5%, respectively, each $p < 0.001$). In an Asian population study, the FIR group had significantly lower 5-year BCR-free survival when compared with the LR group (87.5 vs 93.5%; $P = 0.002$) [29]. These results could be caused by a discrepancy between bGS and pathological Gleason score. Yang et al. reported that 25.5% of patients with bGS 6 FIR PCa and PSA between 10 and 20 ng/ml required PGU and pathological upstaging [2]. Similarly, a report involving 359 men with bGS 6 and PSA between 10 and 20 ng/ml who underwent RP, revealed that 40.4% patients required PGU; among this group, 5% were upgraded into $GS \geq 8$ [30]. Here, 83.3% of patients required PGU after RP, 16.7% had pathologic GS above $4 + 3$. These results suggest that a proportion of patients with Gleason score 6 at preoperative biopsy may always require PGU.

Advances in software and hardware technology has led to the development of multi-parametric MRI for use in the detection of prostate cancer. Validation of this and other MRI-based tools have been summarized in guidelines published by the European Society of Urogenital Radiology (ESUR) along with a scoring system for PCa known as PI-RADS. Seo et al. revealed that PI-RADS can serve as a predictor of GS upgrading, with an estimated accuracy of 0.672–0.685 [1]. Another study of 126 cancer foci demonstrated that: i) PIRAD scores were 90% accurate at predicting Gleason score agreement between biopsy and pathologic GS (OR: 2.64, $p < 0.001$) and ii) MRI findings were capable of predicting PGU. Here, it was revealed that PI-RADS scores were a significant predictor of PGU (OR: 7.407, $p < 0.001$, data not shown) and SPGU (OR: 6.246, $p < 0.001$). Therefore, patients with FIR PCa, a bGS of 6 and a PI-RADS score ≤ 3 may be good candidates for AS. Among them, estimated 10-year BCR-free survival for patients with PCa and a PI-RADS score ≤ 2 was 84.4%, as good or better than the results reported from other studies of patients with LR PCa (66% to 88%) [31, 32]. Therefore, patients with FIR PCa with preoperative MRI (PI-RADS score ≤ 2) appear to be the ideal candidate for AS; furthermore, AS was seven safer in a subset of these patients with smaller biopsy tumor lengths.

This study does have several limitations that should be mentioned, primarily, the limited number of subjects and retrospective nature. Additionally, the PI-RADS score was assigned on biparametric MRI in patients included in earlier period. However, the diagnostic performance of the PI-RADS score of biparametric MRI is not reported to be inferior to that of multiparametric MRI [33]. Another limitation is the relatively high rate of PGU. The single pathologist who has a specialty for uro-oncology reviewed all of the specimens included in this study through International Society of Urological Pathology (ISUP) recommendation of modified Gleason score which announced in 2005 after handling by very thin sectioned. Regardless the extent of tumor, any Gleason pattern 4 was found in any section at radical prostatectomy

specimen with 99% Gleason pattern 3, therefore Gleason score was $3 + 4$. It was reason for high rate of PGU. In our results, 159 patients (79.9%) were pathologically upgraded to Gleason score $3 + 4$ and only 38 patients (15.9%) to Gleason score $4 + 3$ among 203 patients had experienced PGU after RP. The pathologic profiles of our participants appear to be relatively more aggressive (ie, higher PSA level, higher rate of high-grade disease) than those reported in western series. It is important to note that the rate of PSA screening in Asia is still not as high as in Western countries [34].

Conclusions

Among the patients with FIR PCa, a bGS of 6 and a PSA of between 10-20 ng.ml, preoperative MRI was capable of predicting sPGU and BCR. Based on these results, we suggest that patients with FIR PCa who had a negative preoperative MRI and minimal tumor volume as assessed by biopsy are ideal candidates for AS.

Abbreviations

PCa: Prostate cancer; bGS: Biopsy Gleason score; AS: Active surveillance; LR: Low risk; IR: Intermediate risk; SEER: Surveillance, Epidemiology and End Results; NCCN: National Comprehensive Cancer Network; FIR: Favorable intermediate risk; UFIR: Unfavorable intermediate risk; PSA: Prostate specific antigen; BCR: Biochemical recurrence; PGU: Pathologic Gleason score upgrading; MRI: Magnetic resonance imaging; RP: Radical prostatectomy; T2WI: T_2-weighted image; DWI: Diffusion-weighed image; DCE: Dynamic contrast-enhanced; BMI: Body mass index; ECE: Extracapsular extension; SVI: Seminal vesicle invasion; PSM: Positive surgical margin; SPGU: Significant pathologic Gleason score upgrading.

Acknowledgements

This work was supported by Grant Basic Science Research Program through the National Research Foundation of Korea (NRF) funded by the Ministry of Education (2020R1A2C1100011)

Authors' contributions

Protocol/project development: Sung Kyu Hong. Data collection or management: Hyungwoo Ahn, Sung Il Hwang, Hak Jong Lee, Sangchul Lee, Hakmin Lee, Seok-Soo Byun, Gheeyoung Choe. Data analysis: Jong Jin Oh. Manuscript writing/editing: Jong Jin Oh. All authors read and approved the final manuscript.

Author details

[1] Department of Urology, Seoul National University Bundang Hospital, Seongnam, Korea. [2] Department of Urology, Seoul National University College of Medicine, Seoul, Korea. [3] Department of Radiology, Seoul National University Bundang Hospital, Seongnam, Korea. [4] Department of Radiology, Seoul National University College of Medicine, Seoul, Korea. [5] Department of Pathology, Seoul National University Bundang Hospital, Seongnam, Korea.

References

1. Seo JW, Shin SJ, Taik OhY, Jung DC, Cho NH, Choi YD, et al. PI-RADS Version 2: Detection of Clinically Significant Cancer in Patients With Biopsy Gleason Score 6 Prostate Cancer. AJR Am J Roentgenol. 2017;209(1):W1-w9.
2. Yang DD, Mahal BA, Muralidhar V, Vastola ME, Boldbaatar N, Labe SA, et al Pathologic Outcomes of Gleason 6 Favorable Intermediate-Risk Prostate Cancer Treated With Radical Prostatectomy: Implications for Active Surveillance. Clin Genitourin Cancer. 2018;16(3):226–34.
3. Musunuru HB, Yamamoto T, Klotz L, Ghanem G, Mamedov A, Sethukavalan P, et al. Active Surveillance for Intermediate Risk Prostate Cancer: Survival Outcomes in the Sunnybrook Experience. J Urol. 2016;196(6):1651–8.
4. Tsai HT, Philips G, Taylor KL, Kowalczyk K, Huai-Ching K, Potosky AL: Utilization and predictors of expectant management among elderly men with low-and intermediate-risk localized prostate cancer in U.S. urological practice. Urol Pract. 2017;4(2):132–9.
5. Aghazadeh MA, Frankel J, Belanger M, McLaughlin T, Tortora J, Staff I, et al. National Comprehensive Cancer Network(R) Favorable Intermediate Risk Prostate Cancer-Is Active Surveillance Appropriate? J Urol. 2018;199(5):1196–201.
6. Tosoian JJ, Mamawala M, Epstein JI, Landis P, Wolf S, Trock BJ, et al. Intermediate and Longer-Term Outcomes From a Prospective Active-Surveillance Program for Favorable-Risk Prostate Cancer. J Clin Oncol. 2015;33(30):3379–85.
7. Godtman RA, Holmberg E, Khatami A, Pihl CG, Stranne J, Hugosson J. Long-term Results of Active Surveillance in the Goteborg Randomized, Population-based Prostate Cancer Screening Trial. Eur Urol. 2016;70(5):760–6.
8. Grossfeld GD, Latini DM, Lubeck DP, Broering JM, Li YP, Mehta SS, et al. Predicting disease recurrence in intermediate and high-risk patients undergoing radical prostatectomy using percent positive biopsies: results from CaPSURE. Urology. 2002;59(4):560–5.
9. Morris WJ, Keyes M, Palma D, Spadinger I, McKenzie MR, Agranovich A, et al.: Population-based study of biochemical and survival outcomes after permanent 125I brachytherapy for low- and intermediate-risk prostate cancer. Urology 2009;73(4):860–5; discussion 5–7
10. Weiner AB, Patel SG, Etzioni R, Eggener SE. National trends in the management of low and intermediate risk prostate cancer in the United States. J Urol. 2015;193(1):95–102.
11. Abern MR, Aronson WJ, Terris MK, Kane CJ, Presti JC Jr, Amling CL, et al. Delayed radical prostatectomy for intermediate-risk prostate cancer is associated with biochemical recurrence: possible implications for active surveillance from the SEARCH database. Prostate. 2013;73(4):409–17.
12. Iremashvili V, Manoharan M, Parekh DJ, Punnen S. Can nomograms improve our ability to select candidates for active surveillance for prostate cancer? Prostate Cancer Prostatic Dis. 2016;19(4):385–9.
13. Iremashvili V, Pelaez L, Manoharan M, Jorda M, Rosenberg DL, Soloway MS. Pathologic prostate cancer characteristics in patients eligible for active surveillance: a head-to-head comparison of contemporary protocols. Eur Urol. 2012;62(3):462–8.
14. Gandaglia G, Ploussard G, Isbarn H, Suardi N, De Visschere PJ, Futterer JJ, et al. What is the optimal definition of misclassification in patients with very low-risk prostate cancer eligible for active surveillance? Results from a multi-institutional series. Urol Oncol. 2015;33(4):164.e1-9.
15. Morlacco A, Cheville JC, Rangel LJ, Gearman DJ, Karnes RJ. Adverse Disease Features in Gleason Score 3 + 4 "Favorable Intermediate-Risk" Prostate Cancer: Implications for Active Surveillance. Eur Urol. 2017;72(3):442–7.
16. Heidegger I, Ladurner M, Skradski V, Klocker H, Schafer G, Horninger W, et al. Adverse pathological findings in needle biopsy gleason score 6 prostate cancers with low and intermediate preoperative PSA levels following radical prostatectomy. Anticancer Res. 2012;32(12):5481–5.
17. Montironi R, Scarpelli M, Lopez-Beltran A, Cheng L. Editorial comment on: Expression of the endothelin axis in noninvasive and superficially invasive bladder cancer: relation to clinicopathologic and molecular prognostic parameters. Eur Urol. 2009;56(5):846–7.
18. Cookson MS, Fleshner NE, Soloway SM, Fair WR. Correlation between Gleason score of needle biopsy and radical prostatectomy specimen: accuracy and clinical implications. J Urol. 1997;157(2):559–62.
19. Weinreb JC, Barentsz JO, Choyke PL, Cornud F, Haider MA, Macura KJ, et al. PI-RADS Prostate Imaging - Reporting and Data System: 2015, Version 2. Eur Urol. 2016;69(1):16–40.
20. Vargas HA, Hotker AM, Goldman DA, Moskowitz CS, Gondo T, Matsumoto K, et al. Updated prostate imaging reporting and data system (PIRADS v2) recommendations for the detection of clinically significant prostate cancer using multiparametric MRI: critical evaluation using whole-mount pathology as standard of reference. Eur Radiol. 2016;26(6):1606–12.
21. Kim K, Lee JK, Choe G, Hong SK. Intraprostatic locations of tumor foci of higher grade missed by diagnostic prostate biopsy among potential candidates for active surveillance. Sci Rep. 2016;6:36781.
22. Cookson MS, Aus G, Burnett AL, Canby-Hagino ED, D'Amico AV, Dmochowski RR, et al. Variation in the definition of biochemical recurrence in patients treated for localized prostate cancer: the American Urological Association Prostate Guidelines for Localized Prostate Cancer Update Panel report and recommendations for a standard in the reporting of surgical outcomes. J Urol. 2007;177(2):540–5.
23. Raldow AC, Zhang D, Chen MH, Braccioforte MH, Moran BJ, D'Amico AV. Risk Group and Death From Prostate Cancer: Implications for Active Surveillance in Men With Favorable Intermediate-Risk Prostate Cancer. JAMA Oncol. 2015;1(3):334–40.
24. Rodrigues G, Lukka H, Warde P, Brundage M, Souhami L, Crook J, et al. The prostate cancer risk stratification (ProCaRS) project: recursive partitioning risk stratification analysis. Radiother Oncol. 2013;109(2):204–10.
25. Klotz L. Active Surveillance for Intermediate Risk Prostate Cancer. Curr Urol Rep. 2017;18(10):80.
26. Sebastianelli A, Morselli S, Vitelli FD, Gabellini L, Tasso G, Venturini S, et al. The role of prostate-specific antigen density in men with low-risk prostate cancer suitable for active surveillance: results of a prospective observational study. Prostate Int. 2019;7(4):139–42.
27. Yamamoto T, Musunuru HB, Vesprini D, Zhang L, Ghanem G, Loblaw A, et al. Metastatic Prostate Cancer in Men Initially Treated with Active Surveillance. J Urol. 2016;195(5):1409–14.
28. Loeb S, Folkvaljon Y, Bratt O, Robinson D, Stattin P. Defining Intermediate Risk Prostate Cancer Suitable for Active Surveillance. J Urol. 2019;201(2):292–9.
29. Jung JW, Lee JK, Hong SK, Byun SS, Lee SE. Stratification of patients with intermediate-risk prostate cancer. BJU Int. 2015;115(6):907–12.
30. Santok GD, Abdel Raheem A, Kim LH, Chang K, Lum TG, Chung BH, et al. Prostate-specific antigen 10–20 ng/mL: A predictor of degree of upgrading to >/=8 among patients with biopsy Gleason score 6. Investig Clin Urol. 2017;58(2):90–7.
31. Kane CJ, Im R, Amling CL, Presti JC Jr, Aronson WJ, Terris MK, et al. Outcomes after radical prostatectomy among men who are candidates for active surveillance: results from the SEARCH database. Urology. 2010;76(3):695–700.
32. Weight CJ, Reuther AM, Gunn PW, Zippe CR, Dhar NB, Klein EA. Limited pelvic lymph node dissection does not improve biochemical relapse-free survival at 10 years after radical prostatectomy in patients with low-risk prostate cancer. Urology. 2008;71(1):141–5.
33. Monni F, Fontanella P, Grasso A, Wiklund P, Ou YC, Randazzo M, et al. Magnetic resonance imaging in prostate cancer detection and management: a systematic review. Minerva Urol Nefrol. 2017;69(6):567–78.
34. Zhang K, Bangma CH, Roobol MJ. Prostate cancer screening in Europe and Asia. Asian J Urol. 2017;4(2):86–95.

12

Development and internal validation of a prediction model of prostate cancer on initial transperineal template-guided prostate biopsy

Yuliang Chen[1], Zhien Zhou[1], Yi Zhou[1], Xingcheng Wu[1], Yu Xiao[2], Zhigang Ji[1], Hanzhong Li[1] and Weigang Yan[1*]

Abstract

Background: Due to the invasiveness of prostate biopsy, a prediction model of the individual risk of a positive biopsy result could be helpful to guide clinical decision-making. Most existing models are based on transrectal ultrasonography (TRUS)-guided biopsy. On the other hand, transperineal template-guided prostate biopsy (TTPB) has been reported to be more accurate in evaluating prostate cancer. The objective of this study is to develop a prediction model of the detection of high-grade prostate cancer (HGPC) on initial TTPB.

Result: A total of 1352 out of 3794 (35.6%) patients were diagnosed with prostate cancer, 848 of whom had tumour with Grade Group 2–5. Age, PSA, PV, DRE and f/t PSA are independent predictors of HGPC with $p < 0.001$. The model showed good discrimination ability (c-index 0.886) and calibration during internal validation and good clinical performance was observed through decision curve analysis. The external validation of CPCC-RC, an existing model, demonstrated that models based on TRUS-guided biopsy may underestimate the risk of HGPC in patients who underwent TTPB.

Conclusion: We established a prediction model which showed good discrimination ability and calibration in predicting the detection of HGPC by initial TTPB. This model can be used to aid clinical decision making for Chinese patients and other Asian populations with similar genomic backgrounds, after external validations are conducted to further confirm its clinical applicability.

Keywords: Transperineal template-guided prostate biopsy, High-grade prostate cancer, Prediction model, Nomogram

Introduction

According to GLOBOCAN data in 2018, the incidence and mortality of prostate cancer ranked second and fifth, respectively, among all cancers in men [1]. Prostate biopsy is essential for the diagnosis of prostate cancer.

Due to the invasive nature of biopsy, it would be very helpful if the individual risk of a positive biopsy result can be calculated through prediction models and guide clinical decision-making.

The incidence and prevalence of prostate cancer in Asian populations are significantly lower than in individuals of Caucasian and African descent [1, 2], suggesting ethnic differences in the occurrence of prostate cancer. At present, the most widely used and well-validated prediction models for prostate biopsy are the Prostate Cancer Prevention Trial Risk Calculator (PCPT-RC) and the

*Correspondence: ywgpumch@sina.com
[1] The Department of Urology, Peking Union Medical College Hospital, Chinese Academy of Medical Sciences, No. 1 Shuaifuyuan, Dongcheng District, Beijing 100730, China
Full list of author information is available at the end of the article

European Randomized Study of Screening for Prostate Cancer Risk Calculator (ERSPC-RC) [3, 4]. However, the predicted risk of these models was reported to be overestimated by 20% in Chinese patients [5], which highlights the necessity of building a prediction model for Chinese patients, as well as Asian populations with similar genomic backgrounds.

Most of the existing models for the Chinese population, for example, the Chinese Prostate Cancer Risk Calculator (CPCC-RC), are based on transrectal ultrasonography (TRUS)-guided biopsy [6]. However, the transrectal approach has a higher probability of omitting tumours in the anterior prostate than does the transperineal approach [7]. On the other hand, transperineal template-guided prostate biopsy (TTPB) is reported to be effective in detecting prostate cancer in patients with multiple negative transrectal biopsies, mainly due to improved sensitivity for anterior and apical tumours [8, 9]. Risk models based on TRUS-guided biopsy may not appropriately predict the risk of prostate cancer detected by transperineal biopsy.

The main objective of our study was to develop and internally validate a prediction model for the detection of high-grade prostate cancer (HGPC) by TTPB in biopsy-naïve Chinese patients. In addition, we conducted an external validation of CPCC-RC, an existing prediction model based on TRUS-guided biopsy, to evaluate its performance in predicting TTPB results [10].

Patients and methods

Study population and design

We undertook a consecutive cohort study in prostate biopsy-naïve patients in our institution (Peking Union Medical College Hospital, a tertiary hospital in Beijing, China) between December 2003 and July 2019. The included patients met at least one of the following criteria: (1) prostate-specific antigen (PSA) >4.0 ng/mL; (2) abnormal findings on DRE; and (3) imaging results indicating the suspicion of prostate cancer. We excluded patients with PSA levels >100.0 ng/mL or any history of prostate cancer, previous biopsy, endocrine treatment, or perineal surgery. A retrospective analysis of prospectively collected clinical data was performed.

The collection and use of all participant data and biological specimens in this study was ethically approved by the Ethics Committee of Peking Union Medical College Hospital, Chinese Academy of Medical Science. All the patients included in our study signed a written informed consent.

Procedures

As described in our previous study [11], TTPB was conducted in operation room with patients in lithotomy position. Local anesthesia was given to 3643 patients (96.0%), with 10 ml of 1% lidocaine injected intracutaneously and subcutaneously into the perineum, and another 10 mL onto the capsule to the right and left sides of the prostatic apex. The other 151 patients (4.0%) received general anesthesia due to intolerance of pain or personal choice.

A biplanar TRUS probe (SONOLINE Adara SLC Ultrasound; Siemens, Erlangen, Germany) attached to a brachytherapy stepping unit (Computerized Medical System, St. Louis, MO, USA), and a standard 0.5-cm brachytherapy template over the perineum were used to guide the transperineal biopsy. The length, width and height of the prostate were measured by ultrasound, and the prostate volume (PV) was calculated. One to four cores were taken by Bard biopsy gun (C.R. Bard, Covington, GA, USA) from each of the 11 regions [11], with more cores for larger prostates. The pathological assessment of biopsy specimens was conducted by two pathologists in our institution, one of whom has more than 10 years of experience in urological pathology.

Pathological assessment

All the biopsy cores were evaluated by at least 2 experienced urological pathologists in our institution according to the 2014 International Society of Urological Pathology (ISUP) modified Gleason system [12]. Overall GS was assigned after a comprehensive assessment of proportion of different Gleason patterns and distribution of each core. Discordant results from the 2 pathologists were resolved through discussion. Pathology slides and reports of cancerous specimens included in our study before 2015 were reviewed and updated by pathologists.

Outcomes and predictors

The outcome variable was the detection of HGPC, which in our study, was defined as prostate cancer with ISUP Grade Group > 1 (Gleason score > 6) because Grade Group 1 cancer is usually indolent and does not require aggressive treatments [13]. Referring to EAU guidelines [14], the two keynote risk calculators based on the Caucasian population [3, 4] and other prediction models of prostate biopsy [10, 15–17], we selected age, PSA level, PV, DRE, and free-to-total (f/t) PSA as potential predictors.

Statistical analysis

Statistical analysis was performed with R software (http://www.r-project.org/, version 4.0, Vienna, Austria).

The mean ± SD was used to describe data in a normal distribution, while the median and interquartile range were used for data in a skewed distribution. A multivariate logistic regression model was established with the detection of HGPC as the dependent variable. Age, PSA, PV, DRE, and f/t PSA were included as potential predictors. Similar to other prediction models [4, 10], natural logarithm transformation was performed for PSA and PV to achieve better linearity with logit P. Independent variables that have a significant impact on the detection rate in univariate analysis were included in the final models after consideration of their clinical utility. A nomogram was developed based on significant predictors. Internal validation was performed with the concordance index (c-index) calculated and calibration curve depicted for the prediction model by bootstrapping with 1000 resamples. Decision curve analysis was conducted to evaluate the clinical performance of our models. A two-sided P value < 0.05 denoted statistical significance.

Results

Characteristics of participants

A total of 3794 patients were enrolled consecutively from December 2003 to July 2019. The characteristics of all patients are shown in Table 1. An average of 22.2 cores were taken from each patient with a median of 22 cores. 1352 out of 3794 (35.6%) patients were diagnosed with prostate cancer, 848 of whom had tumours categorized as Grade group 2–5 according to ISUP consensus.

Model development

Age, logPSA, logPV, age, f/t PSA and DRE were significantly related to the detection of HGPC in univariate analysis and were also independent predictors of HGPC in multivariate logistic analysis (Table 2). To facilitate clinical use, we established a nomogram based on this prediction model (Fig. 1). The optimal cut-off of risk threshold which maximized Youden index (sensitivity + specificity − 1) was calculated to be 0.244 (sensitivity = 0.839, specificity = 0.748).

Internal validation

The apparent C-index of our model is 0.866. Using 1000-resample bootstrapping, the optimism of our model is calculated to be 0.002, and the bias-corrected C-index to be 0.865, demonstrating good discrimination ability. The calibration curve, also depicted by bootstrapping, is shown in Fig. 2a with excellent calibration between predictions and observations (bias-corrected slope = 0.994, bias-corrected intercept = −0.004).

External validation of an existing model

Using our TTPB data, we conducted external validation of CPCC-RC [10], which was an existing prediction model for the Chinese population based on a transrectal approach. The C-index was 0.826 when predicting HGPC using the CPCC-RC. The upwardly curved calibration curve in Fig. 2b suggests that the CPCC-RC underestimates the risk of HGPC in patients who undergo TTPB.

Table 1 Characteristics of 3794 men in the development cohort

Parameter	Development cohort (n = 3794)
Age (years)*	68 (61–74)
PSA (ng/ml)*	10.00 (6.80–15.78)
Abnormal DRE	831 (21.9%)
f/t PSA*	0.143 (0.098–0.200)
Prostate volume (ml)*	45 (35–60)
PC detected	1352 (35.6%)
ISUP grade group	
1	504
2	279
3	206
4	151
5	212
HGPC detected	848 (22.4%)
In PC patients	587 (43.4%)
In HGPC patients	456 (53.8%)

*Data in skewed distribution described by median and interquartile range

Table 2 Model predicting the detection of high-grade prostate cancer on initial transperineal template-guided prostate biopsy

Predictor	Univariate analysis			Multivariable model		
	OR(95% CI)	β	P	Adjusted OR (95% CI)	β	P
Age	1.0691 (1.0589–1.0794)	0.0668	< 0.001	1.0686 (1.0563–1.0809)	0.0663	< 0.001
DRE	7.9510 (6.6878–9.4529)	2.0733	< 0.001	3.9141 (3.1915–4.8002)	1.3646	< 0.001
logPSA	3.7242 (3.3035–4.1985)	1.3149	< 0.001	2.8486 (2.4842–3.2665)	1.0468	< 0.001
logPV	0.2128 (0.1731–0.2618)	− 1.5470	< 0.001	0.1728 (0.1323–0.2257)	− 1.7556	< 0.001
f/t PSA	0.0006 (0.0002–0.0023)	− 7.2973	< 0.001	0.0305 (0.0073–0.1276)	− 3.4910	< 0.001
Intercept	–	–	–	–	− 1.7803	–

Development and internal validation of a prediction model of prostate cancer on initial transperineal...

83

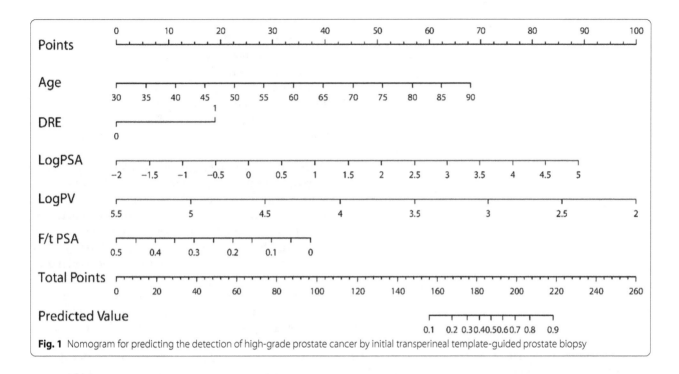

Fig. 1 Nomogram for predicting the detection of high-grade prostate cancer by initial transperineal template-guided prostate biopsy

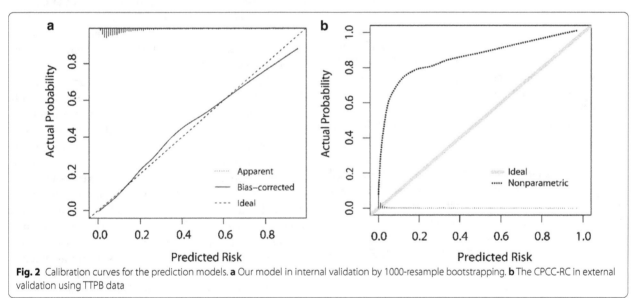

Fig. 2 Calibration curves for the prediction models. **a** Our model in internal validation by 1000-resample bootstrapping. **b** The CPCC-RC in external validation using TTPB data

Decision curve analysis

We performed decision curve analysis for our model. In Fig. 3, the net benefit of conducting biopsy for all or none of the patients, which are two extreme situations, is represented by the grey line and the horizonal black line, respectively. In a wide range of risk thresholds, our model outperformed the two extreme strategies with a much higher net benefit. For example, if we use 0.3 as a risk threshold to determine whether TTPB is required according to our model, after weighing the benefit

and cost, there is a net benefit for 11 out of every 100 people.

Discussion

Although there have been prediction models for the detection of HGPC in Chinese population [10, 16–18], our study is the first to be based on TTPB to the best of our knowledge. Compared with the transrectal approach, transperineal biopsy is less likely to cause rectal bleeding (RR = 0.02, 95% CI 0.01–0.06) and fever (RR = 0.26, 95%

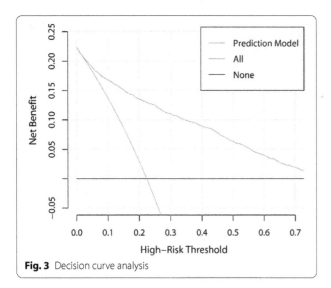

Fig. 3 Decision curve analysis

CI 0.14–0.28) according to a meta-analysis by Xiang et al. [7]. A recent research based on UK National Health Service data demonstrated that from 2017 to 2019, the sepsis rate of transperineal biopsy was significantly lower than that of transrectal approach (0.42% vs. 1.12%, p < 0.001) [19]. On the other hand, transperineal biopsy was reported to be associated with severer pain (VAS score: 4.0 vs. 2.0), higher rate of additional anesthesia (15.0% vs. 1.2%) and extended operation time (17.51 ± 3.33 min vs. 14.73 ± 3.25 min) in comparison with transrectal approach [20].

While no significant difference was observed between the positive rate of transrectal and transperineal biopsy according to a meta-analysis [7], there has been evidence that the transperineal approach exceeds transrectal biopsy in terms of accurate diagnosis and risk assessment of prostate cancer [21–23]. A multi-centre autopsy study revealed that the proportion of anterior tumours did not significantly differ from that of posterior ones [24]. A higher detection rate of TTPB than of TRUS-guided biopsy was observed for anterior prostate cancer, possibly due to the difference in sites where the biopsy cores are taken [23]. When TTPB was given to active surveillance patients within 12 months of diagnosis by TRUS biopsy, histopathological upgrading was observed in 38.8% (83/208) of them by Voss et al. [21]. TTPB also demonstrated better concordance with radical prostatectomy pathology than did TRUS biopsy [22].

Although these two approaches were not directly compared in our study, we conducted external validation of the CPCC-RC. With our data collected from a similar population, the predicted risk of HGPC is underestimated by the CPCC-RC for a wide range of risk thresholds, suggesting that TTPB might be more sensitive in

detecting HGPC. Of course, we must take into account the presence of different operators and pathologists between our cohort and the CPCC-RC, which may have influenced biopsy results.

MRI-targeted biopsy was reported to surpasses systematic biopsy in detecting high-grade prostate cancer [25] but still omits approximately 10% of clinically significant prostate cancer in patients with MRI-visible lesions [26]. As a result, systematic biopsies are typically suggested in addition to the MRI targeted biopsies. Meanwhile, due to the requirement of equipment and the high cost of MRI, patients with poor medical resource or poor financial conditions may not have access to MRI examination at the first visit or simply not be willing to receive one. For them, available clinical data are age, PSA level, prostate volume, and DRE result. Our models can be used during such biopsy counselling, when benefit and harm can be weighed by doctors and patients through the predicted probability of a positive biopsy result. With data from the developing cohort, we estimated the risk threshold for recommending TTPB to be 24.4%, which is in concordance with the empirical threshold of 25% [4]. This threshold can also be personalized during consultation. For patients with low predicted risk, observation might be a choice. Average risk patients might benefit from MRI for further risk assessment and high-risk patients might be recommended for MRI and biopsies.

Our study does have some limitations. First, some significant small tumours may have been missed in TTPB. In our study, this rate is not known, since it is not feasible to compare TTPB result with post prostatectomy or transperineal saturation biopsy results for each patient. Hence, some patients might need some follow up or further investigations even if the predicted risk is low. Second, some novel clinical indicators with better effects, such as Prostate Health Index, 4-Kallikrein Panel Score and Genomic Score [27], were not included in our study. Considering that such indicators are difficult to obtain in areas with general medical conditions, those included in our study are closer to practical applications. Finally, participants of our research were enrolled from a single centre, and further external validation is required to confirm the clinical applicability of our model.

Conclusion

We established and internally validated a prediction model for the detection of HGPC on initial TTPB in a Chinese population. Good clinical performance was indicated by decision curve analysis. External validations are required to further confirm the efficacy of our model.

Acknowledgements

Not applicable.

Authors' contributions

Y Chen: project development, data analysis, manuscript writing; Z Zhou: project development, data collection, manuscript editing; Y Zhou: data collection, manuscript editing; X Wu: data collection and analysis; Y Xiao: data collection and analysis; Z Ji: data collection, manuscript editing; H Li: data collection, manuscript editing; W Yan: project development, data collection, manuscript editing. All authors read and approved the final manuscript.

Author details

[1] The Department of Urology, Peking Union Medical College Hospital, Chinese Academy of Medical Sciences, No. 1 Shuaifuyuan, Dongcheng District, Beijing 100730, China. [2] The Department of Pathology, Peking Union Medical College Hospital, Chinese Academy of Medical Sciences, No. 1 Shuaifuyuan, Dongcheng District, Beijing 100730, China.

References

1. Bray F, Ferlay J, Soerjomataram I, Siegel RL, Torre LA, Jemal A. Global cancer statistics 2018: GLOBOCAN estimates of incidence and mortality worldwide for 36 cancers in 185 countries. CA Cancer J Clin. 2018;68(6):394–424.
2. Rebbeck TR, Haas GP. Temporal trends and racial disparities in global prostate cancer prevalence. Can J Urol. 2014;21(5):7496–506.
3. Roobol MJ, Steyerberg EW, Kranse R, Wolters T, van den Bergh RCN, Bangma CH, et al. A risk-based strategy improves prostate-specific antigen-driven detection of prostate cancer. Eur Urol. 2010;57(1):79–85.
4. Thompson IM, Ankerst DP, Chi C, Goodman PJ, Tangen CM, Lucia MS, et al. Assessing prostate cancer risk: results from the Prostate Cancer Prevention Trial. J Natl Cancer Inst. 2006;98(8):529–34.
5. Zhu Y, Wang JY, Shen YJ, Dai B, Ma CG, Xiao WJ, et al. External validation of the Prostate Cancer Prevention Trial and the European Randomized Study of Screening for Prostate Cancer risk calculators in a Chinese cohort. Asian J Androl. 2012;14(5):738–44.
6. He B-M, Chen R, Sun T-Q, Yang Y, Zhang C-L, Ren S-C, et al. Prostate cancer risk prediction models in Eastern Asian populations: current status, racial difference, and future directions. Asian J Androl. 2020;22(2):158–61.
7. Xiang J, Yan H, Li J, Wang X, Chen H, Zheng X. Transperineal versus transrectal prostate biopsy in the diagnosis of prostate cancer: a systematic review and meta-analysis. World J Surg Oncol. 2019;17(1):31.
8. Gershman B, Zietman AL, Feldman AS, McDougal WS. Transperineal template-guided prostate biopsy for patients with persistently elevated PSA and multiple prior negative biopsies. Urol Oncol. 2013;31(7):1093–7.
9. Pal RP, Elmussareh M, Chanawani M, Khan MA. The role of a standardized 36 core template-assisted transperineal prostate biopsy technique in patients with previously negative transrectal ultrasonography-guided prostate biopsies. BJU Int. 2012;109(3):367–71.
10. Chen R, Xie L, Xue W, Ye Z, Ma L, Gao X, et al. Development and external multicenter validation of Chinese Prostate Cancer Consortium prostate cancer risk calculator for initial prostate biopsy. Urol Oncol. 2016;34(9):416.e1–e7.
11. Mai Z, Yan W, Zhou Y, Zhou Z, Chen J, Xiao Y, et al. Transperineal template-guided prostate biopsy: 10 years of experience. BJU Int. 2016;117(3):424–9.
12. Epstein JI, Egevad L, Amin MB, Delahunt B, Srigley JR, Humphrey PA. The 2014 International Society of Urological Pathology (ISUP) consensus conference on gleason grading of prostatic carcinoma: definition of grading patterns and proposal for a new grading system. Am J Surg Pathol. 2016;40(2):244–52.
13. Epstein JI, Amin MB, Reuter VE, Humphrey PA. Contemporary Gleason Grading of Prostatic Carcinoma: an update with discussion on practical issues to implement the 2014 International Society of Urological Pathology (ISUP) consensus conference on Gleason Grading of Prostatic Carcinoma. Am J Surg Pathol. 2017;41(4):e1–e7.
14. Mottet NPC, den Bergh RCN, Briers E, De Santis M, Fanti S, Gillessen S, Grummet AM, Henry AM, Lam TB, Mason HG, van der Kwast HG, van der Poel HG, Rouvière O, Schoots D, Tilki D, Wiegel T. EAU-EANM-ESTRO-ESUR-SIOG Guidelines on Prostate Cancer: Uropean Association of Urology; 2020. https://uroweb.org/guideline/prostate-cancer/
15. Wu Y-S, Zhang N, Liu S-H, Xu J-F, Tong S-J, Cai Y-H, et al. The Huashan risk calculators performed better in prediction of prostate cancer in Chinese population: a training study followed by a validation study. Asian J Androl. 2016;18(6):925–9.
16. Huang Y, Cheng G, Liu B, Shao P, Qin C, Li J, et al. A prostate biopsy strategy based on a new clinical nomogram reduces the number of biopsy cores required in high-risk patients. BMC Urol. 2014;14:8.
17. Tang P, Chen H, Uhlman M, Lin Y-R, Deng X-R, Wang B, et al. A nomogram based on age, prostate-specific antigen level, prostate volume and digital rectal examination for predicting risk of prostate cancer. Asian J Androl. 2013;15(1):129–33.
18. Kuo SC, Hung SH, Wang HY, Chien CC, Lu CL, Lin HJ, et al. Chinese nomogram to predict probability of positive initial prostate biopsy: a study in Taiwan region. Asian J Androl. 2013;15(6):780–4.
19. Tamhankar AS, El-Taji O, Vasdev N, Foley C, Popert R, Adshead J. The clinical and financial implications of a decade of prostate biopsies in the NHS: analysis of Hospital Episode Statistics data 2008–2019. BJU Int. 2020;126(1):133–41.
20. Guo L-H, Wu R, Xu H-X, Xu J-M, Wu J, Wang S, et al. Comparison between ultrasound guided transperineal and transrectal prostate biopsy: a prospective, randomized, and controlled trial. Sci Rep. 2015;5:16089.
21. Voss J, Pal R, Ahmed S, Hannah M, Jaulim A, Walton T. Utility of early transperineal template-guided prostate biopsy for risk stratification in men undergoing active surveillance for prostate cancer. BJU Int. 2018;121(6):863–70.
22. Marra G, Eldred-Evans D, Challacombe B, Van Hemelrijck M, Polson A, Pomplun S, et al. Pathological concordance between prostate biopsies and radical prostatectomy using transperineal sector mapping biopsies: validation and comparison with transrectal biopsies. Urol Int. 2017;99(2):168–76.
23. Hossack T, Patel MI, Huo A, Brenner P, Yuen C, Spernat D, et al. Location and pathological characteristics of cancers in radical prostatectomy specimens identified by transperineal biopsy compared to transrectal biopsy. J Urol. 2012;188(3):781–5.
24. Breslow N, Chan CW, Dhom G, Drury RA, Franks LM, Gellei B, et al. Latent carcinoma of prostate at autopsy in seven areas the International Agency for Research on Cancer, Lyons, France. Int J Cancer. 1977;20(5):680–8.
25. Siddiqui MM, Rais-Bahrami S, Turkbey B, George AK, Rothwax J, Shakir N, et al. Comparison of MR/ultrasound fusion-guided biopsy with ultrasound-guided biopsy for the diagnosis of prostate cancer. JAMA. 2015;313(4):390–7.
26. Ahdoot M, Wilbur AR, Reese SE, Lebastchi AH, Mehralivand S, Gomella PT, et al. MRI-targeted, systematic, and combined biopsy for prostate cancer diagnosis. N Engl J Med. 2020;382(10):917–28.
27. Srivastava S, Koay EJ, Borowsky AD, De Marzo AM, Ghosh S, Wagner PD, et al. Cancer overdiagnosis: a biological challenge and clinical dilemma. Nat Rev Cancer. 2019;19(6):349–58.

13

Development and head-to-head comparison of machine-learning models to identify patients requiring prostate biopsy

Shuanbao Yu[1†], Jin Tao[1†], Biao Dong[1†], Yafeng Fan[1†], Haopeng Du[1], Haotian Deng[1], Jinshan Cui[1], Guodong Hong[1] and Xuepei Zhang[1,2*]

Abstract

Background: Machine learning has many attractive theoretic properties, specifically, the ability to handle non predefined relations. Additionally, studies have validated the clinical utility of mpMRI for the detection and localization of CSPCa (Gleason score $\geq 3+4$). In this study, we sought to develop and compare machine-learning models incorporating mpMRI parameters with traditional logistic regression analysis for prediction of PCa (Gleason score $\geq 3+3$) and CSPCa on initial biopsy.

Methods: A total of 688 patients with no prior prostate cancer diagnosis and tPSA ≤ 50 ng/ml, who underwent mpMRI and prostate biopsy were included between 2016 and 2020. We used four supervised machine-learning algorithms in a hypothesis-free manner to build models to predict PCa and CSPCa. The machine-learning models were compared to the logistic regression analysis using AUC, calibration plot, and decision curve analysis.

Results: The artificial neural network (ANN), support vector machine (SVM), and random forest (RF) yielded similar diagnostic accuracy with logistic regression, while classification and regression tree (CART, AUC $= 0.834$ and 0.867) had significantly lower diagnostic accuracy than logistic regression (AUC $= 0.894$ and 0.917) in prediction of PCa and CSPCa (all $P < 0.05$). However, the CART illustrated best calibration for PCa (SSR $= 0.027$) and CSPCa (SSR $= 0.033$). The ANN, SVM, RF, and LR for PCa had higher net benefit than CART across the threshold probabilities above 5%, and the five models for CSPCa displayed similar net benefit across the threshold probabilities below 40%. The RF (53% and 57%, respectively) and SVM (52% and 55%, respectively) for PCa and CSPCa spared more unnecessary biopsies than logistic regression (35% and 47%, respectively) at 95% sensitivity for detection of CSPCa.

Conclusion: Machine-learning models (SVM and RF) yielded similar diagnostic accuracy and net benefit, while spared more biopsies at 95% sensitivity for detection of CSPCa, compared with logistic regression. However, no method achieved desired performance. All methods should continue to be explored and used in complementary ways.

Keywords: Prostate cancer, Machine learning, Predictive model, Prostate biopsy

*Correspondence: zhangxuepei@263.net
†Shuanbao Yu, Jin Tao, Biao Dong and Yafeng Fan contributed equally to this work.
[1] Department of Urology, The First Affiliated Hospital of Zhengzhou University, No. 1 Jianshe East Road, Zhengzhou 450052, China
Full list of author information is available at the end of the article

Background

Prostate cancer (PCa) is the most common malignancy of the male reproductive system, with over one million cases and 358 989 deaths in 2018 [1, 2]. Prostate-specific antigen (PSA) testing, introduced in the 1990s, not only increased the incidence of clinically insignificant PCa (CSPCa, defined as Gleason score $\geq 3 + 4$), but also led to an increased number of unnecessary biopsies. This is particularly the case in a PSA gray zone, at which 65–70% of men have a negative biopsy result [3]. In our study, the PCa and CSPCa were detected in 23% and 17%, 27% and 18%, 53% and 47%, 68% and 66%, 73% and 68%, and 93% and 93% of the men with serum total PSA (tPSA) in the range of ≤ 10 ng/ml, 10–20 ng/ml, 20–30 ng/ml, 30–40 ng/ml, 40–50 ng/ml, and > 50 ng/ml, respectively. Therefore, the major challenge is to identify CSPCa among cases with serum tPSA ≤ 50 ng/ml at an early stage.

Studies have validated the clinical utility of multiparametric resonance imaging (mpMRI) in the detection and localization of International Society of Urological Pathology grade ≥ 2 cancers [4, 5]. Additionally, predictive models have the potential to improve diagnostic accuracy to influence disease trajectory and reduce healthcare costs [6, 7]. To reduce unnecessary biopsy and overdiagnosis, a dozen of nomograms have been used to help diagnose PCa and/or CSPCa, including PCPT-RC [8], STHLM3 [9], ERSPC-RC [10], and CRCC-PC [11], which are based on standard statistical technique of logistic regression (LR).

Over the past decade, we have entered the era of big data, and major advancements have emerged in the fields of statistics, artificial intelligence technology and urological medicine [12, 13]. Machine learning-assisted models have been proposed as a supplement or alternative for standard statistical techniques, including artificial neural network (ANN), support vector machine (SVM), classification and regression tree (CART), and random forest (RF). Machine learning has many attractive theoretic characteristics, specifically, the ability to deal with non-predefined relations such as nonlinear effects and/or interactions, at the cost of reducing interpretability and explanation, especially for complex nonlinear models [14, 15]. However, model validation helps to discover domain-relevant models with better generalization ability, and further implies better interpretability. These new algorithms incorporating mpMRI parameters may help improve the diagnosis of CSPCa [16, 17], but available data is limited.

In this study, we sought to develop and evaluate of multiple supervised machine-learning models based on age, PSA derivates, prostate volume, and mpMRI parameters to predict PCa and CSPCa. Additionally, we compare our models with conventional LR analysis to evaluate whether there were improvements in the diagnostic ability, using the same variables and population.

Methods

Study populations

This retrospective study was approved by the Institutional Ethics Review Board, and a waiver of informed consent was obtained. Between April 2016 and March 2020, prostate biopsy and mpMRI examination was done among 903 consecutive patients without a prior prostate biopsy. The 25 patients diagnosed with other types of tumors, 94 patients with incomplete data, and 96 patients with tPSA > 50 ng/ml were excluded leaving 688 cases available for analysis.

Data collection

The clinical variables including the age at prostate biopsy, serum tPSA and free PSA (fPSA) level, reports of mpMRI examination, and results of prostate biopsy were extracted from clinical records. Prostate volume was measured using mpMRI examination, the ratio of fPSA (f/t PSA) was measured by dividing the (fPSA) by the tPSA, and the PSA density (PSAD) was calculated by dividing the tPSA by the prostate volume. All mpMRI examination were performed using the 3.0-T MRI system with a pelvic phased-array coil, complaint with European Society of Urology Radiology guidelines. The scan protocol for all patients included T2-weighted imaging, diffusion-weighted imaging, and dynamic contrast-enhanced imaging. The prostate mpMRI images were interpreted by two experienced genitourinary radiologists with at least three years of prostate mpMRI experience. The mpMRI results were divided into groups according to the reports: "negative", "equivocal", and "suspicious" for the presence of PCa (MRI-PCa), seminal vesicle invasion (MRI-SVI), lymph node invasion (MRI-LNI) according to the mpMRI reports.

All patients underwent transrectal ultrasound-guided systematic 12-point biopsy according to the same protocol by three surgeons. If suspected malignant nodules by mpMRI and/or ultrasound, additional 1–5 needles were performed in regions with cognitive MRI-ultrasound fusion and/or abnormal ultrasound echoes. Biopsy cores were analyzed according to the standards of International Society of Urological Pathology.

Machine learning-assisted methods

Four types of supervised machine learning-based methods (ANN, SVM, CART, and RF) were applied in this study. Nine variables comprising age, PSA derivates (tPSA, f/tPSA, and PSAD), prostate volume, mpMRI results (MRI-PCa, MRI-SVI, and MRI-LNI), and results of prostate biopsy were used to develop the PCa and CSPCa prediction models. Age of patients,

PSA derivates, and prostate volume were normalized [(value − minimum value)/(maximum value − minimum value)] to fall in between 0 and 1, and entered as continuous variables. The mpMRI parameters were entered as dummy variables, and biopsy results were entered as binary variables.

The machine learning models were fit using the packages in R (version 3.6.2). The ANN is based on biological neural networks and composed of interconnected groups of artificial neurons [15]. And it was trained using the function of "Std_Backpropagation" in the package of "RSNNS", and used three hyperparameters: size, learnFuncParams, and maxit. The three hyperparameters for ANN are c(3,3), 0.05 and 100 in the PCa model, and c(4,2), 0,05, and 100 in the CSPCa model. The SVM model is a machine learning model that finds an optimal boundary between the possible outputs. It was trained using the package of "e1071", used a radical kernel and consisted of three hyperparameters: degree, cost, and gamma. The three hyperparameters for SVM are 3, 1, and 0.005 in the PCa model, and 3, 2 and 0.005 in the CSPCa model. The CART is based on the recursive partitioning method and belongs to a family of nonparametric regression methods. It was trained with the package of "rpart" and used three hyperparameters: minsplit, minbucket, and complexity parameter cp. The three hyperparameters for CART are 15, 5, and 0.01 in the PCa model, and 10, 3 and 0.01 in the CSPCa model. The RF is an ensemble learning method which that generating multiple decision trees and forming a "forest" to jointly determine output class [18]. The RF model was trained with using the package of "randomForest" in R, and used two hyperparameters: ntree, and mtry in this study. The two hyperparameters for RF are 500 and 2 in the PCa and CSPCa models.

Statistical analysis

All data cleaning and analyses were conducted using R statistical software (Version 3.6.2). Diagnostic accuracy of the models was evaluated using the area under the ROC curve (AUC). The 95% confidence interval (CI) and comparisons of AUCs were determined using the method of DeLong et al. [19]. Performance characteristics of the models were examined by calibration plots. Calibration was assessed by grouping men in the validation cohort into delices (each of size 20 or 21), and then comparing the mean of predicated probabilities and the observed proportions. The sum squares of the residuals (SSR) was used to assess the deviation of calibration plots from the 45° line [20]. The clinical utility of the models was evaluated with a decision-curve analysis.

Results

Patient characteristics

A total of 688 cases were included in this study. The patients (480, 70%) biopsied before December 31, 2018 were used as training cohort, and the remaining patients (208, 30%) were used as validation cohort. Table 1 summarized the patient characteristics stratified by pathological results. PCa patients displayed higher age (70 vs 66 years, $P < 0.001$), tPSA (20.8 vs 10.5 ng/ml, $P < 0.001$), and PSAD (0.46 vs 0.18, $P < 0.001$), while lower f/tPSA (0.11 vs 0.15, $P < 0.001$) and prostate volume (38 vs 58 ml, $P < 0.001$) compared with no-PCa (Table 1). Additionally, the proportions for suspicious presence of PCa (73% vs 22%), SVI (31% vs 0.7%), and LNI (10% vs 0%) by mpMRI examination were higher among PCa patients than no-PCa (Table 1). The CSPCa patients displayed similar pattern with no-CSPCa patients (Table 1).

Comparison of predictive accuracy between machine-learning models

In our study, four machine-learning models based on age, PSA derivates, prostate volume, and mpMRI parameters were developed to predict initial biopsy results. Among these machine-learning assisted models for PCa and CSPCa, the SVM (AUC = 0.903 for PCa and AUC = 0.925 for CSPCa), RF (AUC = 0.897 for PCa and AUC = 0.916 for CSPCa), LR (AUC = 0.894 for PCa and AUC = 0.917 for CSPCa), and ANN (AUC = 0.891 for PCa and AUC = 0.911 for CSPCa) models outperformed CART (AUC = 0.834 for PCa and AUC = 0.867 for CSPCa) model in diagnostic accuracy (all $P < 0.05$); Whilst the pairwise comparison of AUCs were insignificant amongst ANN, SVM, RF, and LR models for PCa and CSPCa, respectively (each $P > 0.05$) (Fig. 1).

Regarding PCa models, the calibration plot of predicated probabilities against observed proportion of PCa indicated excellent concordance in CART model (SSR = 0.027), followed by SVM (SSR = 0.049), LR (SSR = 0.063), ANN (SSR = 0.091), and RF (SSR = 0.125) (Fig. 2a). For CSPCa models, the calibration plot of CART also had good agreement between the predicated probability and observed ratio of CSPCa on biopsy (SSR = 0.033), followed by LR (SSR = 0.046), ANN (SSR = 0.065), RF (SSR = 0.082), and SVM (SSR = 0.142) models (Fig. 2b).

Impact of machine learning-assisted models on biopsies avoided

To further assess potential clinical benefit of the machine learning-assisted models, we performed DCA using the predicated risk in the validation cohort. It was observed that the ANN, SVM, RF, and LR models for PCa had higher net benefit than CART model across the threshold

Table 1 The clinical characteristics of enrolled patients stratified by pathological results between April 2016 and March 2020

Clinical characteristics	PCa (GS ≥ 3 + 3)			CSPCa (GS ≥ 3 + 4)		
	No (n = 443)[†]	Yes (n = 245)[†]	P	No (n = 488)[†]	Yes (n = 200)[†]	P
Age (years)	66 (61–72)	70 (63–76)	< 0.001	66 (61–72)	70 (63–76)	< 0.001
tPSA (ng/ml)	10.5 (6.65–17.0)	20.8 (9.67–30.3)	< 0.001	10.9 (6.70–17.1)	23.0 (10.9–33.1)	< 0.001
f/tPSA	0.15 (0.10–0.21)	0.11 (0.07–0.17)	< 0.001	0.15 (0.10–0.21)	0.11 (0.07–0.17)	< 0.001
PSAD (ng/ml^2)	0.18 (0.11–0.29)	0.46 (0.25–0.73)	< 0.001	0.19 (0.11–0.30)	0.52 (0.30–0.80)	< 0.001
PV (ml)	58 (39–82)	38 (27–58)	< 0.001	57 (38–81)	37 (27–54)	< 0.001
MRI-PCa, No. (%)			< 0.001			< 0.001
Negative	250 (56)	37 (15)		264 (54)	23 (12)	
Equivocal	95 (21)	29 (12)		104 (21)	20 (10)	
Suspicious	98 (22)	179 (73)		120 (25)	157 (79)	
MRI-SVI, No. (%)			< 0.001			< 0.001
Negative	439 (99)	163 (67)		481 (99)	121 (61)	
Equivocal	1 (0.2)	7 (3)		1 (0.2)	7 (4)	
Suspicious	3 (0.7)	75 (31)		6 (1)	72 (36)	
MRI-LNI, No. (%)			< 0.001			< 0.001
Negative	432 (98)	202 (82)		475 (97)	159 (80)	
Equivocal	11 (2)	18 (7)		12 (2)	17 (9)	
Suspicious	0 (0)	25 (10)		1 (0.2)	24 (12)	

PCa prostate cancer, *CSPCa* clinically significant prostate cancer, *GS* Gleason score, *tPSA* total prostate-specific antigen, *f/tPSA* free/total PSA, *PV* prostate volume, *SVI* seminal vesicle invasion, *LNI* lymph node invasion

[†] Data are presented as median (quartile range) unless other indicated

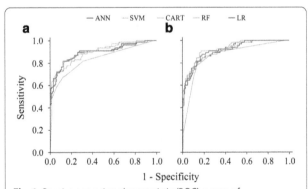

Fig. 1 Receive operating characteristic (ROC) curves of machine-learning and logistic regression models for predicting prostate cancer (PCa) and clinically significant prostate cancer (CSPCa) in the validation cohort. **a** PCa: Gleason score ≥ 3 + 3; **b** CSPCa: Gleason score ≥ 3 + 4. *Abbreviations ANN* artificial neural network, *SVM* support vector machine, *CART* classification and regression tree, *RF* random forest, *LR* logistic regression

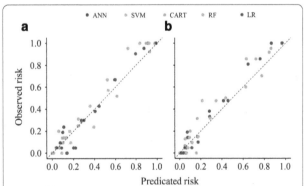

Fig. 2 Calibration plot of observed vs predicted rick of prostate cancer (PCa) and clinically significant prostate cancer (CSPCa) using machine-learning and logistic regression models in the validation cohort. **a**: PCa: Gleason score ≥ 3 + 3; **b** CSPCa: Gleason score ≥ 3 + 4. *Abbreviations ANN* artificial neural network, *SVM* support vector machine, *CART* classification and regression tree, *RF* random forest, *LR* logistic regression

probabilities above 5%, and the five models for CSPCa displayed similar net benefit across the threshold probabilities below 40% (Fig. 3).

Clinical consequences of using machine learning-assisted models at given sensitivity, including the number of biopsies that could be spared and the number of PCa by Gleason score that would be missed were displayed in Table 2. Using the SVM (74/143, 52%) and RF (76/143, 53%) models for PCa, significantly more unnecessary biopsies would be spared at 95% sensitivity for detection of CSPCa, compared with using ANN (53/143, 37%) and LR (50/143, 35%) models (all *P* < 0.05) (Table 2). Additionally, RF (81/143, 57%), SVM (79/143, 55%), and ANN (76/143, 53%) models for CSPCa spared more

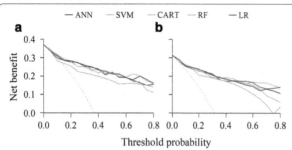

Fig. 3 Decision curve analysis (DCA) of machine-learning and logistic regression models for predicting prostate cancer (PCa) and clinically significant prostate cancer (CSPCa) in the validation cohort. **a** PCa: Gleason score ≥ 3 + 3; **b** CSPCa: Gleason score ≥ 3 + 4. *Abbreviations ANN* artificial neural network, *SVM* support vector machine, *CART* classification and regression tree, *RF* random forest, *LR* logistic regression

unnecessary biopsies than LR (67/143, 47%) model at 95% sensitivity (Table 2). At 95% sensitivity for detection of CSPCa, the RF and SVM models for CSPCa spared more unnecessary biopsies than the corresponding models for PCa (Table 2). However, the differences were insignificant ($P = 0.688$ for RF model, and $P = 0.686$ for SVM model).

Discussion

In our study, we developed, validated, and compared the machine learning-assisted models with LR analysis to predict PCa and CSPCa among patients with serum tPSA ≤ 50 ng/ml, using the same variables and population. The ANN, SVM, and RF models yielded similar diagnostic accuracy and net benefit with LR, and CART had lower diagnostic accuracy than LR in prediction of PCa and CSPCa. However, the CART model illustrated best calibration for PCa and CSPCa. And the SVM and RF models for PCa and CSPCa spared more biopsies than LR at 95% sensitivity for detection of CSPCa.

PCa was detected in 20% of the subjects with serum tPSA in the gray zone (4–10 ng/ml) in our study (data not shown). This was similar with the PCa detection rates of the same group of patients in Singapore (21%) [21], Japan (20%) [22], and Korea (20%) [23], while lower than that in Cleveland Clinic (40%) and Durham VA hospital (43%) [24]. This may suggest that the relationship between PCa risk and PSA level varies between Asian and Western populations, and it is essential to establish area-based risk prediction models. Our study revealed that the rates of PCa and CSPCa increased with tPSA, and CSPCa were detected in 279/301 (93%) of the men with serum tPSA > 50 ng/ml. Therefore, we recommended all cases with tPSA > 50 ng/ml to undergo prostate biopsy, and developed machine learning-assisted models to predict

PCa and CSPCa among patients with tPSA ≤ 50 ng/ml (in accordance with ERSPC-RC) [10].

A growing body of literatures have validated the clinical utility of mpMRI in the detection and localization of CSPCa [4]. However, as far as we know, the knowledge about the performance of risk prediction models incorporating mpMRI parameters is limited. We developed machine learning-assisted models based on age, PSA derivates, prostate volume, and mpMRI parameters in our study. The digital rectal examination and transrectal ultrasound were excluded as risk factors because of potential interobserver variability in its assessment [3, 25]. The ANN, SVM, RF and LR models (AUC = 0.891–0.903 for PCa, and AUC = 0.911–0.925 for CSPCa) incorporating mpMRI parameters developed in our study outperformed CRCC-PC (AUC = 0.80 for PCa, and AUC = 0.83 for CSPCa) and MRI-ERSPC-RC (AUC = 0.85 for CSPCa). This may suggest that the combination of mpMRI parameters including MRI-PCa, MRI-SVI, and MRI-LNI could improve the diagnostic accuracy of prediction model for PCa and CSPCa. The mpMRI parameters included in our models were extracted from the reports of mpMRI examination and were somewhat subjective. Some study showed that mpMRI radiomics features significantly associated with PCa aggressiveness on the histopathological and genomic levels [26, 27]. And addition of mpMRI radiomics may enhance the objectivity and diagnostic accuracy of prediction model.

For prediction of PCa, ANN has become (alongside LR) one of the fastest growing and most effective machine-learning algorithms [15]. Theoretically, ANN has considerable advantages over traditional statistical approaches, which automatically allow no explicit distributional assumptions, arbitrary nonlinear associations, and possible interactions. A systematic review including 28 studies showed that ANN outperformed regression in 10 (36%) cases, ANN and regression tied in 14 (50%) cases, and regression wined in the remaining 4 (14%) cases [14]. In our study, ANN displayed similar diagnostic accuracy and net benefit for prediction of PCa and CSPCa with LR. Based on the available data, ANN does not have significantly advantages in clinical practice compared with LR, and should not replace traditional LR for the classification of medical data.

Another three machine-learning algorithms (SVM, CART, and RF) were developed to predict PCa and CSPCa in our study. Some studies showed that RF algorithms outperformed LR model in the fields of identifying peripheral artery disease and mortality risk [28], predicting clinical outcomes after robot-assisted radical prostatectomy [29], and predicting clinical outcomes of large vessel occlusion before mechanical thrombectomy [30].

Table 2 Percentage of biopsies that would be spared or delayed using machine-learning and logistic regression models at given sensitivity for detection of CSPCa in the validation cohorts

Models	Sensitivity for detection of CSPCa	Cut-off for predicted risk (%)	Biopsies sSpared † (n = 208), n (%)	Unnecessary biopsy avoided		Biopsy delayed		
				GS < 3 + 3 (n = 131), n (%)	GS = 3 + 3 (n = 12), n (%)	GS = 3 + 4 (n = 11), n (%)	GS = 4 + 3 (n = 18), n (%)	GS ≥ 4 + 4 (n = 36), n (%)
Biopsies spared or delayed using PCa models at given sensitivity for detection of CSPCa								
ANN	64/65 (98%)	9	34 (16)	32 (24)	1 (8)	0 (0)	1 (6)	0 (0)
SVM	64/65 (98%)	11	57 (24)	55 (42)	1 (8)	0 (0)	0 (0)	1 (3)
CART	64/65 (98%)	NA	NA	NA	NA	NA	NA	NA
RF	64/65 (98%)	7	61 (29)	57 (44)	3 (25)	1 (9)	0 (0)	0 (0)
LR	64/65 (98%)	7	30 (14)	27 (21)	2 (17)	1 (9)	0 (0)	0 (0)
ANN	62/65 (95%)	11	56 (25)	51 (39)	2 (17)	1 (9)	1 (6)	1 (3)
SVM	62/65 (95%)	14	77 (37)	71 (54)	3 (25)	1 (9)	1 (6)	1 (3)
CART	62/65 (95%)	NA	NA	NA	NA	NA	NA	NA
RF	62/65 (95%)	11	79 (38)	73 (56)	3 (25)	1 (9)	2 (11)	0 (0)
LR	62/65 (95%)	10	53 (25)	47 (36)	3 (25)	1 (9)	1 (6)	1 (3)
ANN	59/65 (91%)	27	109 (52)	99 (76)	4 (33)	3 (27)	1 (6)	2 (6)
SVM	59/65 (91%)	23	110 (53)	100 (76)	4 (33)	4 (36)	1 (6)	1 (3)
CART	57/65 (88%)	10	104 (50)	90 (69)	6 (50)	4 (36)	1 (6)	3 (8)
RF	59/65 (91%)	20	101 (49)	91 (69)	4 (33)	4 (36)	2 (11)	0 (0)
LR	59/65 (91%)	24	107 (51)	97 (74)	4 (33)	4 (36)	1 (6)	1 (3)
Biopsies spared or delayed using CSPCa models at given sensitivity for detection of CSPCa								
ANN	64/65 (98%)	7	60 (29)	58 (44)	1 (8)	0 (0)	0 (0)	1 (3)
SVM	64/65 (98%)	9	69 (33)	65 (50)	3 (25)	0 (0)	0 (0)	1 (3)
CART	64/65 (98%)	NA	NA	NA	NA	NA	NA	NA
RF	64/65 (98%)	7	79 (38)	75 (57)	3 (25)	1 (9)	0 (0)	0 (0)
LR	64/65 (98%)	6	61 (29)	57 (44)	3 (25)	0 (0)	1 (6)	0 (0)
ANN	62/65 (95%)	8	79 (38)	75 (57)	1 (8)	1 (9)	1 (6)	1 (3)
SVM	62/65 (95%)	10	82 (39)	76 (58)	3 (25)	1 (9)	1 (6)	1 (3)
CART	62/65 (95%)	NA	NA	NA	NA	NA	NA	NA
RF	62/65 (95%)	8	84 (40)	78 (60)	3 (25)	1 (9)	2 (11)	0 (0)
LR	62/65 (95%)	7	70 (34)	64 (49)	3 (25)	1 (9)	1 (6)	1 (3)
ANN	59/65 (91%)	9	96 (46)	86 (66)	4 (33)	4 (36)	1 (6)	1 (3)
SVM	59/65 (91%)	18	124 (60)	112 (85)	6 (50)	4 (36)	1 (6)	1 (3)
CART	58/65 (89%)	10	109 (52)	97 (74)	5 (42)	4 (36)	1 (6)	2 (6)
RF	59/65 (91%)	13	102 (49)	92 (70)	4 (33)	3 (27)	3 (17)	0 (0)
LR	59/65 (91%)	14	105 (50)	32 (24)	4 (33)	3 (27)	1 (6)	2 (6)

PCa prostate cancer, *CSPCa* clinically significant prostate cancer, *GS* Gleason score, *ANN* artificial neural network, *SVM* support vector machine, *CART* classification and regression tree, *RF* random forest, *LR* logistic regression, *NA* not applicable

† Number of biopsies spared = number of unnecessary biopsy avoided + number of biopsy delayed

The RF and SVM showed similar diagnostic accuracy with LR model in prediction of PCa and CSPCa in our study, while spared more unnecessary biopsies than LR model at given sensitivity of 98% or 95% (Table 2). Above all, our study did not have enough power to draw conclusion that ANN, SVM, CART and RF models outperformed traditional LR analysis in diagnostic of CSPCa. Now we are entering the era of big data, in which complete patient data including macro-level physiology and

behavior, laboratory and imaging studies, and "-omic" data, are becoming more readily available. Machine learning may become an indispensable tool to handle the complex data [6]. Further validation is required.

Conclusions

Our study developed and compared machine-learning models with LR analysis to predict PCa and CSPCa. The SVM and RF models yielded similar diagnostic accuracy and net benefit with LR, while spared more unnecessary prostate biopsies than LR model at 95% sensitivity for detection of CSPCa. CART model illustrated best calibration for the prediction of PCa and CSPCa. Our study did not have sufficient power to draw conclusion that machine-learning models outperformed traditional LR analysis in prediction of PCa and CSPCa. All methods should continue to be used and explored in complementary ways.

Abbreviations

PCa: Prostate cancer; CSPCa: Clinically significant prostate cancer; PSA: Prostate-specific antigen; tPSA: Total prostate-specific antigen; LR: Logistic regression; ANN: Artificial neural network; SVM: Support vector machine; CART : Classification and regression tree; RF: Random forest; mpMRI: Multiparametric magnetic resonance imaging; f/t PSA: Free/total prostate-specific antigen; SVI: Seminal vesicle invasion; LNI: Lymph node invasion; DCA: Decision curve analysis; AUC: Area under the curve; CI: Confidence interval; SSR: Sum squares of the residuals.

Acknowledgements

Not applicable.

Authors' contributions

X. P. Z., and S. B. Y. conceptualized, designed and supervised the study. J. T., B. D., Y. F. F., H. P. D., H. T. D., J. S. C., G. D. H, and W. G. Q. coordinated and participated data collection. S. B. Y., and J. T. carried out the statistical analysis and drafted the manuscript. X. P. Z., and B. D. provided guidance on the data analysis. X. P. Z., J. T., B. D., and Y. F. F. revised the manuscript. All authors read and approved the final manuscript.

Author details

[1]Department of Urology, The First Affiliated Hospital of Zhengzhou University, No. 1 Jianshe East Road, Zhengzhou 450052, China. [2]Key Laboratory of Precision Diagnosis and Treatment for Chronic Kidney Disease in Henan Province, Zhengzhou 450052, China.

References

1. Ferlay J, Soerjomataram I, Dikshit R, Eser S, Mathers C, Rebelo M, et al. Cancer incidence and mortality worldwide: sources, methods and major patterns in GLOBOCAN 2012. Int J Cancer. 2015;136(5):E359–86.
2. International Agency for Research on Cancer: GLOBAL CANCER OBSERVATORY. 2018. http://gco.iarc.fr/. Cited 15 July 2020.
3. Van Neste L, Hendriks RJ, Dijkstra S, Trooskens G, Cornel EB, Jannink SA, et al. Detection of high-grade prostate cancer using a urinary molecular biomarker-based risk score. Eur Urol. 2016;70(5):740–8.
4. Bratan F, Niaf E, Melodelima C, Chesnais AL, Souchon R, Mege-Lechevallier F, et al. Influence of imaging and histological factors on prostate cancer detection and localisation on multiparametric MRI: a prospective study. Eur Radiol. 2013;23(7):2019–29.
5. Le JD, Tan N, Shkolyar E, Lu DY, Kwan L, Marks LS, et al. Multifocality and prostate cancer detection by multiparametric magnetic resonance imaging: correlation with whole-mount histopathology. Eur Urol. 2015;67(3):569–76.
6. Obermeyer Z, Emanuel EJ. Predicting the future—big data, machine learning, and clinical medicine. N Engl J Med. 2016;375(13):1216–9.
7. Wong NC, Lam C, Patterson L, Shayegan B. Use of machine learning to predict early biochemical recurrence after robot-assisted prostatectomy. BJU Int. 2019;123(1):51–7.
8. Thompson IM, Ankerst DP, Chi C, Goodman PJ, Tangen CM, Lucia MS, et al. Assessing prostate cancer risk: results from the Prostate Cancer Prevention Trial. J Natl Cancer Inst. 2006;98(8):529–34.
9. Gronberg H, Adolfsson J, Aly M, Nordstrom T, Wiklund P, Brandberg Y, et al. Prostate cancer screening in men aged 50–69 years (STHLM3): a prospective population-based diagnostic study. Lancet Oncol. 2015;16(16):1667–76.
10. Roobol MJ, Verbeek JFM, van der Kwast T, Kümmerlin IP, Kweldam CF, van Leenders GJLH. Improving the Rotterdam European randomized study of screening for prostate cancer risk calculator for initial prostate biopsy by incorporating the 2014 International Society of Urological Pathology Gleason Grading and Cribriform growth. Eur Urol. 2017;72(1):45–51.
11. Chen R, Xie L, Xue W, Ye Z, Ma L, Gao X, et al. Development and external multicenter validation of Chinese Prostate Cancer Consortium prostate cancer risk calculator for initial prostate biopsy. Urol Oncol. 2016;34(9):e4161–7.
12. Checcucci E, De Cillis S, Granato S, Chang P, Afyouni AS, Okhunov Z. Applications of neural networks in urology: a systematic review. Curr Opin Urol. 2020;30(6):788–807.
13. Checcucci E, Autorino R, Cacciamani GE, Amparore D, De Cillis S, Piana A, et al. Artificial intelligence and neural networks in urology: current clinical applications. Minerva Urol Nefrol. 2020;72(1):49–57.
14. Sargent DJ. Comparison of artificial neural networks with other statistical approaches: results from medical data sets. Cancer. 2001;91(8 Suppl):1636–42.
15. Hu X, Cammann H, Meyer H-A, Miller K, Jung K, Stephan C. Artificial neural networks and prostate cancer—tools for diagnosis and management. Nat Rev Urol. 2013;10(3):174–82.
16. Alberts AR, Roobol MJ, Verbeek JFM, Schoots IG, Chiu PK, Osses DF, et al. Prediction of high-grade prostate cancer following multiparametric magnetic resonance imaging: improving the Rotterdam European randomized study of screening for prostate cancer risk calculators. Eur Urol. 2019;75(2):310–8.
17. Liu C, Liu SL, Wang ZX, Yu K, Feng CX, Ke Z, et al. Using the prostate imaging reporting and data system version 2 (PI-RIDS v2) to detect prostate cancer can prevent unnecessary biopsies and invasive treatment. Asian J Androl. 2018;20(5):459–64.
18. Liaw A, Wiener M. Classification and regression by RandomForest. Forest. 2001;23:18–22.
19. DeLong ER, DeLong DM, Clarke-Pearson DL. Comparing the areas under two or more correlated receiver operating characteristic curves: a nonparametric approach. Biometrics. 1988;44(3):837–45.
20. Kawakami S, Numao N, Okubo Y, Koga F, Yamamoto S, Saito K, et al. Development, validation, and head-to-head comparison of logistic regression-based nomograms and artificial neural network models predicting prostate cancer on initial extended biopsy. Eur Urol. 2008;54(3):601–11.
21. Lee A, Chia SJ. Contemporary outcomes in the detection of prostate cancer using transrectal ultrasound-guided 12-core biopsy in Singaporean men with elevated prostate specific antigen and/or abnormal digital rectal examination. Asian J Urol. 2015;2(4):187–93.
22. Matsumoto K, Satoh T, Egawa S, Shimura S, Kuwao S, Baba S. Efficacy and morbidity of transrectal ultrasound-guided 12-core biopsy for detection of prostate cancer in Japanese men. Int J Urol. 2005;12(4):353–60.
23. Seo HK, Chung MK, Ryu SB, Lee KH. Detection rate of prostate cancer according to prostate-specific antigen and digital rectal examination in Korean men: a nationwide multicenter study. Urology. 2007;70(6):1109–12.
24. Vickers AJ, Cronin AM, Roobol MJ, Hugosson J, Jones JS, Kattan MW, et al. The relationship between prostate-specific antigen and prostate cancer risk: the Prostate Biopsy Collaborative Group. Clin Cancer Res. 2010;16(17):4374–81.
25. Smeenge M, Barentsz J, Cosgrove D, de la Rosette J, de Reijke T, Eggener S, et al. Role of transrectal ultrasonography (TRUS) in focal therapy of prostate cancer: report from a Consensus Panel. BJU Int. 2012;110(7):942–8.
26. Hectors SJ, Cherny M, Yadav KK, Beksaç AT, Thulasidass H, Lewis S, et al. Radiomics features measured with multiparametric magnetic resonance imaging predict prostate cancer aggressiveness. J Urol. 2019;202(3):498–505.
27. Chaddad A, Niazi T, Probst S, Bladou F, Anidjar M, Bahoric B. Predicting Gleason score of prostate cancer patients using radiomic analysis. Front Oncol. 2018;8:630.

28. Ross EG, Shah NH, Dalman RL, Nead KT, Cooke JP, Leeper NJ. The use of machine learning for the identification of peripheral artery disease and future mortality risk. J Vasc Surg. 2016;64(5):1515-22.e3.

29. Hung AJ, Chen J, Che Z, Nilanon T, Jarc A, Titus M, et al. Utilizing machine learning and automated performance metrics to evaluate robot-assisted radical prostatectomy performance and predict outcomes. J Endourol. 2018;32(5):438–44.

30. Nishi H, Oishi N, Ishii A, Ono I, Ogura T, Sunohara T, et al. Predicting clinical outcomes of large vessel occlusion before mechanical thrombectomy using machine learning. Stroke. 2019;50(9):2379–88.

14

Repurposing FDA approved drugs as radiosensitizers for treating hypoxic prostate cancer

Becky A. S. Bibby[1†], Niluja Thiruthaneeswaran[1,2*†] ⓘ, Lingjian Yang[1], Ronnie R. Pereira[1,3], Elisabet More[1], Darragh G. McArt[4], Paul O'Reilly[4], Robert G. Bristow[1,3], Kaye J. Williams[5], Ananya Choudhury[1] and Catharine M. L. West[1]

Abstract

Background: The presence of hypoxia is a poor prognostic factor in prostate cancer and the hypoxic tumor microenvironment promotes radioresistance. There is potential for drug radiotherapy combinations to improve the therapeutic ratio. We aimed to investigate whether hypoxia-associated genes could be used to identify FDA approved drugs for repurposing for the treatment of hypoxic prostate cancer.

Methods: Hypoxia associated genes were identified and used in the connectivity mapping software QUADrATIC to identify FDA approved drugs as candidates for repurposing. Drugs identified were tested in vitro in prostate cancer cell lines (DU145, PC3, LNCAP). Cytotoxicity was investigated using the sulforhodamine B assay and radiosensitization using a clonogenic assay in normoxia and hypoxia.

Results: Menadione and gemcitabine had similar cytotoxicity in normoxia and hypoxia in all three cell lines. In DU145 cells, the radiation sensitizer enhancement ratio (SER) of menadione was 1.02 in normoxia and 1.15 in hypoxia. The SER of gemcitabine was 1.27 in normoxia and 1.09 in hypoxia. No radiosensitization was seen in PC3 cells.

Conclusion: Connectivity mapping can identify FDA approved drugs for potential repurposing that are linked to a radiobiologically relevant phenotype. Gemcitabine and menadione could be further investigated as potential radiosensitizers in prostate cancer.

Background

The goal of drug repurposing is to find new clinical indications for existing pharmaceuticals that are currently on the market or failed in phase II/III trials. Repurposing is feasible because disease mechanisms are multifactorial and small drug molecules have multiple targets. Drug repurposing is both time and cost effective since the pharmacology and toxicity profile of approved drugs are already established. Approximately 30% of food and drug authority (FDA) applications for repurposed drugs are approved compared with 10% for new drugs [1, 2]. There is also potential for drug radiotherapy combinations to improve therapeutic ratios and enhance efficacy without increasing toxicity [3].

Drug and transcriptomic connectivity mapping can identify drug candidates for repurposing. The most widely used method is CMap (connectivity map project) which connects gene expression profiles to drugs based on data obtained from human cell lines treated with FDA

*Correspondence: nilujat@ausdoctors.net
†BeckyA.S. Bibby and Niluja Thiruthaneeswaran: Joint first author
[1] Translational Radiobiology Group, Division of Cancer Science, School of Medical Sciences, Faculty of Biology, Medicine and Health, University of Manchester, Manchester Academic Health Sciences Centre, The Christie NHS Foundation Trust, Wilmslow Road, Manchester M20 4BX, UK
Full list of author information is available at the end of the article

approved drugs [4]. CMap currently has over one million gene expression profiles from multiple cell lines treated with approximately 20,000 compounds. Since the release of the data sets from the library of integrated cellular signatures (LINCS) program, additional connectivity mapping algorithms have been developed such as the Queens University Belfast Accelerated Drug and Transcriptomic Connectivity (QUADrATiC) program [5]. This software provides an improved and rapid method for calculating connection scores between the LINCS database and FDA approved compounds in order to identify drugs with the potential to reverse the biology or phenotype associated with the genes of interest [6]. Any positive hit from this algorithm has already been identified as a safe therapeutic and can be progressed into a Phase I/II radiotherapy combination trial.

Computation-based approaches to drug repurposing provide an opportunity to identify novel agents to combine with radiotherapy [7]. Prostate cancer is the most common malignancy in men with just under 50,000 new cases diagnosed in the UK and 450,000 in Europe each year [8–10]. The local disease is managed with combinations of surgery, radiotherapy and hormones. The presence of hypoxia increases treatment resistance in prostate cancer patients treated with surgery or radiotherapy [11]. Targeting hypoxia in combination with radiotherapy has not been widely studied in prostate cancer, however, two single arm trials suggest the approach is feasible [12, 13]. To date the most extensive and convincing evidence for hypoxia modification in combination with radiotherapy comes from studies in head and neck cancer and muscle-invasive bladder cancer [14–16]. The retrospective analysis of hypoxia gene signature biomarkers within clinical trials confirmed patients with hypoxic tumors benefit most from hypoxia modification [14, 17]. Hypoxia gene signature biomarkers have been derived for multiple cancers and do not necessarily recapitulate across disease sites hence disease site-specific signatures have been developed [18]. Recently, we derived a gene signature for assessing hypoxia in prostate cancer [19]. The aim of this study was to investigate whether the transcription network associated with our hypoxia gene signature could be used in QUADrATIC to identify FDA approved drugs for potential repurposing for the treatment of hypoxic prostate cancer.

Methods

Identifying hypoxia associated genes

Genes significantly differentially expressed after 24 h exposure to 1% oxygen in more than two cell lines (DU145, PC3, LNCaP, PNT2) were identified previously as seed genes. For each cell line, genes differentially expressed between normoxia and hypoxia conditions

across triplicates were selected using a rank product probability of false positive rate < 0.05 [19]. The 848 seed genes were used to build gene co-expression networks using the publicly available GSE21032 or TCGA cohorts [18, 20]. Gene co-expression networks were assembled and partitioned into gene modules using the Louvain method [19, 21]. Each module was tested for enrichment of the hypoxia seed genes using the Chi-square test. The upregulated genes from the gene module(s) significantly associated with a high percentage of hypoxia seed genes (FDR < 0.01) were used as input for QUADrATiC.

STRING

The STRING database is a free online tool for exploring protein–protein interactions [22]. The user inputs their genes of interest, in this case the 103 GSE21032 and 66 TCGA hypoxia-associated genes, and the STRING database assembles a network of protein–protein interactions based on experimental evidence and predicted function. The associations in STRING include direct physical interactions and predicted indirect functional interactions. The protein–protein interactions are presented as networks, in which nodes represent proteins and the lines associations between proteins. The protein–protein association strength takes the form of a p-value that evaluates multiple channels of evidence as well as the chance of a random interaction between the protein pair [23].

Connectivity mapping

QUADrATiC uses the LINCS database to identify connections between gene expression profiles and FDA-approved drugs [5]. The data in the LINCS database are compiled from in vitro cell line experiments. Two separate gene lists were used in the QUADrATiC software generated from GSE21032 (103 genes; Additional file 1: Table S2) and TCGA (66 genes; Additional file 1: Table S1). Genes were mapped to their corresponding probe(s) in the Affymetrix HG-133UA-na36 annotation (Additional file 1: Tables S3 and S4) and entered into the QUADrATIC software according to the most concordant drug response [24]. In other words, up-regulated genes associated with a poor prognosis (hazard ratio [HR] > 1) comprise the up-regulated set of the signature while up-regulated genes associated with a good prognosis (HR < 1) form the down-regulated set.

Cell lines

Three prostate cancer cell lines were used to test drugs in vitro: DU145 (HTB-81), PC3 (CRL-1435) and LNCaP (CRL-1740). The cell lines were obtained from the American Type Culture Collection and authenticated by short tandem repeat profiling using the Promega Powerplex 21 system. Cell lines were cultured under normal conditions

(37°C, 5% CO_2 in air), screened for mycoplasma and authenticated using short tandem repeat profiling. DU145 and LNCaP cells were cultured in RPMI 1640 (Sigma-Aldrich, UK) with 10% fetal bovine serum (FBS) and 2 mM L-glutamine (Sigma-Aldrich, UK). PC3 cells were cultured in Ham's F12 (Gibco, ThermoFisher, UK) with 10% FBS and 2 mM L-glutamine (Sigma-Aldrich, UK).

Drug preparation

Menadione (Selleck Chem, Texas, USA), gemcitabine (Selleck Chem, Texas, USA) and tirapazamine (APExBIO, Texas, USA) were purchased in lyophilized form. Drugs were reconstituted to a concentration of 50 mM in dimethyl sulfoxide (DMSO) as recommended by the manufacturer. Stock solutions were aliquoted and stored at -80 °C; aliquots were not repeatedly freeze thawed.

Sulforhodamine B (SRB) assays

Cells were seeded into 96 well plates and allowed to adhere overnight in the incubator. The next day plates were treated with 0, 2, 5, 10, 50 or 100 μM of drug or DMSO vehicle control. Following application of the drug, cells were immediately moved into a 0.1% O_2 hypoxia chamber (Don Whitley Scientific, Bingley, UK) or kept in a normoxia incubator for 24 h. The assay endpoint was either 24 h or 4 days post-treatment. For the 24 h time point, the cells were fixed and stained after 24 h incubation with the drug. For the 4-day time point, the drug was removed after 24 h and fresh media added to the cells. Plates were incubated for a further 4 days in normoxia. Cells were fixed and then stained with sulforhodamine B according to the published method [25].

Clonogenic assays

Cells were seeded into plug seal T25 flasks and allowed to adhere overnight in the incubator, with plug seal caps kept loose. The next day media were removed and replaced with fresh media containing the drug (10 μM menadione or 8 nM gemcitabine) or DMSO (vehicle control). Untreated control flasks had fresh media applied. Cells exposed to normoxia, with or without the drug, were incubated with plug seal caps left loose in the incubator for 24 h. Cells exposed to 0.1% oxygen for 24 h, with or without the drug, were incubated with plug seal caps left loose in the H35 hypoxystation (Don Whitley Scientific, Bingley, UK). After 24 h plug seal caps were tightened on the flasks in the hypoxystation to maintain hypoxic conditions during irradiation. Cells were irradiated with x-rays delivered at 0.95 Gy/min using a Faxitron X-ray machine (Tucson, Arizona, USA). After irradiation cells were immediately harvested, counted and seeded onto 6-well plates [26]. Plates were incubated

for 7–21 days until colonies had formed, fixed and stained using crystal violet solution (70% methanol (v/v), 0.1% crystal violet). Plates were imaged on a GelCount machine (Oxford Optronix, Abingdon, UK) and colonies counted using an optimized CHARM algorithm in the GelCount software. The surviving fraction was calculated for each biological repeat (experiments ran on separate days with cells of a different passage) using the mean number of colonies across the six individual wells. The concentration of DMSO was 0.02% (v/v) for menadione and 0.000016% (v/v) for gemcitabine. Sensitizer enhancement ratio (SER) was calculated as the ratio between the doses needed for 1 log kill with or without the drug.

Statistical analysis

Data are presented as mean ± standard error of the mean (SEM). GraphPad PRISM 8 was used to plot graphs, radiation survival curves were fitted with the linear quadratic model. Surviving fractions at 2 Gy (SF2) and SER values were extrapolated from the fit of the linear quadratic model using PRISM 8. GraphPad PRISM 8 was used to perform the F-test and statistical analysis, p values < 0.05 were considered significant.

Results

Hypoxia associated genes

Co-expression networks in the GSE21032 and TCGA cohorts identified hypoxia-associated genes (Additional file 1: Tables S1 and S2). Proteins encoded by the genes in the two networks interacted significantly ($p < 1 \times 10^{-16}$). Figure 1 illustrates the high level of connections between the proteins in the networks. The network plots show only proteins with at least one connection. Sixty-nine of the 103 genes (67%) in the GSE21032 list had at least one connection and there was an average of 3.6 connections per node. The TCGA gene list produced a more highly connected network of protein–protein interactions with 55 of the 66 genes (83%) having at least one connection and an average of 8.2 connections. The gene lists were applied independently to the QUADrATiC connectivity mapping software to identify FDA-approved drugs.

QUADrATiC connectivity mapping

Drugs with negative connections were considered able to target the phenotype of interest, in this case hypoxia in prostate cancer. Using the GSE21032 hypoxia-associated genes there were 5,348 drugs with negative z-scores, of which 2,405 were nominally significant ($p < 0.05$). Using the TCGA hypoxia-associated genes there were 4,827 drugs with negative z-scores, of which 2,270 were nominally significant ($p < 0.05$). The QUADrATiC interface provided summary visualizations of the top connections

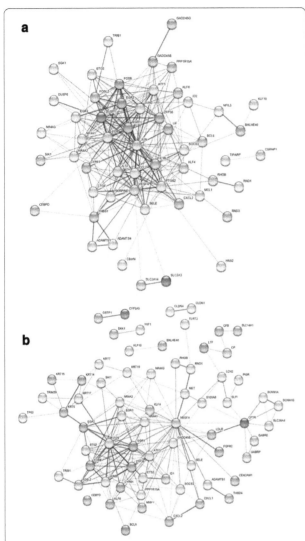

Fig. 1 Prostate cancer hypoxia-associated genes interact at the protein level. The networks, generated using the STRING database, summarize predicted associations between proteins. The nodes represent proteins and only nodes with at least one connection are shown. The edges represent protein–protein interactions and the confidence of the interaction is indicated by the thickness of the edge. **a** Sixty-nine of the 103 hypoxia-associated genes identified in GSE21032 encoded proteins that interacted with at least one other protein in the network. On average each node had 3.6 connections and there are 185 edges representing protein–protein interactions. The observed number of edges in this network was more than expected at random with a protein–protein interaction enrichment value of $p < 1 \times 10^{-16}$, indicating a highly interconnected network of proteins. **b** Fifty-five of the 66 hypoxia-associated genes from the TCGA interacted with at least one other protein in the network and had an average 8.2 connections. There are 271 edges representing protein–protein interactions and number is more than expected at random ($p < 1 \times 10^{-16}$), indicating a highly interconnected network of proteins

as bubble charts and drug and cell line connections (Additional files 2, 3: Figure S1 and S2).

Drug selection

The top 10 drugs from each of the two gene lists were ranked based on Z-score (Table 1). There were two prostate cell lines, PC3 and VCaP, in the connectivity mapping analysis but drug selection was not restricted to the highest ranking drugs identified in these cell lines (Table 2). The strength of the connection between the genes and the drug was considered more important than the cell line in which it was identified because (i) there were only two prostate cancer cell lines in the program and (ii) the importance of hypoxia across solid tumours. Two candidate drugs were selected for in vitro validation, menadione and gemcitabine, because they ranked in the top 10 in the GSE21032 and TCGA datasets in all (Table 1) and the prostate cancer (Table 2) cell lines. Menadione appeared twice in the top 10 ranked drugs in the GSE21032 and TCGA (Table 1) and was the only drug with a strong connection to the VCaP cell line in both datasets (Table 2). Gemcitabine appeared twice in the top 10 ranked drugs in the GSE21032 and once in the TCGA (Table 1) and had a strong connection to the PC3 cell line in both datasets (Table 2). Menadione and gemcitabine also had negative Z-scores in the PC3 and VCaP cell lines (Additional file 1: Table S5). The approved application, mechanism of action and reported peak plasma concentrations for menadione and gemcitabine are summarized in Table 3.

Hypoxia selective cytotoxicity

Menadione and gemcitabine were tested alongside the known bioreductively activated tirapazamine. In the DU145, PC3 and LNCaP cell lines tirapazamine demonstrated hypoxia selective cytotoxicity 24 h (Additional file 4: Figure S3) and 4 days (Fig. 2) following drug exposure. There was no loss in cytotoxicity for menadione and gemcitabine 4 days post-treatment in any of the three cell lines. However, hypoxic PC3 cells were more sensitive to 5 µM menadione and 10 µM gemcitabine than the normoxic cells after 24 h drug exposure (Additional file 4: Figure S3).

Radiosensitization

The radiosensitizing ability of the two FDA approved drugs was studied in DU145 and PC3 cells. The rationale for selecting DU145 in addition to PC3 for the radiosensitization experiments is because this cell line was derived from human tissue, whereas the LNCaP cell line was initially derived from human tissue but cultured in a mouse model. Vehicle control experiments confirmed DMSO did not alter surviving fraction

Table 1 Top 10 FDA-approved drugs identified using connectivity mapping

Ranking	GSE21032			TCGA		
	Drug	Cell line	Z-score[¶]	Drug	Cell line	Z-score[¶]
1	**MENADIONE**	HEPG2	− 15.8	CLADRIBINE	A375	− 17.5
2	**MENADIONE**	A375	− 14.0	**MENADIONE**	A375	− 15.6
3	**GEMCITABINE**	A375	− 13.1	HOMOHARRINGTONINE	PC3	− 15.0
4	NICLOSAMIDE	HEPG2	− 13.0	**MENADIONE**	HEPG2	− 14.6
5	**GEMCITABINE**	HCC515	− 12.1	NICLOSAMIDE	HEPG2	− 14.6
6	CLADRIBINE	A375	− 11.7	DIGITOXIN	A549	− 14.3
7	DIGITOXIN	A549	− 11.4	AZACITIDINE	A375	− 14.0
8	DIGOXIN	PC3	− 11.3	CLOFARABINE	A375	− 13.9
9	PENTAMIDINE	HEPG2	− 11.1	**GEMCITABINE**	HCC515	− 13.5
10	TENIPOSIDE	A375	− 11.1	CLADRIBINE	PC3	− 13.3

[¶] p values < 0.001

Table 2 Top 10 FDA-approved drugs identified using connectivity mapping in the prostate cancer cell lines

Ranking	GSE21032			TCGA		
	Drug	Cell line	Z-score	Drug	Cell line	Z-score
1	DIGOXIN	PC3	− 11.31	HOMOHARRINGTONINE	PC3	− 14.98
2	OUABAIN	PC3	− 10.48	CLADRIBINE	PC3	− 13.29
3	DIGITOXIN	PC3	− 9.83	DIGITOXIN	PC3	− 13.15
4	BISACODYL	PC3	− 9.56	**MENADIONE**	VCAP	− 12.56
5	CLOFARABINE	PC3	− 9.42	DIGOXIN	PC3	− 12.10
6	HOMOHARRINGTONINE	PC3	− 8.86	OUABAIN	PC3	− 11.59
7	ITRACONAZOLE	PC3	− 8.84	**GEMCITABINE**	PC3	− 11.56
8	**MENADIONE**	VCAP	− 8.69	AZACITIDINE	PC3	− 10.16
9	**GEMCITABINE**	PC3	− 8.36	BORTEZOMIB	VCAP	− 10.15
10	TENIPOSIDE	PC3	− 8.35	CEFACLOR	PC3	− 9.92

Table 3 Application, mechanism and peak plasma concentrations for menadione and gemcitabine

	Menadione	Gemcitabine
Approved application	Used in vitamin K deficiency and severe hypoprothrombinemia	Treatment of locally advanced or metastatic cancer
Mechanism of action	Synthetic vitamin K3. It is also an inhibitor of Siah2 (E3 ubiquitin ligase) ligase activity	Inhibition of DNA synthesis and inhibition of enzymes related to deoxynucleotide metabolism
Peak plasma concentration and equivalent in vitro dose	115–407 ng/mL[¶] 668.6 ng–2.3 µM	3–6 µg/mL 11.2–22.4 µM
Equivalent in vitro dose	668.6 ng–2.3 µM	11.2–22.4 µM

[¶] Reported values for phytomenadione, doses up to 200 mg menadione are tolerated in humans

compared to the untreated controls and DMSO plus radiation did not alter surviving fraction compared to radiation alone (Additional file 5: Figure S4). Figure 3 shows survival curves for the cells irradiated in normoxia and hypoxia. Oxygen enhancement ratio (OERs) calculated at the 10% survival level were 1.34 for DU145 and 1.69 for PC3 cells. Figure 4 shows menadione was a weak radiosensitizer in DU145 cells only. The SER for menadione in DU145 cells was 1.02 in normoxia and 1.15 in hypoxia. Figure 5 shows gemcitabine was also a weak radiosensitizer in DU145 cells only. The SER for gemcitabine was 1.27 in normoxia and 1.09 in hypoxia.

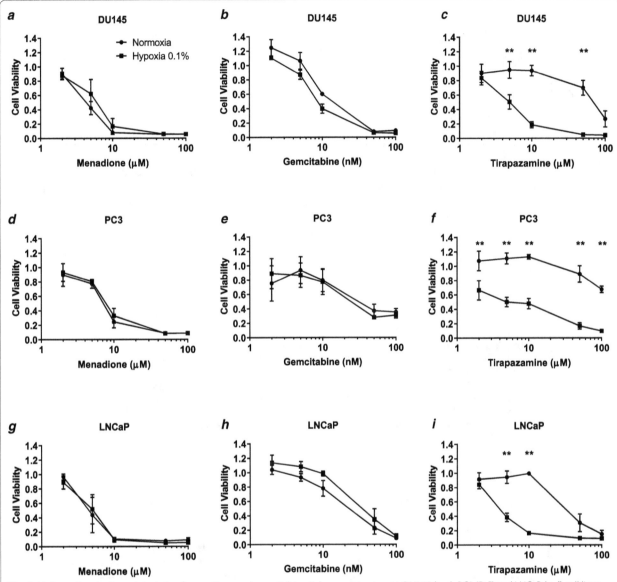

Fig. 2 No hypoxia-selective cytotoxicity of menadione and gemcitabine 4 days post-treatment. DU145 (**a–c**), PC3 (D-F) and LNCaP (**g–i**) cell lines were exposed to menadione, gemcitabine or tirapazamine under normoxia or 0.1% O₂ hypoxia. Only tirapazamine demonstrated hypoxia selective cytotoxicity in the cell lines. The data points represent the mean ± SEM of 2–4 values taken from each biological repeat, within each biological repeat there were 6 intra-assay replicates. Statistical analysis was performed using multiple t-tests with Holm-Sidak correction. **indicates $p < 0.01$

Discussion

Our study demonstrated how a gene expression network associated with hypoxia can be used in the QUADrATIC software to identify FDA approved drugs with the potential to be repurposed. The candidate drugs selected for in vitro validation, menadione and gemcitabine, showed similar cytotoxicity in normoxia and hypoxia in three cell lines. There was also evidence that the drugs were weak radiosensitizers in normoxia and hypoxia in one of the cell lines studied.

Although menadione and gemcitabine did not demonstrate hypoxia-selective cytotoxicity the drugs had similar efficacy in normoxia and hypoxia. In contrast, many chemotherapeutic agents (e.g., cisplatin, 5-FU and doxorubicin) have reduced cytotoxicity in vitro in hypoxia [27–30]. In general, few studies compared the cytotoxicity of chemotherapeutic agents in normoxia and hypoxia in prostate cancer cell lines. Docetaxel, a first line systemic treatment for prostate cancer, has been shown to have reduced cytotoxicity in hypoxia (1% and 0.1%

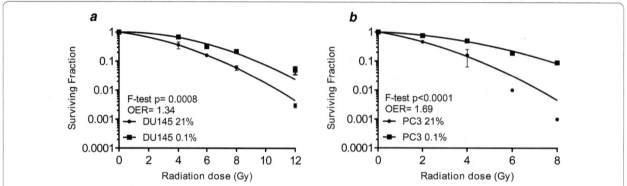

Fig. 3 Hypoxia increased radioresistance in the DU145 and PC3 cell lines. Cell survival curves for DU145 (**a**) and PC3 (**b**) cells, irradiated under normoxia or 0.1% O_2. The data points represent the mean ± SEM of 2–4 values taken from each biological repeat. OERs were calculated at SF10% and statistical analysis was performed using the F-test

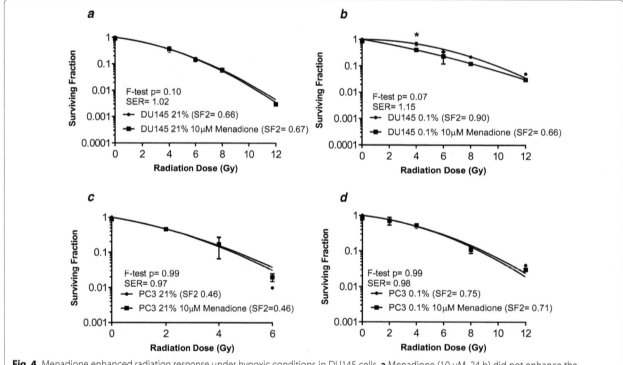

Fig. 4 Menadione enhanced radiation response under hypoxic conditions in DU145 cells. **a** Menadione (10 μM, 24 h) did not enhance the radiosensitivity of normoxic DU145 cells. **b** The SER of hypoxic DU145 cells treated with menadione was 1.15 and at 4 Gy menadione significantly reduced surviving fraction compared to radiation alone. **c** In the PC3 cell line, menadione did not enhance the radiosensitivity of normoxic or **d** hypoxic cells. The data points represent the mean ± SEM of 2–4 values taken from each biological repeat, within each biological repeat there were 6 intra-assay replicates. Statistical analysis was performed using a paired t-test (ns = not significant, * indicates $p < 0.05$). SERs were calculated at SF10% and statistical analysis was performed using the F-test

oxygen) in a range of cell lines [27]. However, a study in DU145 and 22Rv1 cells showed similar docetaxel cytotoxicity in normoxia and hypoxia (0.5% oxygen) [31]. It is uncommon for drugs studied in radiotherapy combination trials to have had their efficacy first tested under hypoxia. In future, pre-clinical testing as a justification for trial design should involve in vitro testing in hypoxia as well as normoxia.

As expected, we have shown the hypoxia selective toxicity of tirapazamine. Although previously studied in PC3 cells, this is the first study of tirapazamine in DU145 and LNCaP cells. The IC_{50} for PC3 was 5 μM (4 days post-treatment after 24 h at 0.1% O_2), which compares with literature reported IC_{50} doses for tirapazamine in PC3 cells of 15 μM [4 h anoxia] and 22 μM (48 h at 3% O_2) [32, 33]. Tirapazamine has been shown to enhance the

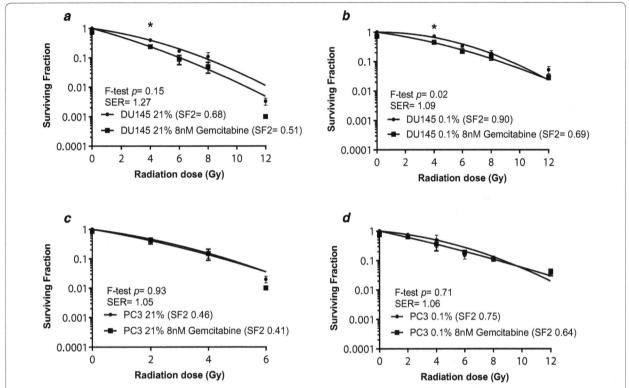

Fig. 5 Gemcitabine enhanced radiation response under normoxic and hypoxic conditions in the DU145 cells. **a** Gemcitabine (8 nM, 24 h) enhanced the radiosensitivity of normoxic DU145 cells, the SER was 1.27 and at 4 Gy gemcitabine significantly reduced surviving fraction compared to radiation alone. **b** Under hypoxia the SER of gemcitabine was 1.09 and at 4 Gy gemcitabine significantly reduced surviving fraction compared to radiation alone. **c** In the PC3 cell line, gemcitabine did not enhance the radiosensitivity of normoxic or **d** hypoxic cells. The data points represent the mean ± SEM of 2–4 values taken from each biological repeat, within each biological repeat there were 6 intra-assay replicates. Statistical analysis was performed using a paired t-test (ns = not significant, * indicates $p < 0.05$). SERs were calculated at SF10% and statistical analysis was performed using the F-test

effect of castration induced hypoxia by inducing apoptosis and subsequently reducing tumor volume [34]. Furthermore, hypoxia induces adaptive androgen independence and confers resistance to androgen deprivation therapy (ADT) [35]. Tirapazamine in combination with ADT has the potential to eliminate hypoxic tumor cells and prevent the development of ADT resistant clones. However, a Phase III trial that randomised head and neck cancer patients to chemoradiotherapy alone or with tirapazamine showed no benefit [36].

To identify gene expression changes in response to hypoxia the cells were exposed to 1% O_2 because the HIF-1 transcription factor is stabilised and changes in gene expression occurs. However, the level of O_2 at which significant resistance to radiation is observed is < 0.13% hence the in vitro experiments were performed at 0.1% O_2 [37]. The physiological level of oxygen in the normal prostate is 3.4–3.9% but oxygen levels in prostate tumor tissue are in the range of 0.3–1.2% [38]. Normoxia in this study is 21% O_2 which is supraphysiological compared to the level of oxygen in the prostate gland. However,

in vitro cell lines are routinely established and cultured in the laboratory under these conditions and have adapted to grow at 21% O_2 and therefore the difference in gene expression may not reflect in vivo changes.

The OERs for the DU145 and PC3 cell lines exposed to 0.1% O_2 for 24 h were low over the dose ranges studied but similar to those previously reported for DU145 and PC3 with the exception of PC3 transfected with mir210 inhibitors giving an OER of ~ 2 [39–42]. Furthermore, in vitro studies have reported varying OERs depending on the duration under hypoxia with OER decreasing with time of exposure under hypoxia for the same cell lines [41].

The guidelines for preclinical and early phase assessment of radiosensitizers state that relatively low SER values in the range 1.2–1.5 may indicate a useful effect, particularly if sensitization occurs at clinically relevant doses of radiation [43]. In the DU145 cell line, the SER for menadione under hypoxia was 1.15 which is comparable to the SER of nimorazole in the head and neck cancer cell lines FaDu (SER 1.14) and UMSCC47 (SER 1.13)

[44]. The SER of 1.27 for gemcitabine in normoxia was comparable to previously reported values in the range of 1.1–3 [45]. This normoxic radiosensitization with gemcitabine is comparable to the radiosensitizing effects of other chemotherapeutic agents such as 5-FU [46].

Menadione, also known as vitamin K_3, is a quinone and synthetic vitamin that can be converted into active vitamin K_2 in the body. Menadione induces the production of reactive oxygen species (ROS) through redox cycling and disrupts the interaction between HIF-1a and its coactivator p300 thus inhibiting HIF-1a transcriptional activity [47–49]. Apatone (menadione and vitamin C) has shown prostate cancer antitumor activity in vitro and the toxicity profile was favorable in a phase I/IIa study [50, 51]. PSA velocity and PSA doubling time decreased in 15 of 17 patients suggesting value in progressing apatone into the Phase III setting.

Gemcitabine is a chemotherapeutic agent used to treat several cancers, it is a nucleoside analogue that is incorporated into the DNA and inhibits DNA synthesis resulting in cell death. Nucleoside analogues such as gemcitabine are considered as potential radiosensitizers because they inhibit the repair of radiation induced DNA damage [52]. In muscle invasive bladder cancer evidence from phase I/II trials supports the concurrent administration of gemcitabine and radiotherapy as a bladder preservation strategy [53, 54]. In the breast cancer cell line MDA-MB-231, the SER for gemcitabine and radiation under hypoxia was 1.59 and under normoxia 1.70 [55]. The radiosensitizing effects of gemcitabine in breast cancer are greater than the effects reported in this study for prostate cancer. However, the radiosensitizing effect of gemcitabine is greater under normoxia agrees with our findings.

A limitation of our study is that radiosensitizing effects were weak and only observed in DU145 cells. This cell line is derived from a central nervous system metastasis of primary prostate adenocarcinoma [56]. In comparison, the PC3 cell line is characteristic of neuroendocrine-like prostate cancer, which represents less than 2% of cases and is biologically distinct from the more common adenocarcinoma subtype [57, 58]. Both patients had prior treatment with hormonal therapy before cell lines were derived. Nonetheless, they are the most commonly used prostate cancer cell lines. Interestingly, a study investigating the radiosensitizing effect of vorinostat in prostate cell lines reported a radiosensitizing effect under normoxia and hypoxia in the DU145 cells but no effect in PC3 cells [59]. A second limitation is that effects were only studied in cell lines grown as monolayers, an in vitro spheroid model may incorporate physiological hypoxia into the model. Although it is worth noting that, the in vitro data utilized by the QUADrATIC connectivity

mapping software was obtained from monolayer cultured under 21% O_2.

Two approaches have been employed to identify FDA-approved drug for repurposing: in silico analytics and experimental screening studies [2]. In a high-throughput oxygen consumption screen, atovaquone was shown to reduce oxygen consumption [60]. Atovaquone is an FDA approved anti-malarial with a similar chemical structure to menadione. Atovaquone was shown to reduce tumor hypoxia and increase radiosensitivity at pharmacological concentrations in spheroids in vitro and in vivo [60]. Interestingly, the drug did not alter the radiosensitivities of hypoxic cells grown as monolayers suggesting that atovaquone affects the tumor microenvironment rather than increasing the intrinsic radiosensitivity of cells [60]. Atovaquone is currently being tested in phase I clinical trial for its ability to alleviate tumor hypoxia in lung cancer (NCT02628080).

Conclusion

In summary, this study highlights how connectivity mapping can be used to identify FDA approved drugs linked to biological phenotypes for potential repurposing. Our work shows the importance of downstream validation and proof-of-principle studies when identifying drugs for repurposing using in silico analytical approaches. Tirapazamine is an effective hypoxia-selective agent in prostate cancer cell lines and could be tested alongside ADT in future studies. In the DU145 cell line, menadione was a hypoxic radiosentiziter and gemcitabine was a normoxic radiosensitizer. Gemcitabine could be further investigated given that the guidelines for preclinical and early phase assessment of radiosensitizers report an SER in the range of 1.2–1.5 could be clinically useful.

Abbreviations

CMap: Connectivity map project; LINCS: Library of integrated cellular signatures; QUADrATIC: Queens University Belfast Accelerated Drug and Transcriptomic Connectivity; TCGA: The Cancer Genome Atlas; OER: Oxygen enhancement ratio; SER: Sensitizer enhancement ratio.

Supplementary Information

Additional file 1. Supplementary Table 1. GSE21032 hypoxia associated genes n = 103. **Supplementary Table 2.** TCGA hypoxia associated genes n = 66. **Supplementary Table 3.** GSE21032 hypoxia associated genes Affymetrix probe IDs. **Supplementary Table 4.** TCGA hypoxia associated genes Affymetrix probe IDs. **Supplementary Table 5.** The Z-scores for menadione and gemcitabine in the prostate cancer cell lines.

Additional file 2. Supplementary Figure 1. Bubble plots representing the strength of the top negative connections identified by QUADrATIC. The larger the bubble the stronger the connection between the identified drug and the input genes. The drug and the cell line, that the connection was derived from, are shown in the bubbles. (**A**) GSE21032 (**B**) TCGA.

Additional file 3. Supplementary Figure 2. Top drug and cell line connections identified by QUADrATiC. The plots represent the top ranked drugs and the cell line that the connection was derived from in the LINCs database. (**A**) GSE21032 (**B**) TCGA.

Additional file 4. Supplementary Figure 3. No loss of cytotoxicity of menadione and gemcitabine in hypoxia versus normoxia after 24 h. DU145 (**A–C**), PC3 (**D–F**) and LNCaP (**G–I**) cell lines were exposed to menadione, gemcitabine or tirapazamine under normoxia or 0.1% O2 hypoxia. Three independent experiments were carried out, with six intra-assay replicates per experiment. Data points represent the mean ± SEM, statistical analysis was performed using a t-test with Holm-Sidak correction; **p < 0.01).

Additional file 5. Supplementary Figure 4. (**A**) Under normoxia DMSO at a concentration of 0.02% (v/v) did not alter the surviving fraction of DU145 cells that were mockirradiated or irradiated with 4 Gy. (**B**) Under hypoxia DMSO at a concentration of 0.02% (v/v) did not alter the surviving fraction of DU145 cells that were mock irradiated or irradiated with 4 Gy. Data points represent the mean ± SEM of 3 biological repeats.

Acknowledgements

Not applicable

Authors' contributions

All authors have read and approved the final manuscript. BB, CW and LJ conceptualization. BB and NT study design and experimental plan. BB, NT, EM conducted the experiments. LY and RP contributed to bioinformatics and data analysis. DM and PO design of QUADrATIC software. BB, NT and CW wrote the manuscript. BB did the figures preparation. CW, AC, RGB, KW review of experimental design, final edits and approval of manuscript. All authors read and approved the final manuscript.

Author details

[1]Translational Radiobiology Group, Division of Cancer Science, School of Medical Sciences, Faculty of Biology, Medicine and Health, University of Manchester, Manchester Academic Health Sciences Centre, The Christie NHS Foundation Trust, Wilmslow Road, Manchester M20 4BX, UK. [2]Sydney Medical School, University of Sydney, Camperdown, Australia. [3]Translational Oncogenomics, CRUK Manchester Institute and CRUK Manchester Centre, Manchester, UK. [4]Centre for Cancer Research and Cell Biology, Queen's University Belfast, Belfast, UK. [5]School of Pharmacy and Pharmaceutical Sciences, University of Manchester, Manchester, UK.

References

1. Graul AI, Sorbera L, Pina P, Tell M, Cruces E, Rosa E, et al. The Year's new drugs & biologics—2009. Drug News Perspect. 2010;23(1):7–36.
2. Cha Y, Erez T, Reynolds IJ, Kumar D, Ross J, Koytiger G, et al. Drug repurposing from the perspective of pharmaceutical companies. Br J Pharmacol. 2018;175(2):168–80.
3. Ahmad SS, Crittenden MR, Tran PT, Kluetz PG, Blumenthal GM, Bulbeck H, et al. Clinical development of novel drug-radiotherapy combinations. Clin Cancer Res. 2019;25(5):1455–61.
4. Lamb J. The Connectivity map: a new tool for biomedical research. Nat Rev Cancer. 2007;7(1):54–60.
5. O'Reilly PG, Wen Q, Bankhead P, Dunne PD, McArt DG, McPherson S, et al. QUADrATiC: scalable gene expression connectivity mapping for repurposing FDA-approved therapeutics. BMC Bioinformatics. 2016;17(1):198.
6. Wen Q, Dunne PD, O'Reilly PG, Li G, Bjourson AJ, McArt DG, et al. KRAS mutant colorectal cancer gene signatures identified angiotensin II receptor blockers as potential therapies. Oncotarget. 2017;8(2):3206–25.
7. Sharma RA, Plummer R, Stock JK, Greenhalgh TA, Ataman O, Kelly S, et al. Clinical development of new drug-radiotherapy combinations. Nat Rev Clin Oncol. 2016;13(10):627–42.
8. Society AC. Cancer facts & figures. Atlanta; 2018.
9. King A BJ. Cancer registration statistics, England: 2016. 2018.
10. Rawla P. Epidemiology of prostate cancer. World J Oncol. 2019;10(2):63–89.
11. Milosevic M, Warde P, Menard C, Chung P, Toi A, Ishkanian A, et al. Tumor hypoxia predicts biochemical failure following radiotherapy for clinically localized prostate cancer. Clin Cancer Res. 2012;18(7):2108–14.
12. Lawton CA, Coleman CN, Buzydlowski JW, Forman JD, Marcial VA, DelRowe JD, et al. Results of a phase II trial of external beam radiation with etanidazole (SR 2508) for the treatment of locally advanced prostate cancer (RTOG Protocol 90–20). Int J Radiat Oncol Biol Phys. 1996;36(3):673–80.
13. Thiruthaneeswaran N YK, Valentine J, Patel U, Choudhury A, Hoskin P, Alonzi R. Prostate radiotherapy in conjunction with carbogen and nicotinamide. A phase Ib/II Study. (PROCON). ASTRO conference 2017.
14. Toustrup K, Sørensen BS, Lassen P, Wiuf C, Alsner J, Overgaard J, et al. Gene expression classifier predicts for hypoxic modification of radiotherapy with nimorazole in squamous cell carcinomas of the head and neck. Radiother Oncol. 2012;102(1):122–9.
15. Janssens GO, Rademakers SE, Terhaard CH, Doornaert PA, Bijl HP, van den Ende P, et al. Accelerated radiotherapy with carbogen and nicotinamide for laryngeal cancer: results of a phase III randomized trial. J Clin Oncol. 2012;30(15):1777–83.
16. Hoskin PJ, Rojas AM, Bentzen SM, Saunders MI. Radiotherapy with concurrent carbogen and nicotinamide in bladder carcinoma. J Clin Oncol. 2010;28(33):4912–8.
17. Yang L, Taylor J, Eustace A, Irlam JJ, Denley H, Hoskin PJ, et al. A gene signature for selecting benefit from hypoxia modification of radiotherapy for high-risk bladder cancer patients. Clin Cancer Res. 2017;23(16):4761–8.
18. Harris BH, Barberis A, West CM, Buffa FM. Gene expression signatures as biomarkers of tumour hypoxia. Clin Oncol (R Coll Radiol). 2015;27(10):547–60.
19. Yang L, Roberts D, Takhar M, Erho N, Bibby BAS, Thiruthaneeswaran N, et al. Development and validation of a 28-gene hypoxia-related prognostic signature for localized prostate cancer. EBioMedicine. 2018;31:182–9.
20. Taylor BS, Schultz N, Hieronymus H, Gopalan A, Xiao Y, Carver BS, et al. Integrative genomic profiling of human prostate cancer. Cancer Cell. 2010;18(1):11–22.
21. Vincent DB, Jean-Loup G, Renaud L, Etienne L. Fast unfolding of communities in large networks. J Stat Mech: Theory Exp. 2008;2008(10):P10008.
22. Szklarczyk D, Morris JH, Cook H, Kuhn M, Wyder S, Simonovic M, et al. The STRING database in 2017: quality-controlled protein-protein association networks, made broadly accessible. Nucleic Acids Res. 2017;45(D1):D362–8.
23. von Mering C, Jensen LJ, Snel B, Hooper SD, Krupp M, Foglierini M, et al. STRING: known and predicted protein-protein associations, integrated and transferred across organisms. Nucl Acids Res. 2005;33(Database issue):D433–7.
24. Zhang SD, Gant TW. A simple and robust method for connecting small-molecule drugs using gene-expression signatures. BMC Bioinformatics. 2008;9:258.
25. Vichai V, Kirtikara K. Sulforhodamine B colorimetric assay for cytotoxicity screening. Nat Protoc. 2006;1(3):1112–6.
26. Franken NA, Rodermond HM, Stap J, Haveman J, van Bree C. Clonogenic assay of cells in vitro. Nat Protoc. 2006;1(5):2315–9.
27. Strese S, Fryknas M, Larsson R, Gullbo J. Effects of hypoxia on human cancer cell line chemosensitivity. BMC Cancer. 2013;13:331.
28. Warren HR, Hejmadi M. Effect of hypoxia on chemosensitivity to 5-fluorouracil in SH-SY5Y neuroblastoma cells. Biosci Horizons Int J Stud Res. 2016;9.
29. Yoshiba S, Ito D, Nagumo T, Shirota T, Hatori M, Shintani S. Hypoxia induces resistance to 5-fluorouracil in oral cancer cells via G(1) phase cell cycle arrest. Oral Oncol. 2009;45(2):109–15.
30. Fujita H, Hirose K, Sato M, Fujioka I, Fujita T, Aoki M, et al. Metformin attenuates hypoxia-induced resistance to cisplatin in the HepG2 cell line. Oncol Lett. 2019;17(2):2431–40.
31. Forde JC, Perry AS, Brennan K, Martin LM, Lawler MP, Lynch TH, et al. Docetaxel maintains its cytotoxic activity under hypoxic conditions in prostate cancer cells. Urol Oncol. 2012;30(6):912–9.
32. Patterson AV, Ferry DM, Edmunds SJ, Gu Y, Singleton RS, Patel K, et al. Mechanism of action and preclinical antitumor activity of the novel

hypoxia-activated DNA cross-linking agent PR-104. Clin Cancer Res. 2007;13(13):3922–32.

33. Jiang F, Yang B, Fan L, He Q, Hu Y. Synthesis and hypoxic-cytotoxic activity of some 3-amino-1,2,4-benzotriazine-1,4-dioxide derivatives. Bioorg Med Chem Lett. 2006;16(16):4209–13.

34. Johansson A, Rudolfsson SH, Kilter S, Bergh A. Targeting castration-induced tumour hypoxia enhances the acute effects of castration therapy in a rat prostate cancer model. BJU Int. 2011;107(11):1818–24.

35. Geng H, Xue C, Mendonca J, Sun XX, Liu Q, Reardon PN, et al. Interplay between hypoxia and androgen controls a metabolic switch conferring resistance to androgen/AR-targeted therapy. Nat Commun. 2018;9(1):4972.

36. Rischin D, Peters LJ, O'Sullivan B, Giralt J, Fisher R, Yuen K, et al. Tirapazamine, cisplatin, and radiation versus cisplatin and radiation for advanced squamous cell carcinoma of the head and neck (TROG 02.02, HeadSTART): a phase III trial of the Trans-Tasman Radiation Oncology Group. J Clin Oncol. 2010;28(18):2989–95.

37. Hammond EM, Asselin MC, Forster D, O'Connor JP, Senra JM, Williams KJ. The meaning, measurement and modification of hypoxia in the laboratory and the clinic. Clin Oncol (R Coll Radiol). 2014;26(5):277–88.

38. McKeown SR. Defining normoxia, physoxia and hypoxia in tumours-implications for treatment response. Br J Radiol. 2014;87(1035):20130676.

39. Quero L, Dubois L, Lieuwes NG, Hennequin C, Lambin P. miR-210 as a marker of chronic hypoxia, but not a therapeutic target in prostate cancer. Radiother Oncol. 2011;101(1):203–8.

40. Stewart GD, Nanda J, Katz E, Bowman KJ, Christie JG, Brown DJ, et al. DNA strand breaks and hypoxia response inhibition mediate the radiosensitisation effect of nitric oxide donors on prostate cancer under varying oxygen conditions. Biochem Pharmacol. 2011;81(2):203–10.

41. Zölzer F, Streffer C. Increased radiosensitivity with chronic hypoxia in four human tumor cell lines. Int J Radiat Oncol Biol Phys. 2002;54(3):910–20.

42. Thompson HF, Butterworth KT, McMahon SJ, Ghita M, Hounsell AR, Prise KM. The impact of hypoxia on out-of-field cell survival after exposure to modulated radiation fields. Radiat Res. 2017;188(6):636–44.

43. Harrington KJ, Billingham LJ, Brunner TB, Burnet NG, Chan CS, Hoskin P, et al. Guidelines for preclinical and early phase clinical assessment of novel radiosensitisers. Br J Cancer. 2011;105(5):628–39.

44. Sorensen BS, Busk M, Olthof N, Speel EJ, Horsman MR, Alsner J, et al. Radiosensitivity and effect of hypoxia in HPV positive head and neck cancer cells. Radiother Oncol. 2013;108(3):500–5.

45. Pauwels B, Korst AE, Lardon F, Vermorken JB. Combined modality therapy of gemcitabine and radiation. Oncologist. 2005;10(1):34–51.

46. Valdes G, Iwamoto KS. Re-evaluation of cellular radiosensitization by 5-fluorouracil: high-dose, pulsed administration is effective and preferable to conventional low-dose, chronic administration. Int J Radiat Biol. 2013;89(10):851–62.

47. Gerasimenko JV, Gerasimenko OV, Palejwala A, Tepikin AV, Petersen OH, Watson AJ. Menadione-induced apoptosis: roles of cytosolic Ca(2+) elevations and the mitochondrial permeability transition pore. J Cell Sci. 2002;115(Pt 3):485–97.

48. Loor G, Kondapalli J, Schriewer JM, Chandel NS, Vanden Hoek TL, Schumacker PT. Menadione triggers cell death through ROS-dependent mechanisms involving PARP activation without requiring apoptosis. Free Radical Biol Med. 2010;49(12):1925–36.

49. Na YR, Han KC, Park H, Yang EG. Menadione and ethacrynic acid inhibit the hypoxia-inducible factor (HIF) pathway by disrupting HIF-1alpha interaction with p300. Biochem Biophys Res Commun. 2013;434(4):879–84.

50. Jamison JM, Gilloteaux J, Taper HS, Summers JL. Evaluation of the in vitro and in vivo antitumor activities of vitamin C and K-3 combinations against human prostate cancer. J Nutr. 2001;131(1):158s-s160.

51. Tareen B, Summers JL, Jamison JM, Neal DR, McGuire K, Gerson L, et al. A 12 week, open label, phase I/IIa study using apatone for the treatment of prostate cancer patients who have failed standard therapy. Int J Med Sci. 2008;5(2):62–7.

52. Ruiz van Haperen VW, Veerman G, Vermorken JB, Peters GJ. 2',2'-Difluorodeoxycytidine (gemcitabine) incorporation into RNA and DNA of tumour cell lines. Biochem Pharmacol. 1993;46(4):762–6.

53. Oh KS, Soto DE, Smith DC, Montie JE, Lee CT, Sandler HM. Combined-modality therapy with gemcitabine and radiation therapy as a bladder preservation strategy: long-term results of a phase I trial. Int J Radiat Oncol Biol Phys. 2009;74(2):511–7.

54. Choudhury A, Swindell R, Logue JP, Elliott PA, Livsey JE, Wise M, et al. Phase II study of conformal hypofractionated radiotherapy with concurrent gemcitabine in muscle-invasive bladder cancer. J Clin Oncol. 2011;29(6):733–8.

55. Wouters A, Pauwels B, Burrows N, Baay M, Deschoolmeester V, Vu TN, et al. The radiosensitising effect of gemcitabine and its main metabolite dFdU under low oxygen conditions is in vitro not dependent on functional HIF-1 protein. BMC Cancer. 2014;14:594.

56. Stone KR, Mickey DD, Wunderli H, Mickey GH, Paulson DF. Isolation of a human prostate carcinoma cell line (DU 145). Int J Cancer. 1978;21(3):274–81.

57. Tai S, Sun Y, Squires JM, Zhang H, Oh WK, Liang CZ, et al. PC3 is a cell line characteristic of prostatic small cell carcinoma. Prostate. 2011;71(15):1668–79.

58. Nadal R, Schweizer M, Kryvenko ON, Epstein JI, Eisenberger MA. Small cell carcinoma of the prostate. Nat Rev Urol. 2014;11(4):213–9.

59. Jonsson M, Ragnum HB, Julin CH, Yeramian A, Clancy T, Frikstad KM, et al. Hypoxia-independent gene expression signature associated with radiosensitisation of prostate cancer cell lines by histone deacetylase inhibition. Br J Cancer. 2016;115(8):929–39.

60. Ashton TM, Fokas E, Kunz-Schughart LA, Folkes LK, Anbalagan S, Huether M, et al. The anti-malarial atovaquone increases radiosensitivity by alleviating tumour hypoxia. Nat Commun. 2016;7:12308.

15

Carbon ion radiotherapy for prostate cancer with bladder invasion

Yuhei Miyasaka[1,2], Hidemasa Kawamura[1,2*] ⓘ, Hiro Sato[1,2], Nobuteru Kubo[1,2], Tatsuji Mizukami[1,3], Hiroshi Matsui[2,4], Yoshiyuki Miyazawa[4], Kazuto Ito[4,5], Takashi Nakano[1,6], Kazuhiro Suzuki[2,4] and Tatsuya Ohno[1,2]

Abstract

Background: The optimal management of clinical T4 (cT4) prostate cancer (PC) is still uncertain. At our institution, carbon ion radiotherapy (CIRT) for nonmetastatic PC, including tumors invading the bladder, has been performed since 2010. Since carbon ion beams provide a sharp dose distribution with minimal penumbra and have biological advantages over photon radiotherapy, CIRT may provide a therapeutic benefit for PC with bladder invasion. Hence, we evaluated CIRT for PC with bladder invasion in terms of the safety and efficacy.

Methods: Between March 2010 and December 2016, a total of 1337 patients with nonmetastatic PC received CIRT at a total dose of 57.6 Gy (RBE) in 16 fractions over 4 weeks. Among them, seven patients who had locally advanced PC with bladder invasion were identified. Long-term androgen-deprivation therapy (ADT) was also administered to these patients. Adverse events were graded according to the Common Terminology Criteria for Adverse Event version 5.0.

Results: At the completion of our study, all the patients with cT4 PC were alive with a median follow-up period of 78 months. Grade 2 acute urinary disorders were observed in only one patient. Regarding late toxicities, only one patient developed grade 2 hematuria and urinary urgency. There was no grade 3 or worse toxicity, and gastrointestinal toxicity was not observed. Six (85.7%) patients had no recurrence or metastasis. One patient had biochemical and local failures 42 and 45 months after CIRT, respectively. However, the recurrent disease has been well controlled by salvage ADT.

Conclusions: Seven patients with locally advanced PC invading the bladder treated with CIRT were evaluated. Our findings seem to suggest positive safety and efficacy profiles for CIRT.

Keywords: Carbon ion radiotherapy, Prostate cancer, Bladder invasion

Background

Localized prostate cancer (PC) is generally treated with radical prostatectomy, external beam radiotherapy (EBRT), and brachytherapy, with or without androgen-deprivation therapy (ADT) [1]. Although favorable clinical outcomes following these treatments are well known, in the case of locally advanced PC invading adjacent structures, that is, clinical T4 (cT4) PC, the prognosis is not satisfactory [2]. A recent study reported that the addition of local therapy, such as surgery and radiotherapy (RT) to systemic therapy, including ADT, provides a survival benefit even for cT4 PC [3]. Therefore, optimization of these local therapies is of importance in the management of cT4 PC.

Carbon ion radiotherapy (CIRT), which is one of the modalities of EBRT initiated at the National Institute of Radiological Sciences in 1994 in Japan, provides a sharp dose distribution with minimal penumbra and has biological advantages due to its high relative biological

*Correspondence: kawa@gunma-u.ac.jp
[1] Department of Radiation Oncology, Gunma University Graduate School of Medicine, 3-39-22, Showa-machi, Maebashi, Gunma 371–8511, Japan
Full list of author information is available at the end of the article
This article belongs to the Topical Collection: Urological oncology.

effectiveness (RBE) in the Bragg Peak, resulting from a high linear energy transfer [4]. At our institution, the Gunma University Heavy Ion Medical Center, CIRT for localized PC, including tumors invading bladder, has been performed since March 2010. Previous studies showed that CIRT for localized PC was a safe and effective treatment [5–9], but these studies did not include cT4 disease. Considering that CIRT has physical and biological advantages over photon radiotherapy, CIRT may provide therapeutic benefits even for the progressive PC. To evaluate this, we retrospectively reviewed patients with locally advanced PC with bladder invasion treated with CIRT.

Methods
Patients

Between March 2010 and December 2016, a total of 1337 patients with clinically nonmetastatic PC received CIRT at our institution. All the patients were pathologically diagnosed with adenocarcinoma. All pre-treatment biopsy specimens were re-evaluated by a central pathologist at Gunma University Hospital. Tumor grades were decided according to the modified Gleason grading system proposed by the International Society of Urological Pathology [10]. Urological examination, trans-rectal ultrasonography, computed tomography (CT), magnetic resonance imaging (MRI), and bone scintigraphy were performed for staging. Cystoscopic examination was performed when the diagnosis of bladder invasion and/or the invaded regions was difficult to confirm by radiographic examinations. Assessing these findings, the institutional cancer board with urological oncologists, radiologists, and radiation oncologists participated in diagnosing clinical stages of PC according to the International Union Against Cancer TNM classification (2002). In this study, we evaluated patients who had locally advanced PC with bladder invasion and without invasion to the rectum, pelvic floor muscles, and pelvic wall. Bladder invasion was diagnosed based on cystoscopic findings in principle; in cases when cystoscopy was not performed before ADT and when there were no apparent cystoscopic findings after ADT, MRI findings before ADT were used for the diagnosis. All the treatment plans were approved by the institutional conference before carrying out the actual treatment.

Carbon ion radiotherapy

CIRT was performed at a total dose of 57.6 Gy (RBE) in 16 fractions over 4 weeks, with a fractional dose of 3.6 Gy (RBE) at four treatment sessions per week. The prescribed dose was according to previous studies on CIRT [7, 8]. Details of CIRT techniques have been previously reported [9]. The patients were positioned in a customized cradle (Moldcare; Alocare, Tokyo, Japan) with a low-temperature thermoplastic sheet (Shellfitter; Kuraray, Co., Ltd., Osaka, Japan). The bladder was filled with 100 mL 0.9% sterile saline, and the rectum was emptied using an enema just before CT simulation. Treatment planning was performed with Xio-N (Elekta, Stockholm, Sweden and Mitsubishi Electric, Tokyo, Japan) using a set of images of 2-mm-thick CT fused with MRI. Clinical target volume (CTV) included whole prostate, proximal seminal vesicle (SV), and bladder wall, which tumors invaded before ADT. For the tumor invading SV, CTV was expanded to include at least the invaded SV. The planning target volume (PTV1) for the initial nine fractions included CTV plus anterior and lateral margins of 10 mm, cranial and caudal margins of 6 mm, posterior margin of 5 mm, and lateral margins to seminal vesicle of 3 mm. The second PTV (PTV2) for the latter seven fractions was generated by cutting the posterior PTV margin in front of the anterior wall of the rectum [7]. Each field was using a spread-out Bragg peak, which was shaped with multi-leaf collimators and compensation bolus for each patient. Three radiation ports were used in the bilateral and anterior directions. At each treatment session using the anterior port, the bladder was filled with 100 mL 0.9% sterile saline.

Androgen deprivation therapy

ADT was administered to all the patients for a minimum of 24 months. Patients recieved combined androgen blockade therapy (CAB) consisting of luteinizing hormone-releasing hormone (LH-RH) agonist or antagonist, and antiandrogen for at least 5 months before CIRT and during CIRT. After completing CIRT, all the patients recieved an adjuvant LH-RH agonist or antagonist monotherapy.

Followup and clinical evaluation

All patients were followed up by physical examination and blood test, including PSA and urine test, at 3-month intervals; CT, MRI, bone scintigraphy, and trans-rectal ultrasonography were performed once a year for 5 years. Adverse events (AE) were evaluated according to the Common Terminology Criteria for Adverse Events (CTCAE) version 5.0 [11]. Biochemical failure was defined in accordance with the Radiation Therapy Oncology Group-Association of Therapeutic Radiation Oncology Phoenix Consensus Conference definition [12].

Results
Patients' characteristics

Seven patients who had locally advanced PC with bladder invasion were identified from the medical record. The patients' characteristics are summarized in Table 1. The

Table 1 Summary of the patients' characteristics.

Patient number	1	2	3	4	5	6	7
Seminal vesicle invasion	+	+	−	+	−	+	+
Gleason score	5+4	4+3	4+3	5+4	4+5	5+4	4+5
Positive cores	8/8	10/10	4/8	6/10	8/8	10/12	10/12
Initial PSA (ng/mL)	11.6	87	37.3	32.1	73.7	7.8	9.39
ADT duration before CIRT (months)	12	5	6	6	6	6	12
Total ADT duration (months)	40	24	28	32	25	46	33

PSA Prostate-specific antigen, *ADT* Androgen deprivation therapy, *CIRT* Carbon ion radiotherapy

median follow-up period was 78 months (range 37–109). The median age at diagnosis was 65 years (range 53–81). The median initial prostate-specific antigen (PSA) level was 32.1 ng/ml (range 7.8–87.0). Three patients (42.9%) had primary Gleason pattern 5. Five patients (71%) had seminal vesicle invasion. Three patients were diagnosed with bladder invasion by cystoscopic findings, while four patients were diagnosed by MRI findings. The median total duration of the ADT was 32 months (range 24–46).

Clinical outcomes

The clinical courses of the patients with locally advanced PC are summarized in Table 2. All the patients are alive and being followed-up. There was no grade 3 or worse AE. Acute urinary disorder was seen in four patients (#2, #3, #6, #7). One of these patients (#3) needed an alpha-blocker for urinary frequency. As for late toxicity, one patient (#6) complained about urinary urgency; thus, requiring medication. The patient took aspirin and developed hematuria 16 months after receiving CIRT. However, this AE was easily dealt with using a hemostatic agent (carbazochrome sodium sulfonate hydrate) and was never observed again. Two other patients have also taken medication, which increased the risk of bleeding (cilostazol and ethyl icosapentate), but they had no hematuria induced by CIRT. There were no gastrointestinal AE in these seven patients. After the termination of ADT, six patients were tested for serum testosterone, and the recoveries to the standard value were observed. One patient who was not tested for testosterone presented with a slight increase in PSA within the Phoenix definition and thus was considered to recover from the castration status. Only one patient had a recurrence. A patient (#2) had biochemical and local failure 42 and 45 months after CIRT, respectively. The serum testosterone level was 2.28 ng/mL when there was a clinical failure. The recurrent tumor was detected at the original site, and there was no metastatic disease. Salvage CAB was administered to the patient, after which the recurrent disease was undetected on MRI, and serum PSA level monotonically decreased to less than 0.1 ng/ml and remained low

thereafter. The other patients have had no evidence of the disease.

A representative case: Patient #1

In July of 20XX, a Japanese man in his 50 s diagnosed with PC was referred to our institution since he desired to receive CIRT. At that time, approximately 10 months of CAB consisting of leuprorelin acetate and bicalutamide had already reduced serum PSA from 11.8 ng/mL (September of 20XX-1) to <0.01 ng/mL (August of 20XX), but cystoscopic findings clearly showed tumor invading the bladder neck. The institutional cancer board diagnosed the clinical stage as cT4N0M0 by checking the CT images, MRI, bone scintigraphy, and cystoscopic findings (Fig. 1a, d). The tumor also invaded the right seminal vesicle. Pre-treatment biopsy specimens were reviewed by a central pathologist. Tumor cells were found in all the cores (8/8), and the Gleason score was diagnosed as 5+4=9.

CIRT was performed at a total dose of 57.6 Gy (RBE) in 16 fractions over 4 weeks from October to November of 20XX. Figure 2 shows the dose distribution. During this treatment period, dermatitis (grade 1) was observed in the irradiated region. There was no other acute toxicity.

After completion of CIRT, bicalutamide was discontinued. Blood and urine tests were performed every 3 months, and CT, MRI, bone scintigraphy, and transrectal ultrasonography were performed once a year for 5 years. Chronological changes in MRI findings are shown in Fig. 1b, c. Serum PSA levels were kept under 0.01 ng/mL till ADT was finished. The cystoscopic findings on April of 20XX+2 showed that the bladder lesion shrank but remained (Fig. 1e). Six months later, as similar findings were found in the cystoscopic examination, a transurethral resection biopsy was performed. The biopsy findings showed urothelial mucosa with xanthogranulomatous lesions and no malignant cells (Fig. 1f). After discussion with urological oncologists in Gunma University Hospital, leuprorelin acetate was discontinued on December of 20XX+2. Thereafter, the serum PSA level was still well controlled. Approximately 9 years after

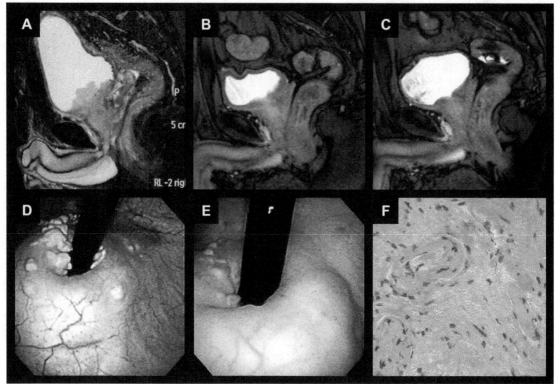

Fig. 1   Magnetic resonance imaging (MRI), cystoscopic, and pathological findings of the representative case. Fat-saturated T2-weighted images **a** before ADT, **b** just before carbon ion radiotherapy (CIRT), and **c** 2 years after CIRT. Cystoscopic findings **d** just before CIRT and **e** one and half a year after CIRT. **f** Hematoxylin-Eosin stain of biopsy sample from the bladder lesion 2 years after CIRT in a high-power field. There were no malignant cells

CIRT, there have been no findings suggesting recurrence or metastasis. No late toxicity was observed.

Discussion

In the management of cT4 PC, the addition of local therapy to systemic therapy was associated with improved survival compared to systemic therapy alone [3], but the optimal local therapy has not yet been established. We have treated locally advanced PC invading the bladder with CIRT with long-term ADT, expecting that the physical and biological advantages of CIRT over photon RT would yield therapeutic benefits. Thus, we evaluated the safety and efficacy of the CIRT in the current study. To the best of our knowledge, this is the first report describing CIRT with long-term ADT for locally advanced PC with bladder invasion. Our findings showed that none of the seven patients had severe toxicity, and six (85.7%) patients had no recurrence or metastasis with a median follow-up period of 78 months.

There are limited literature on the surgery for cT4 PC [13]. Hajili et al. showed that the prostate cancer-specific survival (PCSS) rates for cT4 PC at 150 months after inductive ADT and subsequent RP were 82%,

and 10.3% of the patients had complications requiring surgical intervention [14]. Kumazawa et al. reported cystoprostatectomy followed by immediate hormone therapy for cT4N0M0 disease. In their study, the PCSS rate at 5 years after the surgery was 87.1% [15]. These findings showed relatively favorable survival despite the advanced disease, although it should be noted that these surgical indications were limited to patients with good general conditions.

EBRT, which is a less invasive treatment modality compared to surgery, is also recommended for very high-risk PC, including cT4 disease [1]. Furthermore, intensity-modulated radiotherapy (IMRT) and image-guided radiotherapy enable higher doses to tumors with lower doses to organs at risk, resulting in the lower incidence of AE and improved biochemical relapse-free survival (bRFS) [16]. In addition, EBRT with high-dose-rate brachytherapy boost may improve bRFS [17]. To our knowledge, little is known regarding the outcomes of patients with cT4 PC treated with EBRT, although a clinical trial to analyze whether surgical treatment or EBRT using photons is the better treatment for cT4 PC is undergoing [18].

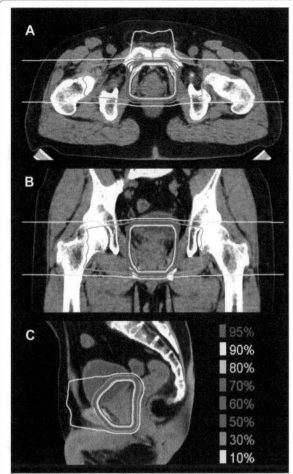

Fig. 2 Dose distribution of carbon ion radiotherapy. **a** Axial, **b** coronal, and **c** sagittal images. Highlighted are 95% (red), 90% (yellow), 80% (green), 70% (blue), 60% (pink), 50% (purple), 30% (light purple), and 10% (cyan) isodose curves

CIRT, a kind of EBRT, contributes to favorable outcomes, especially in advanced PC. Kasuya et al. reported that the prostate cancer-specific mortality at 5 years after CIRT with long-term ADT was 1.5% for high-risk PC [19]. We previously reported that the 5-year biochemical relapse-free rate of high-risk PC was 92.0% in a single-institutional prospective study [9]. The present study showed that 85.7% (6/7) of the patients had no biochemical failure, and all the patients were alive at the median follow-up period of 78 months. We cannot compare these results with those of EBRT due to the lack of available literature specific to cT4 PC, but when compared with the surgical treatment options, our results seem to be favorable, although we acknowledge that the number of patients included in our study is extremely small.

In general, CIRT is also remarkable for the low incidence of late toxicity because of the superior dose accumulation. We previously demonstrated that 9% of the patients had grade 2 late toxicities after CIRT [9], while Cahlon et al. showed that up to 23% of the patients had grade 2 late toxicities after photon-based IMRT [20]. In CIRT for PC with bladder invasion, the irradiated volume of the bladder was larger than that in PC without bladder invasion, which potentially increases the incidence and severity of urinary toxicity. However, with the careful management of inter-fractional displacements mentioned above, there was only one patient with grade 2 late urinary disorder in the current study; thus, supporting that CIRT is tolerable for patients with locally advanced PC with bladder invasion.

These favorable outcomes of the present study may be due to the physical and biological advantages of CIRT over photon RT, which may have provided therapeutic benefits for locally advanced PC. Although our findings provide only the weakest evidence, we are encouraged to further explore the safety and efficacy of CIRT for PC with bladder invasion in larger cohorts.

Table 2 Summary of the clinical course

Patient number	1	2	3	4	5	6	7
Follow-up (months)	109	96	96	78	66	66	37
Alive/ Dead	Alive	Alive	Alive	Alive	Alive	Alive	Alive
Biochemical failure	−	+	−	−	−	−	−
Local failure	−	+	−	−	−	−	−
Distant failure	−	−	−	−	−	−	−
Acute toxicity (max grade)							
Genitourinary	0	1	2	0	0	1	1
Gastrointestinal	0	0	0	0	0	0	0
Late toxicity (max grade)							
Genitourinary	0	0	1	0	0	2	1
Gastrointestinal	0	0	0	0	0	0	0

The present study has some limitations. As mentioned above, this is a case series report with an extremely small number of patients; thus, some potential sources of bias were not excluded. In addition, the effects of clinical and pathological factors, such as age, initial PSA level, Gleason score, the number of positive cores in biopsy samples, and the duration of ADT, were not evaluated in this study. Larger cohort is required to evaluate these factors.

Conclusions

In summary, we report seven patients with locally advanced PC with bladder invasion who received CIRT with long-term ADT, with well tolerable toxicity and favorable prognoses. Our study only provides the weakest evidence because of the extremely small study population without control, but CIRT with long-term ADT seems to be a potential treatment option. For more reliable evidence, further studies are required.

Abbreviations

AE: Adverse event; ADT: Androgen-deprivation therapy; bRFS: Biochemical relapse-free survival; CT: Computed tomography; CAB: Combined androgen blockade; CIRT: Carbon ion radiotherapy; CTCAE: The Common Terminology Criteria for Adverse Event; CTV: Clinical target volume; cT4: Clinical T4; EBRT: External beam radiotherapy; IMRT: Intensity-modulated radiotherapy; PC: Prostate cancer; LH-RH: Luteinizing hormone-releasing hormone; MRI: Magnetic resonance imaging; RBE: Relative biological effectiveness; RT: Radiotherapy; PCSS: Prostate cancer-specific survival; PSA: Prostate-specific antigen; PTV: Planning target volume; SV: Seminal vesicle.

Acknowledgements

Not applicable.

Authors' contributions

HK, TN, KS, and TO designed, directed, and coordinated this study. YM (Yuhei Miyasaka), HS, and TM performed data collecting. YM (Yuhei Miyasaka) wrote the draft. HK, HS, NK, YM (Yoshiyuki Miyazawa), HM, KI, and KS suggested corrections and/or improvements. All authors have read and approved the manuscript.

Author details

[1]Department of Radiation Oncology, Gunma University Graduate School of Medicine, 3-39-22, Showa-machi, Maebashi, Gunma 371–8511, Japan. [2]Gunma University Heavy Ion Medical Center, Maebashi, Japan. [3]Division of Radiation Oncology, Department of Radiology, Faculty of Medicine, Academic Assembly, University of Toyama, Toyama, Japan. [4]Department of Urology, Gunma University Graduate School of Medicine, Maebashi, Japan. [5]Kurosawa Hospital, Takasaki, Japan. [6]Quantum Medical Science Directorate, National Institutes for Quantum and Radiological Science and Technology, Chiba, Japan.

References

1. National Comprehensive Cancer Network (NCCN) Guidelines; Prostate Cancer version 2. 2019. https://www.nccn.org/professionals/physician_gls/pdf/prostate.pdf. Accessed 18 Jul 2019.
2. Hsiao W, Moses KA, Goodman M, Jani AB, Rossi PJ, Master VA. Stage IV prostate cancer: Survival differences in clinical t4, nodal and metastatic disease. J Urol. 2010;184:512–8.
3. Kim AH, Konety B, Chen Z, Schumacher F, Kutikov A, Smaldone M, et al. Comparative Effectiveness of Local and Systemic Therapy for T4 Prostate Cancer. Urology. 2018;120:173–9.
4. Kanai T, Endo M, Minohara S, Miyahara N, Koyama-Ito H, Tomura H, et al. Biophysical characteristics of HIMAC clinical irradiation system for heavy-ion radiation therapy. Int J Radiat Oncol Biol Phys. 1999;44:201–10.
5. Tsuji H, Yanagi T, Ishikawa H, Kamada T, Mizoe JE, Kanai T, et al. Hypofractionated radiotherapy with carbon ion beams for prostate cancer. Int J Radiat Oncol Biol Phys. 2005;63:1153–60.
6. Ishikawa H, Tsuji H, Kamada T, Yanagi T, Mizoe JE, Kanai T, et al. Carbon ion radiation therapy for prostate cancer: Results of a prospective phase II study. Radiother Oncol. 2006;81:57–64.
7. Okada T, Tsuji H, Kamada T, Akakura K, Suzuki H, Shimazaki J, et al. Carbon Ion Radiotherapy in Advanced Hypofractionated Regimens for Prostate Cancer: From 20 to 16 Fractions Radiation Oncology. Int J Radiat Oncol Biol Phys. 2012;84:968–72.
8. Nomiya T, Tsuji H, Maruyama K, Toyama S, Suzuki H, Akakura K, et al. Phase I/II trial of definitive carbon ion radiotherapy for prostate cancer: evaluation of shortening of treatment period to 3 weeks. Br J Cancer. 2014;110:2389–95.
9. Kawamura H, Kubo N, Sato H, Mizukami T, Katoh H, Ishikawa H, et al. Moderately hypofractionated carbon ion radiotherapy for prostate cancer: a prospective observational study "GUNMA0702." BMC Cancer. 2020;20:75.
10. Epstein JI, Allsbrook WC, Amin MB, Egevad LL, Bastacky S, López Beltrán A, et al. The 2005 International Society of Urological Pathology (ISUP) consensus conference on Gleason grading of prostatic carcinoma. Am J Surg Pathol. 2005;29:1228–42.
11. NCI Common Terminology Criteria for Adverse Events (CTCAE) v5.0 data files. 2020. https://evs.nci.nih.gov/ftp1/CTCAE/About.html. Accessed 31 May 2020.
12. Roach M, Hanks G, Thames H, Schellhammer P, Shipley WU, Sokol GH, et al. Defining biochemical failure following radiotherapy with or without hormonal therapy in men with clinically localized prostate cancer: Recommendations of the RTOG-ASTRO Phoenix Consensus Conference. Int J Radiat Oncol. 2006;65:965–74.
13. Yuan P, Wang S, Liu X, Wang X, Ye Z, Chen Z. The role of cystoprostatectomy in management of locally advanced prostate cancer: A systematic review. World J Surg Oncol. 2020;18:1–7.
14. Hajili T, Ohlmann CH, Linxweiler J, Niklas C, Janssen M, Siemer S, et al. Radical prostatectomy in T4 prostate cancer after inductive androgen deprivation: results of a single-institution series with long-term follow-up. BJU Int. 2019;123:58–64.
15. Kumazawa T, Tsuchiya N, Saito M, Inoue T, Narita S, Horikawa Y, et al. Cystoprostatectomy as a treatment of prostate cancer involving the bladder neck. Urol Int. 2009;83:141–5.
16. Hatano K, Tohyama N, Kodama T, Okabe N, Sakai M, Konoeda K. Current status of intensity-modulated radiation therapy for prostate cancer: History, clinical results and future directions. Int J Urol. 2019;26:775–84.
17. Hoskin PJ, Rojas AM, Bownes PJ, Lowe GJ, Ostler PJ, Bryant L. Randomised trial of external beam radiotherapy alone or combined with high-dose-rate brachytherapy boost for localised prostate cancer. Radiother Oncol. 2012;103:217–22.
18. Ranasinghe WKB, Reichard CA, Bathala T, Chapin BF. Management of cT4 Prostate Cancer. Eur Urol. 2020;6:221–6.
19. Kasuya G, Ishikawa H, Tsuji H, Nomiya T, Makishima H, Kamada T, et al. Significant impact of biochemical recurrence on overall mortality in patients with high-risk prostate cancer after carbon-ion radiotherapy combined with androgen deprivation therapy. Cancer. 2016;122:3225–31.
20. Cahlon O, Hunt M, Zelefsky MJ. Intensity-Modulated Radiation Therapy: Supportive Data for Prostate Cancer. Semin Radiat Oncol. 2008;18:48–57.

16

Usefulness of the prostate health index in predicting the presence and aggressiveness of prostate cancer among Korean men

Jae Yoon Kim[1†], Ji Hyeong Yu[1†], Luck Hee Sung[1], Dae Yeon Cho[1], Hyun-Jung Kim[2] and Soo Jin Yoo[3*]

Abstract

Background: We aimed to evaluate the usefulness of the Beckman Coulter prostate health index (PHI) and to compare it with total prostate-specific antigen (PSA) levels and related derivatives in predicting the presence and aggressiveness of prostate cancer (PCa) in the Korean population.

Methods: A total of 140 men who underwent their first prostate biopsy for suspected PCa were included in this prospective observational study. The diagnostic performance of total PSA, free PSA, %free PSA, [–2] proPSA (p2PSA), %p2PSA, and PHI in detecting and predicting the aggressiveness of PCa was estimated using the receiver operating characteristic curve (ROC) and logistic multivariate regression analyses.

Results: Of 140 patients, PCa was detected in 63 (45%) of participants, and 48 (76.2%) of them had significant cancer with a Gleason score (GS) $\geq$ 7. In the whole group, the area under the curve (AUC) for ROC analysis of tPSA, free PSA, %fPSA, p2PSA, %p2PSA, and PHI were 0.63, 0.57, 0.69, 0.69, 0.72, and 0.76, respectively, and the AUC was significantly greater in the PHI group than in the tPSA group ($p = 0.005$). For PCa with GS $\geq$ 7, the AUCs for tPSA, free PSA, %fPSA, p2PSA, %p2PSA, and PHI were 0.62, 0.58, 0.41, 0.79, 0.86, and 0.87, respectively, and the AUC was significantly greater in the PHI group than in the tPSA group ($p < 0.001$). In the subgroup with tPSA 4–10 ng/mL, both %p2PSA and PHI were strong independent predictors for PCa ($p = 0.007$, $p = 0.006$) and significantly improved the predictive accuracy of a base multivariable model, including age, tPSA, fPSA and %fPSA, using multivariate logistic regression analysis. ($p = 0.054$, $p = 0.048$). Additionally, at a cutoff PHI value > 33.4, 22.9% (32/140) of biopsies could be avoided without missing any cases of aggressive cancer.

Conclusions: This study shows that %p2PSA and PHI are superior to total PSA and %fPSA in predicting the presence and aggressiveness (GS $\geq$ 7) of PCa among Korean men. Using PHI, a significant proportion of unnecessary biopsies can be avoided.

Keywords: Prostate health index, Prostate-specific antigen, Prostate cancer, Korean

*Correspondence: sjyoo@paik.ac.kr
†Jae Yoon Kim and Ji Hyeong Yu contributed equally to this work as first authors
3 Department of Laboratory Medicine, Sanggye Paik Hospital, Inje University College of Medicine, 1342 Dongil-ro, Nowon-gu, Seoul 01757, Republic of Korea
Full list of author information is available at the end of the article

Background

Prostate cancer (PCa) is the second most common cancer in the Western population [1].

In Korea, the incidence of PCa has steadily increased, and it is now the fifth most common cancer among men [2]. Several studies have demonstrated that PCa in Korean men shows worse disease characteristics [3]. Kang and colleagues demonstrated that Koreans had higher T stages compared to their American counterparts ($p = 0.021$) and higher Gleason scores compared to Americans in all age groups. Moreover, Koreans also had higher Gleason scores compared to Americans for PSA > 10 ng/mL ($p < 0.05$) in their study.

A large proportion of PCa cases diagnosed in the Korean population show poor differentiation compared to their American counterparts [4]. Therefore, the accuracy of diagnosis and risk stratification of PCa using appropriate biomarkers may be more important for suitable treatment in the Korean population.

Total prostate-specific antigen (tPSA) is a widely used tumour marker for the screening, diagnosis, monitoring, and prognosis of PCa worldwide [5]. The introduction of tPSA has resulted in increased early detection of PCa and reduced mortality [6]. In the early diagnosis of PCa using tPSA, the main problem was that the low positive predictive value (PPV) of tPSA resulted in unnecessary biopsies [7]. The positive rate for cancer at biopsy was approximately 25% among the population with PSA levels of 2–10 µg/L.

In addition, PSA cannot accurately identify aggressive PCa, which has clinical significance for treatment. Consequently, the wide application of PSA in detecting PCa has increased concerns about over-diagnosis and over-treatment [8].

Therefore, the development of new biomarkers is needed to improve the detection of PCa and to discriminate clinically significant and insignificant PCa.

Several studies have performed PSA isoform assays to overcome the limitations of PSA. Free PSA (fPSA) consists of three different forms: benign PSA, intact inactive PSA, and proPSA. The subfraction of proPSA has several molecular isoforms, [−2], [−4], and [−5, −7] proPSA [9].

Previous studies have demonstrated a significantly increased detection rate for PCa by measuring [−2] proPSA (p2PSA), especially the derivatives %p2PSA (p2PSA/fPSA) and prostate health index (PHI), which is a mathematical combination of tPSA, fPSA, and p2PSA [10, 11]. Additionally, recent studies demonstrated that %p2PSA and PHI showed superior performance to tPSA or %fPSA (fPSA/tPSA) in predicting PCa aggressiveness [12].

The aim of this prospective, observational study was to investigate the usefulness of p2PSA and its derived %p2PSA and PHI in the detection of PCa and to discriminate clinically significant PCa in Korean patients by estimating its ability to avoid unnecessary biopsies.

Methods

The study included consecutive men who underwent their first prostate biopsy between April 2016 and July 2019. The indications for prostate biopsies were any one

of the following: serum tPSA > 3.0 ng/mL, presence of a palpable nodule on prostate digital rectal examination, and observation of hypoechoic findings on transrectal prostate ultrasonography. Exclusion criteria were medical therapies or procedures that might affect PSA levels, acute prostate inflammation, or urinary tract infection in the 3 months prior to biopsy. Patients who underwent prostate biopsy or were treated with any 5-alpha-reductase inhibitors were excluded.

Blood samples were collected to measure the pre-biopsy tPSA, fPSA, and p2PSA levels prior to prostate biopsy. The blood was processed to clot for 1 h at room temperature, followed by centrifugation for 15 min. The sera were aliquoted and frozen at -80° C and processed on an Access 2 immunoassay system (Beckman Coulter, Brea, CA, USA) using dedicated Access tPSA, fPSA, and p2PSA reagents. %p2PSA was calculated using the formula [(p2PSA pg/mL)/ (fPSA ng/mL × 1000)] × 100, and PHI using the formula [(p2PSA pg/ mL)/(fPSA ng/mL] × $\sqrt{tPSA}$.

The patients then underwent transrectal ultrasound-guided prostate biopsies following a standardised extended scheme with at least 12 biopsy cores obtained from the prostate gland and additional cores taken when other areas were suspected. The specimens were inspected by a genitourinary pathologist who was blinded to the results of the blood test. PCa was confirmed and graded according to the definitions of the International Society of Urological Pathology.

The primary endpoint was comparison of accuracy of the diagnostic performance of %p2PSA and PHI with that of tPSA and %fPSA, which are currently widely used biomarkers in detecting PCa at biopsy. The secondary endpoint was the predictive ability of these biomarkers to discriminate aggressive PCa with a Gleason score (GS) ≥ 7.

Quantitative data are presented as median (interquartile range) and categorical data as numbers (n) and percentages. The normal distribution of variables was assessed using the Kolmogorov-Smirnov test. Student's t-test was used for comparisons of parametric variables, and the Mann-Whitney U-test for non-parametric continuous variables. Bivariate and multivariate logistic regression analyses were used to determine the association between the biomarkers and the presence of PCa in the whole group and subgroup with PSA 4–10 and PCa with GS ≥ 7 at biopsy.

These markers were added to the base multivariate model, including age, tPSA, fPSA and %fPSA, to evaluate the usefulness of %p2PSA and PHI in predicting the presence of PCa. The improvement in predictive accuracy was measured as the area under the curve (AUC) of the receiver operating characteristic (ROC) analysis. The

DeLong method was used to compare the statistical differences between the AUCs. Odds ratios (ORs) with 95% confidence intervals were determined.

Statistical analyses were conducted using SPSS Statistics version 26 (IBM Corp., Armonk, NY, USA). Statistical significance was set at $p < 0.05$. AUC comparisons were conducted using MedCalc software 19.4 (MedCalc Software, Mariakerke, Belgium).

The study protocol was approved by the Institutional Review Board (IRB) of the Sanngye Paik Hospital, Inje University. All participants provided written informed consent before participation in the study. All methods were carried out in accordance with relevant guidelines and regulations.

Results

A total of 140 men who underwent their first prostate biopsy with positive or negative prostate biopsy between April 2016 and July 2019 were included in this study. The demographic and clinical characteristics of the study participants are summarised in Table 1. The range of tPSA levels was 0.82–23.9 ng/mL for those without cancer and 1.63–91.7 ng/mL for those with cancer. Among all patients, 77 men had a tPSA level between 4 and 10 ng/mL. PCa at the initial biopsy was detected in 45% (63/140) of the patients. Among 63 patients diagnosed with PCa, 15 (23.8%) had GS 6 disease, 18 (28.6%) had GS 7 disease, and 30 (47.6%) had GS $\geq$ 8 disease.

Patients with PCa showed significantly higher age, tPSA, %p2PSA, and PHI compared to those without PCa

Table 1 Demographic and clinical characteristics of all study subjects who underwent the first prostate biopsy

	Total	No cancer	Cancer	P value
	N, 140	N, 77 (55%)	N, 63 (45%)	–
Age, yr	69.0 (10.0)	67.0 (9.0)	72.0 (10.0)	**0.001**
tPSA, ng/mL	6.93 (6.05)	6.45 (3.8)	8.18 (15.3)	**0.010**
fPSA	1.03 (0.92)	0.92 (0.8)	1.07 (1.4)	0.160
%fPSA	14.55 (9.29)	17.13 (8.0)	11.16 (9.0)	**0.003**
p2PSA, pg/mL	19.18 (30.97)	15.54 (16.7)	31.06 (58.6)	**<0.001**
%p2PSA	2.02 (2.21)	1.57 (1.5)	2.83 (2.6)	**<0.001**
PHI	45.90 (82.72)	39.54 (38.0)	91.18 (147.9)	**<0.001**
Positive core number	–	–	5.0 (7.0)	–
Number (percentage)				
GS 6%	–	–	15 (23.8%)	–
GS 7			18 (28.6%)	–
GS $\geq$ 8			30 (47.6%)	–

Data are shown as median (interquartile range), or number (%)

PSA, prostate-specific antigen; tPSA, total PSA; fPSA, free PSA; p2PSA, [2]proPSA; PHI, prostate health index; GS, Gleason score

P value to be statiscally significant with bolditalics

Table 2 Descriptive characteristics of subjects with tPSA 4–10 ng/mL

	Total	No cancer	Cancer	P value
	N, 77	N, 48 (62.3%)	N, 29 (37.7%)	–
Age, yr	68.0 (12.0)	66.5 (11.0)	71.0 (12.0)	**0.010**
tPSA, ng/mL	6.41 (2.5)	6.42 (2.3)	6.13 (2.8)	0.877
fPSA	0.92 (0.5)	0.97 (0.6)	0.92 (2.4)	0.185
%fPSA	15.49 (8.6)	16.83 (7.5)	13.04 (7.1)	0.284
p2PSA, pg/mL	16.86 (17.5)	15.34 (16.1)	17.09 (23.7)	0.189
%p2PSA	1.61 (1.6)	1.50 (1.0)	2.35 (2.6)	**0.015**
PHI	41.35 (37.9)	39.65 (28.9)	53.72 (56.8)	**0.018**
Positive core number	–	–	4.0 (7.0)	–
Number (percentage)				
GS 6	–	–	9 (31%)	–
GS 7			10 (34.5%)	–
GS $\geq$ 8			10 (34.5%)	–

Data are shown as median (interquartile range), or number (%)

PSA, prostate-specific antigen; tPSA, total PSA; fPSA, free PSA; p2PSA, [2]proPSA; PHI, prostate health index; GS, Gleason score

P value to be statiscally significant with bolditalics

at biopsy. Conversely, %fPSA levels were significantly higher in patients without PCa. However, the fPSA concentration did not differ between the two groups.

In 77 patients with a tPSA level between 4 and 10 ng/mL, %p2PSA and PHI were significantly different between groups with and without PCa (Table 2). However, the median tPSA, %fPSA, and p2PSA levels did not differ between the two groups.

In the PCa group, 48 (76.2%) patients with GS $\geq$ 7 showed significantly higher %p2PSA (3.17% vs. 1.26%, $p < 0.001$) and PHI (120.8 vs. 35.4, $p < 0.001$) compared to those with GS 6 disease (Table 3). Patients with GS $\geq$ 7 had a more positive core number (6.0 vs. 3.0, $p = 0.032$)

In 140 patients, the AUC for tPSA, fPSA, %fPSA, p2PSA, %p2PSA, and PHI were 0.63, 0.57, 0.69, 0.69, 0.72, and 0.76, respectively (Fig. 1)

Additionally, we analysed the predictive value of individual markers for predicting the probability of PCa for different age groups. Using %p2PSA and PHI had similar predictive values for different age groups, although there were some differences in the predictive value among markers for different age groups (Additional file 1: Table S1).

Using tPSA as a standard, the AUC was significantly greater in the PHI group ($p = 0.005$). Both %p2PSA and PHI were strong independent predictive markers ($p < 0.001, p < 0.001$) and significantly increased the predictive accuracy of a base multivariable model, including age, tPSA, fPSA and %fPSA, using multivariate logistic regression analysis (Table 4).

Table 3 Comparison between GS 6 disease and more aggressive disease in PCa patients

	GS 6	GS ≥ 7	P value
	N, 15 (23.8%)	N, 48 (76.2%)	–
Age, yr	73.0 (9.0)	72.0 (12.0)	*0.520*
tPSA, ng/mL	7.47 (4.6)	9.75 (23.6)	*0.156*
fPSA	0.97 (0.6)	1.13 (1.7)	*0.358*
%fPSA	13.08 (8.0)	10.98 (9.2)	*0.302*
p2PSA, pg/mL	13.9 (13.4)	45.3 (72.6)	***0.001***
%p2PSA	1.26 (1.0)	3.17 (2.2)	***< 0.001***
PHI	35.4 (28.0)	120.8 (148.6)	***< 0.001***
Positive core number	3.0 (4.0)	6.0 (6.0)	***0.032***

Data are shown as median (interquartile range), or number (%)

PSA, prostate-specific antigen; tPSA, total PSA; fPSA = free PSA; p2PSA, [2] proPSA; PHI, prostate health index; GS, Gleason score

P value to be statiscally significant with bolditalics

Similarly, in the subgroup of patients with tPSA 4–10 ng/mL, both %p2PSA and PHI were strong independent predictors ($p = 0.007$, $p = 0.005$) and showed significantly improved predictive accuracy in addition to a base multivariable model using multivariate logistic regression analysis (Table 5).

In Table 6, the results of univariate and multivariable logistic regression analyses identifying the predictors of PCa with a Gleason score ≥ 7 are presented. %p2PSA and PHI significantly improved the predictive accuracy of a base multivariable model. ($p = 0.002$, $p = 0.001$).

Table 7 shows the number of patients in whom unnecessary biopsies could be avoided and the number and pathologic characteristics of cancers that would be missed using %fPSA, p2PSA, %p2PSA, and PHI at a cutoff level with 90% sensitivity in the subgroup with tPSA 4–10 ng/mL and the entire population, respectively.

At a cutoff PHI value of 33.4, 22.9% (32/140) of patients could have avoided unnecessary biopsies without missing any significant aggressive cancers (GS ≥ 7). In the subgroup with tPSA 4–10 ng/mL, the use of %p2PSA (12/77, 15.5%) and PHI (9/77, 11.7%) could have avoided unnecessary biopsies without missing patients with aggressive cancers.

Patients with aggressive cancers had higher PHI scores. Compared to the other markers, the median values of the PHI score showed a more obvious stepwise increase along the Gleason score (Fig. 2).

Discussion

This study evaluated the usefulness of %p2PSA and PHI in 140 subjects, and our findings support previous results regarding both biomarkers. %p2PSA and PHI showed higher predictive performance in the detection of PCa compared to standard reference methods, and they were

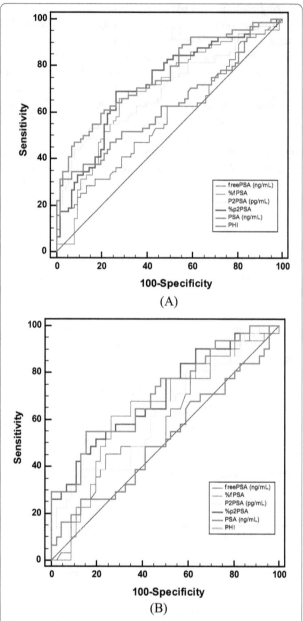

Fig. 1 ROC curves depicting the accuracy of individual predictors of prostate cancer. **A** ROC curves in all subjects. **B** ROC curves in subjects with tPSA 4–10 ng/mL. PSA, prostate-specific antigen; fPSA, free PSA; p2PSA, [-2]proPSA; PHI, prostate health index; ROC, receiver operating characteristic; tPSA, total PSA

better able to distinguish aggressive (GS ≥ 7) from clinically indolent PCa. Thus, their use could avoid unnecessary biopsies without missing clinically significant cancers.

Currently, PSA is widely used for PCa screening, but the limitations of PSA as a biomarker for PCa detection have been well demonstrated. It is necessary to distinguish PCa from benign prostatic disease and to clarify

Table 4 Logistic regression analyses predicting the probability of prostate cancer

Predictors	AUC of individual predictor variable (95% CI); P value*	Bivariate analysis OR(95%CI); P value	Multivariate analysis		
			Base model ** OR (95%CI); P value	Base model + %p2PSA OR (95%CI); P value	Base model + PHI OR (95%CI); P value
Age	0.66 (0.57–0.74) *0.470*	1.077 (1.03–1.13); *0.002*	**1.063 (1.01–1.12); 0.014**	**1.070 (1.02–1.13); 0.011**	**1.068 (1.01–1.13); 0.013**
tPSA, ng/mL	0.63 (0.54 – 0.71) -	1.100 (1.04–1.16); *0.001*	1.064 (0.96–1.18); *0.252*	1.049 (0.95 – 1.16); *0.335*	1.013 (0.93–1.10); *0.761*
fPSA	0.57 (0.48–0.65) *0.117*	1.543 (1.06–2.25); *0.024*	1.036 (0.51–2.10); *0.921*	1.012 (0.52–1.97); *0.971*	0.886 (0.48–1.65); *0.701*
%fPSA	0.69 (0.61–0.77) *0.203*	0.927 (0.88–0.98); *0.004*	0.943 (0.87–1.03); *0.181*	0.947 (0.87–1.03); *0.193*	0.959 (0.89–1.04); *0.294*
p2PSA, pg/mL	0.69 (0.60–0.76) *0.157*	1.021 (1.01–1.04); *0.001*	–	–	–
%p2PSA	0.72 (0.63–0.78) *0.109*	1.708 (1.31–2.22); *< 0.001*	–	**1.550 (1.18–2.04); 0.002**	–
PHI	**0.76 (0.67–0.82) 0.005**	1.017 (1.01–1.02); *< 0.001*	–	–	**1.015 (1.01–1.02); 0.002**
AUC of multivariate models (95% CI);	–	–	0.736 (0.66–0.81) *< 0.001*	0.793 (0.72–0.86) *< 0.001*	0.796 (0.72–0.86) *< 0.001*
Gain in predictive accuracy (95% CI); P value	–	–	–	**0.056 (− 0.0–0.11); 0.058**	**0.060 (0.00–0.12); 0.037**

AUC, area under the receiver operating characteristic curve; PSA, prostate-specific antigen; fPSA, free PSA; p2PSA, [-2]proPSA; PHI, prostate health index; tPSA, total PSA; OR, odds ratio; CI, confidence interval

*P value: Comparison of AUC using tPSA as standard

**Base model includes age, tPSA, fPSA and %fPSA

P value to be statiscally significant with bolditalics

the aggressiveness of cancers, but PSA cannot completely predict the presence and biological behaviour of PCa [13]. The early detection of PCa using PSA results in a large number of negative biopsies and a high proportion of patients diagnosed with clinically low aggressive tumours (over-diagnosis) followed by unnecessary treatment (over-treatment) and morbidity related to complications [14, 15]. Thus, a more specific biomarker that could increase predictive accuracy and risk stratification properties is needed to identify patients who may have PCa and reduce morbidity due to unnecessary diagnosis and treatment.

The usefulness of %p2PSA and PHI in the detection of PCa has been studied extensively in recent years. The biomarkers improve the specificity of tPSA for PCa detection and are associated with a more aggressive state of disease [5, 13].

Catalona et al. demonstrated that high PHI levels were associated with an increased detection rate of PCa in subjects with a tPSA level between 2 and 10 ng/ml in a prospective multi-institutional study [16]. Jansen et al. showed that PHI showed significantly superior performance compared to PSA and %fPSA for PCa prediction,

and the involvement of p2PSA in a base multivariable model significantly improved the predictive value and specificity of PCa [17].

Several studies have also validated the usefulness of PHI in Asian countries. Chiu et al., in their prospective study, showed that PHI improved the diagnostic accuracy compared with PSA-based predictive models in 569 subjects with PSA levels between 4 and 10 ng/mL in Hong Kong [18]. In a multicentre study in Shanghai, Na et al. demonstrated the superior diagnostic accuracy of PHI compared to tPSA both in subjects with a PSA level between 2.1 and 10 ng/mL and in those with a PSA level > 10 ng/mL [19].

One meta-analysis showed that %p2PSA and PHI consistently improved diagnostic performance compared to tPSA and %fPSA in detecting PCa and could reduce unnecessary biopsies [20]. In addition, a European prospective study showed that PHI showed improved predictive performance for GS ≥ 7 PCa [21]. The 2016 guidelines of the European Association of Urology suggested that PHI could be considered as an additional diagnostic method for patients with PSA levels of 2–10 ng/mL and a negative DRE [22].

Table 5 Logistic regression analyses predicting probability of prostate cancer in subjects with tPSA 4–10 ng/mL

Predictors	AUC of individual predictor variable (95% CI); P value*	Bivariate analysis OR(95%CI); P value	Multivariate analysis		
			Base model ** OR (95%CI); P value	Base model + %p2PSA OR (95% CI); P value	Base model + PHI OR(95%CI); P value
Age	0.63 (0.51–0.74) 0.235	1.069 (1.01–1.13); 0.031	**1.081 (1.02–1.15); 0.013**	**1.084 (1.01–1.16); 0.018**	**1.084 (1.01–1.16); 0.018**
tPSA, ng/mL	0.50 (0.38–0.61) –	1.024 (0.76–1.38); 0.875	1.615 (0.66–3.86); 0.281	1.384 (0.49 – 3.88); 0.536	1.243 (0.44–3.48); 0.679
fPSA	0.59 (0.47–0.70) 0.418	0.529 (0.18–1.53); 0.240	0.038 (0.00–11.2); 0.261	0.070 (0.00–53.9); 0.433	0.071 (0.00–56.5); 0.437
%fPSA	0.63 (0.52–0.74) 0.090	0.961 (0.89–1.03); 0.284	1.155 (0.80–1.66); 0.448	1.108 (0.73–1.69); 0.631	1.108 (0.73–1.69); 0.632
p2PSA, pg/mL	0.59 (0.47–0.70) 0.286	1.023 (1.00–1.05); 0.089	–	–	–
%p2PSA	**0.70 (0.59–0.81) 0.038**	1.020 (1.00–1.04); 0.007	–	**1.022 (1.01–1.04); 0.007**	–
PHI	**0.70 (0.59–0.81) 0.020**	1.743 (1.19–2.56); 0.005	–	–	**1.760 (1.17–2.64); 0.006**
AUC of multivariate models (95% CI);	–	–	0.682 (0.57–0.78) 0.003	0.784 (0.68–0.87) <0.001	0.787 (0.68–0.87) <0.001
Gain in predictive accuracy (95% CI); P value	–	–	–	0.102 (− 0.00–0.21); 0.054	0.104 (0.00–0.21); 0.048

AUC, area under the receiver operating characteristic curve; PSA, prostate-specific antigen; fPSA, free PSA; p2PSA, [-2]proPSA; PHI, prostate health index; tPSA, total PSA, OR, odds ratio; CI, confidence interval

*P value: Comparison of AUC using tPSA as standard

**Base model includes age, tPSA, fPSA and %fPSA

P value to be statiscally significant with bolditalics

In the current study, the addition of %p2PSA or PHI to a predictive base multivariate regression model significantly increased its predictive accuracy. Moreover, %p2PSA and PHI were associated with aggressiveness of PCa and could improve the predictive performance of the base model for detecting GS ≥ 7 PCa. The proportion of aggressive cancer was mostly associated with the PHI level among these markers. At a cutoff PHI value of 33.4, 22.9% (32/140) of biopsies could have been avoided without missing any significant aggressive cancers (GS ≥ 7). In the same context, at a cutoff PHI value of 26.3, 11.7% (9/77) of biopsies would have been avoided without missing any significant aggressive cancers (GS ≥ 7) in subjects with a tPSA 4–10 ng/mL. Similarly, another study demonstrated that 15.5–45.2% of their group could have avoided unnecessary biopsies at a cut-off of PHI score 25–32, although they would have missed 1.1–3.8% of significant aggressive cancers [23, 24].

The European population had a fourfold higher incidence of PCa than the Asian population, while age and PSA level showed a tendency to be higher among Asians in a previous study [25]. Korean men also have a lower incidence of PCa compared to the Western population, but PCa in the Korean population shows worse characteristics of the disease compared to Western men [3, 4]. Most of the previously reported data regarding %p2PSA and PHI have been collected mainly in Western groups; therefore, it is necessary to verify the usefulness of these biomarkers in Korean groups. Kim et al. evaluated the clinical predictive value of %p2PSA and PHI in Korean men [26]. Similar to previous studies, they suggested that the diagnostic accuracy of PHI was better than that of tPSA in the Korean population.

Recently, multiparametric magnetic resonance imaging (MRI) has improved the detection rate of potentially significant PCa [27], but it generally requires higher costs and radiological expertise. It has been reported that MRI and PHI are complementary to each other for detecting significant PCa [28]. PHI is a blood test that can be performed simply and is ordered by general practitioners, and there is no need for radiologic interpretation. In the future, as the cost of a blood test will probably decrease, PHI will be widely used as a screening tool for PCa.

Table 6 Logistic regression analyses predicting the probability of Gleason score ≥ 7 disease

Predictors	AUC of individual predictor variable (95% CI);) P value*	Bivariate analysis OR(95%CI); P value	Multivariate analysis		
			Base model ** OR(95% CI); P value	Base model + %p2PSA OR (95% CI); P value	Base model + PHI OR(95%CI); P value
Age	0.55 (0.42–0.67) 0.508	1.028 (0.95–1.12); 0.513	1.005 (0.92–1.09); 0.913	1.050 (0.95–1.16); 0.357	1.028 (0.93–1.13); 0.577
tPSA, ng/mL	0.62 (0.48–0.77) –	1.064 (0.99–1.14); 0.086	1.031 (0.92–1.16); 0.602	1.016 (0.940–1.098); 0.688	0.974 (0.90–1.05); 0.498
fPSA	0.58 (0.44–0.72) 0.358	1.818 (0.84–3.94); 0.129	1.399 (0.39–5.04); 0.608	0.943 (0.36–2.46); 0.904	0.727 (0.28–1.88); 0.511
%fPSA	0.41 (0.26–0.57) 0.302	0.973 (0.91–1.04); 0.440	0.977 (0.88–1.09); 0.675	0.978 (0.86–1.11); 0.731	1.010 (0.90–1.13); 0.869
p2PSA, pg/mL	**0.79 (0.68–0.91) 0.004**	1.047 (1.01–1.09); 0.017	–	–	–
%p2PSA	**0.86 (0.75–0.93) 0.001**	1.020 (1.01–1.04); 0.007	–	**1.029 (1.01–1.05); 0.015**	–
PHI	**0.87 (0.76–0.94) < 0.001**	3.887 (1.73–8.74); 0.001	–	–	**3.833 (1.56–9.40); 0.003**
AUC of multivariate models (95% CI)	–	–	0.629 (0.50–0.75) 0.086	**0.861 (0.75–0.94) < 0.001**	**0.886 (0.78–0.95) < 0.001**
Gain in predictive accuracy (95% CI); P value	–	–	–	**0.232 (0.08–0.38); 0.002**	**0.257 (0.11–0.40); 0.001**

AUC, area under the receiver operating characteristic curve; PSA, prostate-specific antigen; fPSA, free PSA; p2PSA, [-2]proPSA; PHI, prostate health index; tPSA, total PSA; OR, odds ratio; CI, confidence interval

*P value: Comparison of AUC using tPSA as standard

**Base model includes age, tPSA, fPSA and %fPSA

P value to be statiscally significant with bolditalics

Table 7 Cut-off of 90% sensitivity of the markers in subjects with tPSA 4–10 ng/mL

Marker	Cut-off at 90% sensitivity	% Specificity	Unnecessary biopsy avoided	Missed cancer			
				Total	Missed GS 6	Missed GS 7	Missed GS ≥ 8
Total PSA 4–10 ng/mL							
%fPSA	≤ 7.86	9%	4 (5.2%)	3 (10.3%)	0 (0%)	1 (3.5%)	2 (6.8%)
p2PSA (pg/mL)	≥ 8.08	17%	7 (9.1%)	3 (10.3%)	2 (6.8%)	0 (0%)	1 (3.5%)
% p2PSA	**≥ 1.20**	**27%**	**12 (15.5%)**	**3 (10.3%)**	**3 (10.3%)**	**0 (0%)**	**0 (0%)**
PHI	**≥ 26.33**	**25%**	**9 (11.7%)**	**2 (6.8%)**	**2 (6.8%)**	**0 (0%)**	**0 (0%)**
All study subjects							
%fPSA	≤ 6.42	7%	6 (4.3%)	7 (11.1%)	0 (0%)	2 (3.2%)	5 (7.9%)
p2PSA (pg/mL)	≥ 8.07	20%	16 (11.4%)	7 (11.1%)	4 (6.3%)	2 (3.2%)	1 (1.6%)
% p2PSA	≥ 1.22	31%	24 (17.1%)	7 (11.1%)	7 (11.1%)	0 (0%)	0 (0%)
PHI	**≥ 33.40**	**40%**	**32 (22.9%)**	**5 (7.9%)**	**5 (7.9%)**	**0 (0%)**	**0 (0%)**

PSA, prostate-specific antigen; fPSA, free PSA; p2PSA, [-2]proPSA; PHI, prostate health index

Bold types to represent clinical significance could avoid unnessasary biopsies for %p2SPA and PHI

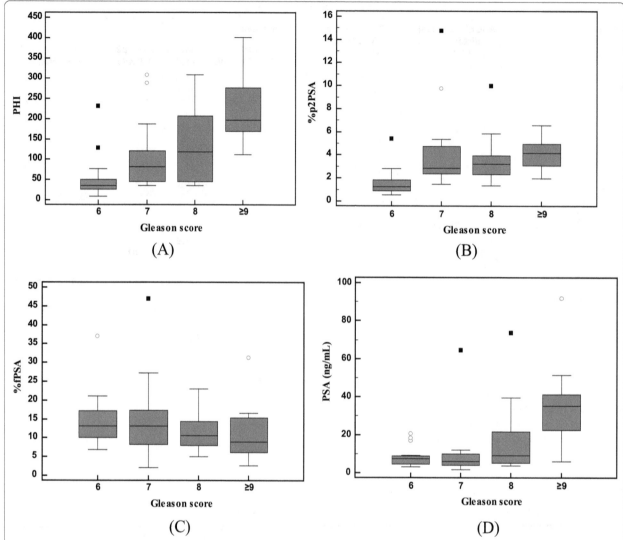

Fig. 2 Box plots comparing PHI (**A**), %p2PSA (**B**), %fPSA (**C**) and tPSA (**D**) in relation to a biopsy Gleason score. PSA, prostate-specific antigen; fPSA, free PSA; p2PSA, [-2]proPSA; PHI, prostate health index; tPSA, total PSA

This study has several limitations. First, it was performed in a single tertiary centre and had a relatively small sample size. Second, not all patients in our study underwent radical prostatectomy; therefore, we could not inspect the occurrence of Gleason upgrading after prostatectomy. In addition, we did not inspect the percentage of tumour involvement in each biopsy core and tumour size. Finally, we did not use multiparametric MRI. MRI could help guide more accurate localisation for biopsy and increase the performance for detecting significant PCa.

Conclusions
Our findings suggest that the diagnostic performance of %p2PSA and PHI to predict the presence and aggressiveness of PCa was superior to that of PSA and %fPSA in

the Korean population. Using PHI, a high proportion of unnecessary biopsies could be avoided. Further research is needed to support these results.

Abbreviations
AUC: Area under the curve; fPSA: Free PSA; GS: Gleason score; p2PSA: [− 2] proPSA; PCa: Prostate cancer; PHI: Prostate health index; PSA: Prostate-specific antigen; ROC: Receiver operating characteristic; tPSA: Total PSA.

Supplementary Information

Additional file 1: Table S1. Predictive value of individual markers predicting the probability of prostate cancer for different age groups.

Acknowledgements

The authors thank all our participants for their gracious participation in this study.

Authors' contributions

SJY, JYK, JHY have made substantial contributions to the conception and design or acquisition of data. JYK, LHS, and DYC performed the analysis and interpretation of data. JYK and SJY have been involved in drafting the manuscript or revising it critically for important intellectual content. HJK performed the histological examination of the specimens. All authors have given final approval for the manuscript to be published. All authors read and approved the final manuscript.

Author details

[1]Department of Urology, Sanggye Paik Hospital, Inje University College of Medicine, 1342 Dongil-ro, Nowon-gu, Seoul 01757, Republic of Korea. [2]Department of Pathology, Sanggye Paik Hospital, Inje University College of Medicine, 1342 Dongil-ro, Nowon-gu, Seoul 01757, Republic of Korea. [3]Department of Laboratory Medicine, Sanggye Paik Hospital, Inje University College of Medicine, 1342 Dongil-ro, Nowon-gu, Seoul 01757, Republic of Korea.

References

1. Siegel RL, Miller KD, Jemal A. Cancer statistics, 2020. CA Cancer J Clin. 2020;70(1):7–30.
2. Han HH, Park JW, Na JC, Chung BH, Kim CS, Ko WJ. Epidemiology of prostate cancer in South Korea. Prostate Int. 2015;3(3):99–102.
3. Kang DI, Chung JI, Ha HK, Min K, Yoon J, Kim W, Seo WI, Kang P, Jung SJ, Kim IY. Korean prostate cancer patients have worse disease characteristics than their American counterparts. Asian Pac J Cancer Prev. 2013;14(11):6913–7.
4. Song C, Kang T, Ro JY, Lee MS, Kim CS, Ahn H. Nomograms for the prediction of pathologic stage of clinically localized prostate cancer in Korean men. J Korean Med Sci. 2005;20(2):262–6.
5. Saini S. PSA and beyond: alternative prostate cancer biomarkers. Cell Oncol (Dordr). 2016;39(2):97–106.
6. Center MM, Jemal A, Lortet-Tieulent J, Ward E, Ferlay J, Brawley O, Bray F. International variation in prostate cancer incidence and mortality rates. Eur Urol. 2012;61(6):1079–92.
7. Etzioni R, Penson DF, Legler JM, di Tommaso D, Boer R, Gann PH, Feuer EJ. Overdiagnosis due to prostate-specific antigen screening: lessons from U.S. prostate cancer incidence trends. J Natl Cancer Inst. 2002;94(13):981–90.
8. McGrath S, Christidis D, Perera M, Hong SK, Manning T, Vela I, Lawrentschuk N. Prostate cancer biomarkers: are we hitting the mark? Prostate Int. 2016;4(4):130–5.
9. Mikolajczyk SD, Catalona WJ, Evans CL, Linton HJ, Millar LS, Marker KM, Katir D, Amirkhan A, Rittenhouse HG. Proenzyme forms of prostate-specific antigen in serum improve the detection of prostate cancer. Clin Chem. 2004;50(6):1017–25.
10. Hori S, Blanchet JS, McLoughlin J. From prostate-specific antigen (PSA) to precursor PSA (proPSA) isoforms: a review of the emerging role of proPSAs in the detection and management of early prostate cancer. BJU Int. 2013;112(6):717–28.
11. Filella X, Gimenez N. Evaluation of [-2] proPSA and Prostate Health Index (phi) for the detection of prostate cancer: a systematic review and meta-analysis. Clin Chem Lab Med. 2013;51(4):729–39.
12. Lazzeri M, Haese A, Abrate A, de la Taille A, Redorta JP, McNicholas T, Lughezzani G, Lista G, Larcher A, Bini V, et al. Clinical performance of serum prostate-specific antigen isoform [-2]proPSA (p2PSA) and its derivatives, %p2PSA and the prostate health index (PHI), in men with a family history of prostate cancer: results from a multicentre European study, the PROMEtheuS project. BJU Int. 2013;112(3):313–21.
13. Hatakeyama S, Yoneyama T, Tobisawa Y, Ohyama C. Recent progress and perspectives on prostate cancer biomarkers. Int J Clin Oncol. 2017;22(2):214–21.
14. Borghesi M, Ahmed H, Nam R, Schaeffer E, Schiavina R, Taneja S, Weidner W, Loeb S. Complications after systematic, random, and image-guided prostate biopsy. Eur Urol. 2017;71(3):353–65.
15. Heijnsdijk EA, Wever EM, Auvinen A, Hugosson J, Ciatto S, Nelen V, Kwiatkowski M, Villers A, Paez A, Moss SM, et al. Quality-of-life effects of prostate-specific antigen screening. N Engl J Med. 2012;367(7):595–605.
16. Catalona WJ, Partin AW, Sanda MG, Wei JT, Klee GG, Bangma CH, Slawin KM, Marks LS, Loeb S, Broyles DL, et al. A multicenter study of [-2]pro-prostate specific antigen combined with prostate specific antigen and free prostate specific antigen for prostate cancer detection in the 2.0 to 10.0 ng/ml prostate specific antigen range. J Urol. 2011;185(5):1650–5.
17. Jansen FH, van Schaik RH, Kurstjens J, Horninger W, Klocker H, Bektic J, Wildhagen MF, Roobol MJ, Bangma CH, Bartsch G. Prostate-specific antigen (PSA) isoform p2PSA in combination with total PSA and free PSA improves diagnostic accuracy in prostate cancer detection. Eur Urol. 2010;57(6):921–7.
18. Chiu PK, Roobol MJ, Teoh JY, Lee WM, Yip SY, Hou SM, Bangma CH, Ng CF. Prostate health index (PHI) and prostate-specific antigen (PSA) predictive models for prostate cancer in the Chinese population and the role of digital rectal examination-estimated prostate volume. Int Urol Nephrol. 2016;48(10):1631–7.
19. Na R, Ye D, Qi J, Liu F, Helfand BT, Brendler CB, Conran CA, Packiam V, Gong J, Wu Y, et al. Prostate health index significantly reduced unnecessary prostate biopsies in patients with PSA 2–10 ng/mL and PSA > 10 ng/mL: results from a Multicenter Study in China. The Prostate. 2017;77(11):1221–9.
20. Wang W, Wang M, Wang L, Adams TS, Tian Y, Xu J. Diagnostic ability of %p2PSA and prostate health index for aggressive prostate cancer: a meta-analysis. Sci Rep. 2014;4:5012.
21. Guazzoni G, Nava L, Lazzeri M, Scattoni V, Lughezzani G, Maccagnano C, Dorigatti F, Ceriotti F, Pontillo M, Bini V, et al. Prostate-specific antigen (PSA) isoform p2PSA significantly improves the prediction of prostate cancer at initial extended prostate biopsies in patients with total PSA between 2.0 and 10 ng/ml: results of a prospective study in a clinical setting. Eur Urol. 2011;60(2):214–22.
22. Mottet N, Bellmunt J, Bolla M, Briers E, Cumberbatch MG, De Santis M, Fossati N, Gross T, Henry AM, Joniau S, et al. EAU-ESTRO-SIOG guidelines on prostate cancer. Part 1: screening, diagnosis, and local treatment with curative intent. Eur Urol. 2017;71(4):618–29.
23. Lazzeri M, Haese A, de la Taille A, Palou Redorta J, McNicholas T, Lughezzani G, Scattoni V, Bini V, Freschi M, Sussman A, et al. Serum isoform [-2] proPSA derivatives significantly improve prediction of prostate cancer at initial biopsy in a total PSA range of 2–10 ng/ml: a multicentric European study. Eur Urol. 2013;63(6):986–94.
24. Filella X, Foj L, Augé JM, Molina R, Alcover J. Clinical utility of %p2PSA and prostate health index in the detection of prostate cancer. Clin Chem Lab Med. 2014;52(9):1347–55.
25. Wong C, Yip C, Li H, Tan T, Kanesvaran R, Chowbay B, Tan PH, Tan MH, Wong FY. Assessment of the American Joint Committee on Cancer 7th edition staging for localised prostate cancer in Asia treated with external beam radiotherapy. Ann Acad Med Singapore. 2014;43(10):484–91.
26. Park H, Lee SW, Song G, Kang TW, Jung JH, Chung HC, Kim SJ, Park CH, Park JY, Shin TY, et al. J Korean Med Sci. 2018;33(11):e94.
27. Ahmed HU, El-Shater Bosaily A, Brown LC, Gabe R, Kaplan R, Parmar MK, Collaco-Moraes Y, Ward K, Hindley RG, Freeman A, et al. Diagnostic accuracy of multi-parametric MRI and TRUS biopsy in prostate cancer (PROMIS): a paired validating confirmatory study. Lancet. 2017;389(10071):815–22.
28. Druskin SC, Tosoian JJ, Young A, Collica S, Srivastava A, Ghabili K, Macura KJ, Carter HB, Partin AW, Sokoll LJ, et al. Combining Prostate Health Index density, magnetic resonance imaging and prior negative biopsy status to improve the detection of clinically significant prostate cancer. BJU Int. 2018;121(4):619–26.

17

Efficacy of additional periprostatic apex nerve block on pain in each of 12 transrectal prostate core biopsies

Jeong Woo Yoo, Kyo Chul Koo, Byung Ha Chung and Kwang Suk Lee[*]

Abstract

Background: We identified pain variation according to prostate biopsy sites and compared differences in pain relief according to the site of periprostatic nerve block (PNB).

Methods: This retrospective study collected data from 312 patients who underwent transrectal prostate biopsies between January 2019 and August 2020. Patients were stratified into two groups according to the site of local anesthesia (base vs. base and apex PNB), with each block achieved with 2.5 cm^3 of 2% lidocaine. Pain scores were assessed using the visual analog scale at the following time points: probe insertion, PNB at base, PNB at apex, each of the 12 core biopsy sites, and 15 min after biopsy. The results were analyzed using a linear mixed model.

Results: The average pain scores were significantly higher in the base-only PNB group than were those in the base and apex PNB group (3.88 vs 2.82, $p < 0.001$). In the base-only PNB group, the pain scores increased from base to apex ($p < 0.001$), and the pain at each site also gradually increased as the biopsy proceeded ($p < 0.001$). In contrast, in the base and apex PNB group, there was minor change in pain scores throughout the procedure.

Conclusions: The pain scores varied at each site during the prostate biopsy. The provision of a base and apex PNB provided greater pain relief than does base-only PNB during prostate biopsy.

Keywords: Biopsy, Nerve block, Pain, Prostate

Background

Systematic random prostate biopsy is generally performed via a transrectal or transperineal approach for the diagnosis of prostate cancer [1, 2]. The transrectal ultrasound (TRUS)-guided random prostate biopsy may cause severe pain, hematuria, urinary retention, infection, and even septic shock [3–5]. As the experience of pain during prostate biopsy lowers patient compliance, this procedure should be performed under local anesthesia, in accordance with the guidelines provided by the National Comprehensive Cancer Network (NCCN).

The availability of various anesthetic techniques greatly enhances patients' acceptability of prostate biopsy. Active pain relief was not previously adopted; however, for pain relief, general anesthesia, intrarectal local anesthesia, pudendal and caudal nerve block, periprostatic local anesthesia, intravenous conscious sedation (propofol, midazolam), and intravenous analgesics (fentanyl) have been attempted [6]. Among these, intrarectal lidocaine gel (IRLG), pelvic plexus block (PPB), and periprostatic nerve block (PNB) using prilocaine or lidocaine are generally used in the clinical setting [7–11].

A previous meta-analysis reported the usefulness of both the PPB and PNB for pain relief during prostate biopsy, while a recent randomized clinical trial conducted by our research group found no difference between the

*Correspondence: calmenow@yuhs.ac
Department of Urology, Gangnam Severance Hospital, Yonsei University College of Medicine, 211 Eonju-ro, Gangnam-gu, Seoul 06273, Republic of Korea

efficacy of the PPB and base PNB [6, 8]. However, in the latter study, the PNB was stratified according to the nerve block site. The administration of a base PNB and an additional apex PNB relieve overall pain as it blocks a sensitive somatic nerve branch of the pudendal nerve [12].

With the consideration that the level of pain differs according to the site at which the PNB is administered, we speculated that pain levels would also differ among random biopsy sites, and that the degree of pain relief would vary at each site following the administration of an additional nerve block. To the best of our knowledge, no prior studies have investigated these issues. Therefore, we aimed to evaluate differences in pain levels among 12 core biopsy sites, and assess pain relief according to the site of PNB administration.

Methods

Patient selection

This retrospective study collected data from 312 consecutive patients who underwent TRUS-guided prostate biopsies at single institution (Gangnam Severance Hospital, Yonsei University Health System) between January 2019 and August 2020. The indication for prostate biopsy was persistent clinical suspicion of prostate cancer due to an elevated prostate-specific antigen (PSA) level (>2.5 ng/mL) and/or a positive digital rectal examination (DRE) and continuous rise in PSA level during the follow-up period. The exclusion criteria comprised the following: (1) hemorrhoid grade $\geq$ III (n = 3), which indicated that the hemorrhoid tissue prolapsed beyond the dentate line; (2) history of hemorrhoidectomy (n = 1); and (3) inability to communicate (n = 4; two were foreigners and two were old men with communication difficulties). None of the 312 patients had neurological disease such as paraplegia or hemiplegia and none routinely used analgesics for chronic pain or other reasons. Finally, a total of 304 (97.4%) patients were included in the analysis (Fig. 1). This study was approved by the institutional ethics committee (Yonsei University Health System, Seoul, Korea, 3-2019-0418), and all procedures were conducted in accordance with the ethical standards of the 1964 Helsinki declaration and its later amendments. The requirement for informed consent was waived for this study as it was based on retrospective, anonymous patient data and did not involve patient intervention or the use of human tissue samples.

Data collection

The collected patient data included age, PSA level, prostate volume, history of prostate biopsy, DRE (positive; hard surface, nodular lesions or mass-like lesion), pathologic results, time of PNB and biopsies, adverse events (vasovagal syncope, allergic reaction, acute urine retention, clot retention, fever), and visual analog scale (VAS; ranging from 0 [no pain] to 10 [worst pain]) score measured at various time points: probe insertion, PNB at base, PNB at apex, each of the 12 core biopsy sites, and 15 min after prostate biopsy.

TRUS-guided prostate biopsy technique

All patients were hospitalized for half a day. Antibiotics (third generation cephalosporin) were administered prophylactically via intravenous injection 1 h before the biopsy and upon discharge (100 mg orally, three times a day for 2 days).

The patients assumed a left lateral decubitus position during the biopsy. All biopsies were performed by the same experienced urologist. After povidone iodine rectal preparation, all patients received 10 cm^3 of 2% IRLG (Instillagel®, Farco-Farma GmbH, Köln, Germany). After 5 min, a transrectal probe was inserted to measure the prostate volume, and the PNB procedure was performed with a Chiba needle (A & A M.D. Inc., Seongnam, Korea).

Biopsies were performed with the BK 3000 ultrasound system (Analogic Corporation, Peabody, MA, USA) using a 7.5–12-MHz multiplanar probe at each of the 12 biopsy sites, in the following order: right lateral base, right lateral mid, right lateral apex, right medial base, right medial mid, right medial apex, left lateral base, left lateral mid, left lateral apex, left medial base, left medial mid, and left medial apex. A 20-cm, 18-gauge disposable core biopsy instrument (Max-Core®, CR Bard Inc., Covington, GA, USA) was used in all cases.

Site of injection

The two methods of local anesthesia (base PNB and base and apex PNB) were alternately administered—(1) odd days (base-only PNB group: the PNB was administered on both sides of the prostate base) and (2) even days (base and apex PNB group: an additional PNB was administered on both sides of the prostate apex). The site of base injections was aimed at the major neurovascular bundle, after confirming the triangular echogenic "Mount Everest sign" between the base of the prostate and seminal vesicle in the parasagittal longitudinal view of the TRUS [6]. PNB administration at this site was considered to have anesthetized a large portion of the prostate gland. The site for apex injections was aimed at a smaller triangular echogenicity between the puborectalis muscles and the apex of the prostate gland. Each PNB injection utilized 2.5 cm^3 of 2% lidocaine [6]. The base and apex PNB group received the base injection before the apex injection.

Study endpoints

The primary study endpoint was the pain scale score for the two PNB methods in each of the 12 core biopsy sites.

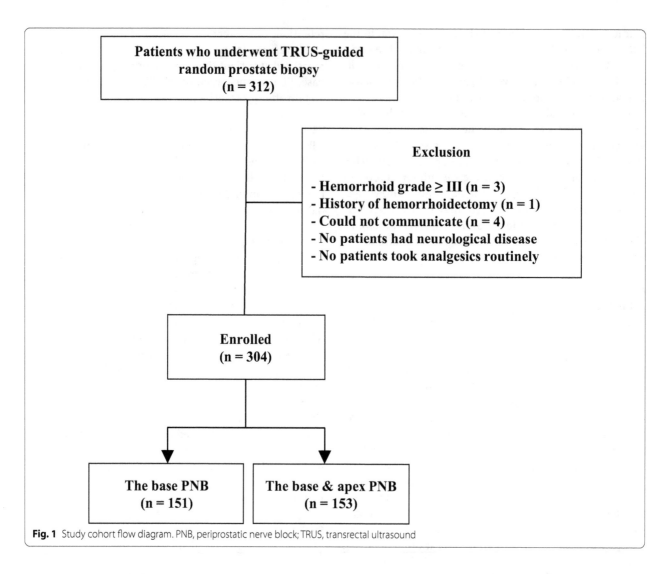

Fig. 1 Study cohort flow diagram. PNB, periprostatic nerve block; TRUS, transrectal ultrasound

The secondary endpoint was the comparison of pain scores between the PNB methods.

Statistical analysis

VAS pain scores in the base and apex PNB were defined as the average of the VAS scores for base and apex injections, respectively. Average pain was defined as the mean (±standard deviation [SD]) of the individual VAS pain scores at the 12 sites. Average pain at the base, mid, and apex of the prostate was defined as the mean (±SD) of the individual VAS pain scores at the base, mid, apex sites, respectively.

Continuous variables are expressed as either the mean±SD or median (interquartile range). Categorical variables were reported as the number of occurrences and frequency. Comparisons between the base-only PNB group and the base and apex PNB group were performed with the independent t-test for continuous variables, and the chi-square test (Fisher's exact test) for two or more

variables. The results were also analyzed using a linear mixed model and illustrated with a mean profile graph. The correlation matrix structure of the linear mixed model was used to determine the relationship between the measured data at various points in time via the application of compound symmetry. Statistical analyses were performed using SAS (version 9.4.; SAS Institute, Cary, NC, USA) and PASS (version 15; NCSS, LLC. Kaysville, Utah, USA). The level of statistical significance was set at $p < 0.05$.

Results

Baseline characteristics and VAS pain scores according to PNB sites

Patient characteristics and VAS pain scores according to PNB sites are presented in Table 1. No differences in PSA concentrations (7.56 ng/mL vs. 6.76 ng/mL), prostate volume (36.55 mL vs. 36.79 mL), or prostate cancer detection rate (62.9% vs. 62.1%) were observed between

Table 1 Baseline characteristics and VAS pain scores according to the PNB sites

	Base	Base and apex	p
N	151 (49.7)	153 (50.3)	
Age (years)	67.86 ± 15.74	68.19 ± 8.59	0.740
PSA (ng/mL)	7.56 (5.40–11.59)	6.76 (4.47–10.19)	0.074
Prostate volume (mL)	36.55 ± 15.74	36.79 ± 16.78	0.900
History of prostate biopsy (n, %)	27 (17.9)	19 (12.4)	0.186
Positive DRE (n, %)	35 (35.7)	25 (28.4)	0.287
Prostate cancer detection rate (n, %)	95 (62.9)	95 (62.1)	0.882
Gleason score			0.171
6 (n, %)	18 (18.9)	26 (27.4)	
≥ 7 (n, %)	77 (81.1)	69 (72.6)	
Pain			
Probe insertion	3.39 ± 2.12	3.36 ± 2.43	0.905
PNB at base	2.91 ± 1.83	2.79 ± 1.94	0.591
PNB at apex		4.60 ± 2.50	
At 15 min post prostate biopsy	0.14 ± 0.58	0.16 ± 0.74	0.749
Time			
Periprostatic nerve block (min)	2.42 ± 0.77	2.59 ± 0.88	0.084
Prostate biopsy (min)	4.20 ± 2.59	4.66 ± 5.41	0.343
Adverse events			
Vasovagal syncope (n, %)	2 (1.3)	0 (0.0)	0.246
Allergic reaction (n, %)	0 (0.0)	0 (0.0)	–
AUR (n, %)	0 (0.0)	0 (0.0)	–
Urinary retention because of blood clot (n, %)	0 (0.0)	0 (0.0)	–
Fever (n, %)	0 (0.0)	0 (0.0)	–

Data are expressed as number (%), mean ± standard deviation, and median (IQR range)

AUR, acute urinary retention; DRE, digital rectal exam; IQR, interquartile; PNB, periprostatic nerve block; PSA, prostate specific antigen; VAS, visual analog scale

the base-only PNB group and the base and apex PNB group. There were no significant differences in VAS pain scores among the different time points (probe insertion, PNB at base, and 15 min after prostate biopsy). Average pain scores at the base, mid, and apex sites are presented in Table 2. The average VAS pain score across all regions (overall, base, mid, and apex) in the base and apex PNB group was lower than that in the base-only PNB group.

Mean profile plots

Older age ($p = 0.029$) and higher VAS scores at probe insertion ($p = 0.002$) were correlated with higher individual VAS scores in each of the 12 core biopsy sites, but a history of prostate biopsy ($p = 0.616$) and DRE ($p = 0.131$) were not. The mean profile plots show the results before and after adjustment for age and VAS pain scores at probe insertion; the VAS pain scores for each of the 12 core biopsies were not significantly different pre- and post-correction for these confounding variables (Fig. 2). The VAS pain scores were significantly higher in the base-only PNB group than in the base and apex PNB group ($p < 0.001$; Fig. 2). A comparison across biopsy

Table 2 Mean VAS pain scores in TRUS-guided random prostate biopsy groups according to PNB sites

	Base	Base and apex	p
12 core VAS pain scores			
Average pain[a]	3.88 ± 2.27	2.82 ± 2.17	< 0.001
Average pain at base[b]	3.74 ± 2.27	2.81 ± 2.20	< 0.001
Average pain at mid[c]	3.82 ± 2.29	2.81 ± 2.17	< 0.001
Average pain at apex[d]	4.08 ± 2.32	2.83 ± 2.18	< 0.001

Data are expressed as mean ± standard deviation

PNB, periprostatic nerve block; SD, standard deviation; TRUS, transrectal ultrasound; VAS, visual analog scale

[a] Mean and SD of the average of 12 sites for each individual VAS pain scores

[b] Mean and SD of the average of 4 base sites for each individual VAS pain scores

[c] Mean and SD of the average of 4 mid sites for each individual VAS pain scores

[d] Mean and SD of the average of 4 apex sites for each individual VAS pain scores

locations in the base-only PNB group (after categorization of the 12 sites into the base, mid, and apex regions) indicated that VAS pain scores increased from the base to apex ($p < 0.001$; Fig. 3). The biopsy of the medial sites

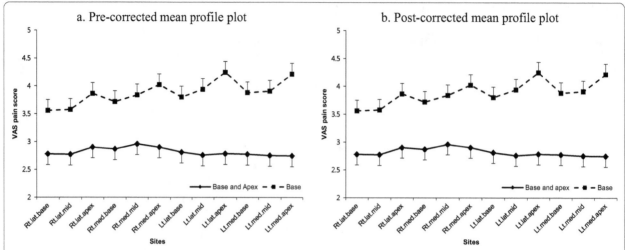

Fig. 2 Mean profile plot of VAS pain scores for each of the 12 core biopsy sites. **a** VAS pain score before adjustment for age and VAS pain score at probe insertion. **b** VAS pain score after adjustment for age and VAS pain score at probe insertion. Lat, lateral; Lt, left; Med, medial; Rt, right; TRUS, transrectal ultrasound; VAS, visual analog scale

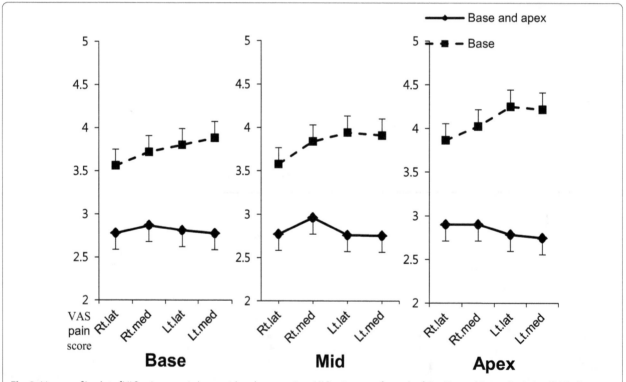

Fig. 3 Mean profile plot of VAS pain scores in base, mid, and apex regions. VAS pain scores for each of the 12 core biopsy sites were divided into base, mid, and apex regions. Adjustments were made for age and the VAS pain score at probe insertion. Lat, lateral; Lt, left; Med, medial; Rt, right; TRUS, transrectal ultrasound; VAS, visual analog scale

was marginally, but significantly, more painful than that of the lateral sites within the base region in the base-only PNB group ($p=0.091$); no significant differences were observed between the medial and lateral sites in the mid ($p=0.134$) or apex ($p=0.392$) regions. Pain scores at each site also gradually increased as the biopsy proceeded in the base-only PNB group ($p<0.001$).

Complications

There were two cases (1.3%) of vasovagal syncope in the base-only PNB group, and both the cases recovered without medical therapy. No major complications were observed in the base and apex PNB group (Table 1).

Discussion

The main factors related to pain during prostate biopsy were identified as age, procedure duration, prostate volume, and lithotomy position [6, 13–15]. Our results confirmed that age and procedure duration are associated with pain due to TRUS-guided prostate biopsy. The administration of a base PNB in addition to an apex PNB resulted in lower VAS pain scores when compared to the base-only PNB, and this result is consistent with that reported in previous studies [6]. We compared VAS pain scores for the base-only PNB across the 12 individual core biopsy sites and observed higher levels of pain at the medial and apex sites than at the lateral and base sites. This novel finding suggests that a potential strategy for the mitigation of severe pain during the biopsy procedure is the administration of an apex PNB, in addition to the base PNB.

The conventional method for pain control during a TRUS-guided prostate biopsy consists of the combination of a PNB and IRLG. A meta-analysis of 26 articles (comprising 36 randomized controlled trials) concluded that the combination of IRLG and PNB is effective and safe [16]. The PNB achieves different degrees of pain control depending on the lidocaine injection site. Previous studies have reported the VAS pain score collected after the procedure to range between 3.37 and 4.97 for the base-only PNB [9, 17, 18]. The VAS pain score of 3.88, as observed in our study, was the mean value of scores collected at each 12 core biopsy sites and was consistent with previously reported values.

The prostate apex is known to be a particularly painful site in TRUS-guided prostate biopsies because of the dominant somatic nerve supply to the region below the dentate line [6]. Our results indicated that the apex PNB was more painful than the prostate base PNB. The apex injection blocks the sensitive somatic nerve branch of the inferior rectal nerve (arising from the pudendal nerve), which is contained in the distal part of the dentate line; this region is penetrated by the needle during PNB or biopsy [19]. Thus, the anatomy of this region may explain the results of a prior study, which reported the increased efficacy of an additional apex lidocaine injection for the PNB method [6]. This previous study reported that the administration of both a base and apex PNB reduced the overall VAS pain score, which is consistent with our results.

Rafael et al. reported that pain in each core biopsy site became more severe as the procedure proceeded [14]. The patients experienced pain when the first puncture was performed, which made them more nervous. This, in turn, resulted in their tendency to physically avoid the pain upon expectation of an ensuing puncture, which potentially led to more severe pain during the subsequent core biopsy [6, 20]. In our study, the base-only PNB group showed similar results. Interestingly, a correlation between procedure progression and VAS pain scores was not observed in the base and apex PNB group. Thus, our results demonstrate the potential benefit of the base and apex PNB, in terms of pain control over the duration of the biopsy procedure.

The results of the present study indicated that the degree of pain relief was also dependent on the site of the lidocaine injection. In the base-only PNB group, the VAS pain score during the apex biopsy was higher than that during the base biopsy. When VAS pain scores were compared between the lateral and medial sites, a marginally significant difference was observed only during the base biopsy. Since the prostatic base is broader than the apex, it can be inferred that a greater distance between the biopsy location and lidocaine injection site is associated with increased pain for the base-only PNB. Our results are consistent with those reported by previous studies that investigated the relationship between prostate volume and the efficacy of local anesthesia [15, 16].

The most recent NCCN guidelines have recommended that prostate magnetic resonance imaging (MRI) should be performed before biopsy to reduce unnecessary prostate biopsies based on the efficacy of radiologic diagnosis [21–24]. Prostate MRI is often effective in identifying cancerous lesions at the anterior and apex sites, which are usually not supported in random prostate biopsies [25]. However, the optimal local anesthetic methods for MRI-/TRUS-guided biopsy in the anterior and apex sites are unknown due to the lack of previous studies on pain variation across different regions. Nevertheless, our results may aid the determination of appropriate local anesthetic protocols in patients with apex lesions during MRI-/TRUS-guided biopsy.

The present study has some limitations that should be acknowledged. First, a retrospective design was used, and the study was conducted at a single center; therefore, the results are sensitive to selection bias. Second, the apex PNB was more painful than the base PNB, and may have adverse events. The results may also have been affected by different total doses of lidocaine injection. We are currently in the process of conducting a prospective, well-controlled, randomized multicenter trial to confirm the results of this study.

Conclusions

Prostate cancer is one of the most prevalent cancers, with rapidly increasing incidence worldwide. TRUS-guided random prostate biopsy is a painful procedure and requires appropriate local anesthesia. The results of this study indicated that core biopsy of the apex site was more painful than was the base site in patients who received the base-only PNB. The administration of an additional apex PNB provided better overall pain control.

Abbreviations

DRE: Digital rectal exam; IRLG: Intrarectal lidocaine gel; MRI: Magnetic resonance imaging; NCCN: National Comprehensive Cancer Network; PNB: Periprostatic nerve block; PPB: Pelvic plexus block; PSA: Prostate-specific antigen; SD: Standard deviation; TRUS: Transrectal ultrasound; VAS: Visual analog scale.

Acknowledgements

Not applicable.

Authors' contributions

Protocol/project development: JWY, KSL, KCK. Data collection and management: JWY, KCK, BHC, KSL. Data analysis: JWY, KSL. Manuscript writing/editing: JWY, KSL. All authors read and approved the final manuscript.

References

1. Sivaraman A, Sanchez-Salas R, Barret E, Ahallal Y, Rozet F, Galiano M, Prapotnich D, Cathelineau X. Transperineal template-guided mapping biopsy of the prostate. Int J Urol. 2015;22(2):146–51.
2. Xiang J, Yan H, Li J, Wang X, Chen H, Zheng X. Transperineal versus transrectal prostate biopsy in the diagnosis of prostate cancer: a systematic review and meta-analysis. World J Surg Oncol. 2019;17(1):31.
3. Borghesi M, Ahmed H, Nam R, Schaeffer E, Schiavina R, Taneja S, Weidner W, Loeb S. Complications after systematic, random, and image-guided prostate biopsy. Eur Urol. 2017;71(3):353–65.
4. Forsvall A, Jönsson H, Wagenius M, Bratt O, Linder A. Rate and characteristics of infection after transrectal prostate biopsy: a retrospective observational study. Scand. J. Urol. 2021;1–7.
5. Li M, Wang Z, Li H, Yang J, Rao K, Wang T, Wang S, Liu J. Local anesthesia for transrectal ultrasound-guided biopsy of the prostate: a meta-analysis. Sci Rep. 2017;7:40421.
6. Nazir B. Pain during transrectal ultrasound-guided prostate biopsy and the role of periprostatic nerve block: what radiologists should know. Korean J Radiol. 2014;15(5):543–53.
7. Wang J, Wang L, Du Y, He D, Chen X, Li L, Nan X, Fan J. Addition of intrarectal local analgesia to periprostatic nerve block improves pain control for transrectal ultrasonography-guided prostate biopsy: a systematic review and meta-analysis. Int J Urol. 2015;22(1):62–8.
8. Kim DK, Hah YS, Kim JW, Koo KC, Lee KS, Hong CH, Chung BH, Cho KS. Is Pelvic Plexus block superior to periprostatic nerve block for pain control during transrectal ultrasonography-guided prostate biopsy? A double-blind, randomized controlled trial. J Clin Med. 2019;8(4).
9. Cantiello F, Cicione A, Autorino R, Cosentino C, Amato F, Damiano R. Pelvic plexus block is more effective than periprostatic nerve block for pain control during office transrectal ultrasound guided prostate biopsy: a single center, prospective, randomized, double arm study. J Urol. 2012;188(2):417–21.
10. Lee MS, Moon MH, Kim CK, Park SY, Choi MH, Jung SI. Guidelines for transrectal ultrasonography-guided prostate biopsy: Korean Society of urogenital radiology consensus statement for patient preparation, standard technique, and biopsy-related pain management. Korean J Radiol. 2020;21(4).
11. Nakai Y, Tanaka N, Matsubara T, Anai S, Miyake M, Hori S, Fujii T, Ohbayashi C, Fujimoto K. Effect of prolonged duration of transrectal ultrasound-guided biopsy of the prostate and pre-procedure anxiety on pain in patients without anesthesia. Res Rep Urol. 2021;13:111–20.
12. Lv Z, Jiang H, Hu X, Yang C, Chand H, Tang C, Li Y. Efficacy and safety of periprostatic nerve block combined with perineal subcutaneous anaesthesia and intrarectal lidocaine gel in transrectal ultrasound guided transperineal prostate biopsy: a prospective randomised controlled trial. Prostate Cancer Prostatic Dis. 2020;23(1):74–80.
13. Song PH, Ko YH. Lateral decubitus position vs. lithotomy position: which is the best way to minimize patient's pain perception during transrectal prostate biopsy? Int Braz J Urol. 2017;43(3):462–9.
14. Rodriguez-Patron Rodriguez R, Mayayo Dehesa T, Lennie Zucharino A, Gonzalez Galan A, Peral Amoros M. Complications of prostatic echo-guided transrectal biopsy and tolerance depending on the patient and the operator. Study of 205 patients. Arch Esp Urol. 2002;55(5):509–21.
15. Gomez-Gomez E, Ramirez M, Gomez-Ferrer A, Rubio-Briones J, Iborra I, Carrasco-Valiente J, Campos JP, Ruiz-Garcia J, Requena-Tapia MJ, Solsona E. Assessment and clinical factors associated with pain in patients undergoing transrectal prostate biopsy. Actas Urol Esp. 2015;39(7):414–9.
16. Yan P, Wang XY, Huang W, Zhang Y. Local anesthesia for pain control during transrectal ultrasound-guided prostate biopsy: a systematic review and meta-analysis. J Pain Res. 2016;9:787–96.
17. Jindal T, Mukherjee S, Sinha RK, Kamal MR, Ghosh N, Saha B, Mitra N, Sharma PK, Mandal SN, Karmakar D. Transrectal ultrasonography (TRUS)-guided pelvic plexus block to reduce pain during prostate biopsy: a randomised controlled trial. BJU Int. 2015;115(6):892–6.
18. Akpinar H, Tufek I, Atug F, Esen EH, Kural AR. Doppler ultrasonography-guided pelvic plexus block before systematic needle biopsy of the prostate: a prospective randomized study. Urology. 2009;74(2):267-271 e261.
19. Kim SJ, Lee J, An DH, Park CH, Lim JH, Kim HG, Park JY. A randomized controlled comparison between periprostatic nerve block and pelvic plexus block at the base and apex of 14-core prostate biopsies. World J Urol. 2019;37(12):2663–9.
20. Chesnut GT, Zareba P, Sjoberg DD, Mamoor M, Carlsson S, Lee T, Fainberg J, Vertosick E, Manasia M, Schoen M, et al. Patient-reported pain, discomfort, and anxiety during magnetic resonance imaging-targeted prostate biopsy. Can Urol Assoc J. 2020;14(5):E202–8.
21. Kuru TH, Roethke MC, Seidenader J, Simpfendorfer T, Boxler S, Alammar K, Rieker P, Popeneciu VI, Roth W, Pahernik S, et al. Critical evaluation of magnetic resonance imaging targeted, transrectal ultrasound guided transperineal fusion biopsy for detection of prostate cancer. J Urol. 2013;190(4):1380–6.
22. Lamb BW, Tan WS, Rehman A, Nessa A, Cohen D, O'Neil J, Green JS, Hines JE. Is prebiopsy MRI good enough to avoid prostate biopsy? A cohort study over a 1-year period. Clin Genitourin Cancer. 2015;13(6):512–7.
23. Pokorny MR, de Rooij M, Duncan E, Schroder FH, Parkinson R, Barentsz JO, Thompson LC. Prospective study of diagnostic accuracy comparing prostate cancer detection by transrectal ultrasound-guided biopsy versus magnetic resonance (MR) imaging with subsequent MR-guided biopsy in men without previous prostate biopsies. Eur Urol. 2014;66(1):22–9.
24. Tonttila PP, Lantto J, Paakko E, Piippo U, Kauppila S, Lammentausta E, Ohtonen P, Vaarala MH. Prebiopsy multiparametric magnetic resonance imaging for prostate cancer diagnosis in biopsy-naive men with suspected prostate cancer based on elevated prostate-specific antigen values: results from a randomized prospective blinded controlled trial. Eur Urol. 2016;69(3):419–25.
25. Carroll PR, Parsons JK, Carlsson S, Castle EP, Catalona WJ, Dahl DM, et al. NCCN guidelines insights: prostate cancer early detection, version 2.2020. J Natl Comp Cancer Netw. 2020.

18

Isolation and characterization of urine microvesicles from prostate cancer patients: Different approaches, different visions

María García-Flores[1,2†] ⓘ, Christian M. Sánchez-López[3,4†] ⓘ, Marta Ramírez-Calvo[1] ⓘ, Antonio Fernández-Serra[1] ⓘ, Antonio Marcilla[3,4*] ⓘ and José Antonio López-Guerrero[1,2,5*] ⓘ

Abstract

Background: Because of their specific and biologically relevant cargo, urine extracellular vesicles (EVs) constitute a valuable source of potential non-invasive biomarkers that could support the clinical decision-making to improve the management of prostate cancer (PCa) patients. Different EV isolation methods differ in terms of complexity and yield, conditioning, as consequence, the analytical result.

Methods: The aim of this study was to compare three different isolation methods for urine EVs: ultracentrifugation (UC), size exclusion chromatography (SEC), and a commercial kit (Exolute® Urine Kit). Urine samples were collected from 6 PCa patients and 4 healthy donors. After filtered through 0.22 μm filters, urine was divided in 3 equal volumes to perform EVs isolation with each of the three approaches. Isolated EVs were characterized by spectrophotometric protein quantification, nanoparticle tracking analysis, transmission electron microscopy, AlphaScreen Technology, and whole miRNA Transcriptome.

Results: Our results showed that UC and SEC provided better results in terms of EVs yield and purity than Exolute®, non-significant differences were observed in terms of EV-size. Interestingly, luminescent AlphaScreen assay demonstrated a significant enrichment of CD9 and CD63 positive microvesicles in SEC and UC methods compared with Exolute®. This heterogeneity was also demonstrated in terms of miRNA content indicating that the best correlation was observed between UC and SEC.

Conclusions: Our study highlights the importance of standardizing the urine EV isolation methods to guaranty the analytical reproducibility necessary for their implementation in a clinical setting.

Keywords: Extracellular microvesicles, Exosomes, Ultracentrifugation, Size exclusion chromatography, miRNA

Background

The diagnosis of prostate cancer (PCa) is currently made by histological confirmation from a prostate biopsy guided by altered serum prostate-specific antigen (PSA) values (≥ 4 ng/ml) and/or a suspicious digital rectal examination (DRE) [1 3]. However, this approach presents many limitations including low specificity of PSA and DRE and the molecular heterogeneity of PCa that at the end determines tumour behavior [4]. For this reason, there is an urgent need in developing

*Correspondence: antonio.marcilla@uv.es; jalopez@fivo.org
†María García-Flores and Christian M. Sánchez-López have contributed equally
[1] Laboratory of Molecular Biology, Fundación Instituto Valenciano de Oncología, 46009 Valencia, Spain
[3] Àrea de Parasitologia, Departament de Farmàcia i Tecnologia Farmacèutica i Parasitologia, Universitat de València, 46000 Burjassot, Valencia, Spain
Full list of author information is available at the end of the article

more targeted and non-invasive diagnostic tools, based on the molecular characterization of body fluids, that provide information about the malignant potential of PCa and allowing the monitoring of the disease into the different clinical scenarios.

Urine, due to the anatomic proximity of the prostate gland to the urethra, constitutes a valuable source of PCa biomarkers particularly derived from exfoliated prostatic cells, excreted proteins, circulating nucleic acids or extracellular vesicles (EVs) [5]. EVs are small membrane vesicles that are classified according to their size, cellular origin and biogenesis into microvesicles, exosomes, and apoptotic bodies [6, 7]. They are released by most cell types in physiological and pathological conditions [7] and can be isolated from all body fluids (including urine, blood, saliva, milk, semen, cerebrospinal fluid, etc.) [8, 9]. EVs contains a variety of molecules including nucleic acids, proteins, lipids, and some other metabolites [10–12], and their composition is affected by different environmental factors and health status [13, 14]. Given their ability to horizontally transfer genetic material and signaling moieties between different cells in the organism, EVs have recently emerged as powerful mediators of cell–cell communication [7].

Currently, EVs-cargo represents a doubtless source of biomarkers that may represent the different PCa progression stages [15, 16] and constitute promising tools for the development of minimally invasive diagnostic approaches. Hence, because of their increasing potential for their use in clinical scenarios, it has become vitally important to improve the isolation methods for maximum purity, yield, and assay reproducibility [17]. The most common approaches for EVs isolation include size exclusion chromatography (SEC); classical ultracentrifugation (UC) [17]; sucrose density-gradient centrifugation; affinity chromatography using antibodies against EVs markers (such as CD9, CD81, CD63) [18]; or commercial kits [8, 19–21]. Despite their importance, EVs isolation and characterization are still considered major scientific challenges [22, 23], and identifying the best techniques for their isolation is crucial for further biomarker discoveries.

The aim of this study was to compare three different EVs isolation methods: UC, SEC, and a commercial kit (Exolute® Urine Kit) using urine from a series of PCa patients and healthy donors (HDs). The outperformance of the three methods was evaluated by using different analytic approaches, including NanoDrop protein quantification, nanoparticle tracking analysis (NTA), transmission electron microscopy (TEM), AlphaScreen Technology, and HTG EdgeSeq miRNA Whole Transcriptome Assay (miRNA WTA).

Methods

Sample collection and ethical considerations

Urine samples from six PCa patients and four HDs (men with no history of cancer or other prior chronical diseases), were retrieved from the archives of the Biobank of the Fundación Instituto Valenciano de Oncología (FIVO). Written informed consent for sample donation for research purposes was obtained from all patients prior to sample collection, and the study was approved by the Clinical Research Ethics Committee (CREC) and the Institutional Ethics Committee (Ref. PROMETEO 2016/103), at the meeting held on May 28, 2015. All methods used during the study were performed in accordance with the relevant guidelines and regulations.

Urine processing

A median of 72 mL (range: 54–90 mL) of urine were collected in sterile urine containers (Ref. 409726 Deltalab, Barcelona, Spain). Protease Inhibitor Cocktail (P8340-5 mL, Sigma Aldrich, San Luis, MO, USA) was added to preserve exosomes (50 μL cocktail in 100 mL urine sample) [24]. Each sample was centrifuged at $1000 \times g$, 10 min at 4 °C, and supernatant were frozen at −80 °C until use. The pre-analytical variables of the samples with SPREC code [25–27] are shown in Table 1.

Briefly, urine samples were thawed at 4 °C before use. Samples were centrifuged at $1000 \times g$, 15 min at room temperature (RT) to remove cell debris, and the collected supernatants were then centrifuged at $3000 \times g$, 15 min

Table 1 Preanalytical variables included in the Standard PREanalytical Code (SPREC), applied to urine samples

Sample ID	Type of sample	SPREC code[a]
127	PCa patient	URN-PIX-D-D-N-N-J
129	PCa patient	URN-PIX-D-D-N-N-J
132	PCa patient	URN-PIX-A-D-N-N-J
144	PCa patient	URN-PIX-B-D-N-N-J
146	PCa patient	URN-PIX-B-D-N-N-J
148	PCa patient	URN-PIX-B-D-N-N-J
161	HDs	URN-PIX-A-D-N-N-J
163	HDs	URN-PIX-A-D-N-N-J
164	HDs	URN-PIX-A-D-N-N-J
167	HDs	URN-PIX-A-D-N-N-J

[a] Each biospecimen is assigned a seven-element-long code that corresponds to seven preanalytical variables. First code element: type of sample (URN: urine). Second code element: type of primary container (PIX: with Protease inhibitors). Third code element: precentrifugation (A: RT < 2 h, B: 3–7 °C < 2 h, D: 3–7 °C 2–4 h). Fourth code element: centrifugation (D: 3–7 °C 10 min < 3000 g with braking). Fifth code element: second centrifugation (N: No centrifugation). Sixth code element: postcentrifugation (N: Not applicable). Seventh code element: storage condition [J: PP (Poly propylene) tube ≥ 5 mL (−85) to (−60) °C. If the preanalytical option used is unknown or inconstant, the letter "X" is used. If the preanalytical option used is known but does not correspond to any of the standard options, the letter "Z" is used. (RT: room temperature 18–25 °C) [25]

at 4 °C. The major urinary contaminant, mucoprotein (the Tamm-Horsfall protein), was removed by adding NaCl to a final concentration of 0.58 M and incubated for 2 h at RT, as previously described [28]. Samples were then centrifuged at $16,000 \times g$, for 20 min at 4 °C, and the supernatant was collected and filtered through 0.22 μm membrane filters (Thermo Fisher Scientific, Waltham, MA, USA). Finally, the total volume of urine from each sample was divided into 3 equal parts, to perform the 3 different EVs isolation methods.

Isolation methods

EVs enrichment by ultracentrifugation (UC) Urine supernatants were centrifuged at $100,000 \times g$, 2 h at 4 °C (in a 50.2 Ti Titanium rotor, Beckman coulter, using a CP100NX ultracentrifuge, Hitachi). The $100,000 \times g$ pellet was resuspended in 150 μL of filtered Phosphate-Buffered Saline (PBS).

Size exclusion chromatography (SEC) EVs isolation was performed as described by Böing et al. [29]. Briefly, up to 12 mL of Sepharose-CL2B (Sigma-Aldrich, San Luis, MO, USA) were stacked in a 15 mL syringe (Sigma-Aldrich, San Luis, MO, USA), and washed 3 times with PBS, previously filtered through 0.22 μm membrane filters, and used as elution buffer. Samples were concentrated using Amicon® Ultra-4 Centrifugal Filter Devices (EMD Millipore, Burlington, MA, USA) by centrifugation at $3200 \times g$, 20 min at 4 °C. Then, up to 0.75 mL of concentrated urine was loaded into the column, and a total of 20 fractions of 0.5 mL were collected from each sample. Fractions 8 and 9 were pooled and selected for further EVs analysis.

ExoLutE® Urine Kit Urine supernatants were concentrated to a final volume of 7 mL using Amicon® Ultra-4 Centrifugal Filter Devices (EMD Millipore Burlington, Ma, USA), and then processed with ExoLutE® Urine Kit (Rosetta Exosome® Inc., Seoul, Republic of Korea) following the manufacturer's instructions. A total of 130 μL of EVs-enriched samples were obtained.

Characterization methods

NanoDrop quantification The protein concentration in each sample was measured at 280 nm absorbance using a NanoDrop 1000 spectrophotometer (Thermo Scientific, Waltham, MA, USA).

Nanoparticle tracking analysis (NTA) Size distribution of particles was determined by NTA in a NanoSight LM10 (Malvern Instrument Ltd, Malvern, UK), using a 405 nm laser and sCMOS camera. Data were analyzed with using the NTA software version 3.3 (Dev Build 3.3.104), with Min track Length, Max Jump Distance, and Blur set to auto, and detection threshold set to 5. Camera level was set to 15, and 5 readings of

30 s at 30 frames per second were taken with manual monitoring of temperature. Samples were diluted with filtered PBS to reach the concentration (20–120 particles/frame) recommended by the manufacturer.

Transmission electron microscopy (TEM) Sample preparation was performed as already described [30] with modifications. Briefly, 8 μL of EVs-containing samples were fixed in 2% paraformaldehyde (PFA) for 30 min, and deposited on Formvar-carbon coated EM grids for 15 min. Then, samples were washed with PBS 0, 1 M, and post-fixed with 1% Glutaraldehyde for 5 min, washed with distilled water, and then contrasted in a mixture of uranyl acetate (1%) and methyl cellulose (0.5%). Samples were analyzed with a Jeol JEM1010 TEM, operating at 80 kV. Four different samples were analyzed for each of the isolation methods, and 100 vesicles were counted in each sample. Images were recorded on a MegaView III digital camera, and EVs size was determined using the Olympus Image Analysis Software. The sample analysis was performed at the Microscopy facility of the Central Service for Experimental Research (SCSIE) from the University of Valencia.

AlphaScreen™ Technology Five μL of EVs resuspended in PBS were transferred to a 96-well white 1/2 area microplate (Perkin Elmer, Madrid, Spain). Samples were incubated overnight at 4 °C with 10 μL/well of anti-human CD9 antibody (SHI-EXO-M01-50; CosmoBio Co, Tokyo, Japan) conjugated to AlphaLisa acceptor beads (10 μg/mL; 6,772,001, Perkin Elmer, Madrid, Spain), and 10 μL/well of biotinylated human anti-CD63 antibody (3 nM, SHI-EXO-M02-50, CosmoBio Co, Tokyo, Japan) previously biotinylated. Then, 25 μL/well of AlphaScreenTM streptavidin-coated donor beads (40 μg/mL; 6,760,002, Perkin Elmer, Madrid, Spain) were added and incubated in the dark for another 30 min at RT. A signal appears (excitation spectra at 680 nm, emission spectra at 615 nm) if the distance between both beads is less than 200 nm (compatible with exosomes size and other small EVs) thanks to the reactivity of O2, and is detected using a Multifunctional microplate reader CLARIOstar® (BMG LABTECH, Ortenberg, Germany). Assays were carried out at Centro de Investigación Principe Felipe (CIPF), Valencia, Spain.

HTG EdgeSeq miRNA Whole Transcriptome Assay (miRNA WTA) Whole miRNA transcriptome expression analysis was performed with urine derived EVs of PCa patients and HDs using the HTG EdgeSeq System (HTG Molecular Diagnostics, Inc., Tucson, AZ, USA) with the HTG EdgeSeq miRNA Whole Transcriptome Assay (miRNA WTA). This assay quantified the expression of 2083 human RNA transcripts (https://www.htgmolecular.com/assays/mirna-wta).

The same amount of EVs ($3,6 \times 10^9$) from each patient were digested with proteinase K following the manufacturer's instructions. miRNAs of interest were then selected by a protection nuclease assay (qNPA) in the HTG EdgeSeq processor using miRNA Whole Transcriptome Assay (miRNA WTA) panel (HTG Molecular Diagnostics, Inc., Tucson, AZ, USA). Library prepared with the miRNA selected was amplified by PCR using adapters for NextSeq 550 System sequencer (Illumina, San Diego, CA, USA). Samples were purified using Agencourt AMPure XP beads kit (Beckman Coulter, Brea, CA, USA), and then quantified by ABI 7500 Fast Real-Time PCR System (qPCR) using KAPA Library Quant Kit Universal qPCR Mix (KAPA Biosystems, Wilmington, MA, USA). For the qPCR, six standards were used in triplicate. Negative controls for PCR and qPCR were also used. After library quantification, all samples were normalized to a concentration of 20 pM. Library sequencing was performed using Next Generation Sequencing (NGS) in a NextSeq 550 System, High Output, 75 cycle v2.5 (Illumina, San Diego, CA, USA). Sequenced data were processed in HTG Parser Software using Bowtie2 for sequenced reads alignment.

Statistical analysis

Kruskal–Wallis non-parametric test and U- Mann Whitney test for post-hoc pairwise comparisons were used to perform a statistical analysis of the different characterization methods. All statistical inference was performed with two-tailed tests with a significance level of 5%.

Additionally, in the processing of HTG EdgeSeq data, Principal Component Analysis was used for data visualization and DESeq2 method for the study of differentially expressed miRNAs. The IBM SPSS Statistics V22.0 package (SPSS, Chicago, IL), R v. 4.0.1 and GraphPad Prism 7 (GraphPad Software Inc.) were used for statistical analysis [31].

Results

Spectrophotometric quantification and NTA

To compare protein and particle yields between the three EVs-isolation procedures, a spectrophotometric quantification at 280 nm, as well as the determination of particle concentration and size distribution by NTA, was performed. Absorbance measurements showed similar protein concentrations in UC (7.57 ± 8.2 µg/mL) and SEC (7.468 ± 3.77 µg/mL), but a significant increase was noted in Exolute® samples (25.99 ± 19.25 µg/mL) (Additional file 1: Figure S1A). Additional file 1: Figure S1B shows the amount of protein divided into PCa patients and HDs, no significant differences were found between the two groups in any of the three isolation methods.

NTA measurements revealed that UC provide the highest number of particles per mL ($4.13 \pm 3 \times 10^{11}$ particles/mL) in comparison with Exolute® ($1.78 \pm 1.03 \times 10^{11}$ particles/mL) p-value $= 0.021$, and SEC ($8.1 \pm 3.54 \times 10^{10}$ particles/mL) p-value $= 0.0011$ (Fig. 1A). However, whereas Exolute® and UC particles had a similar size distribution (modes of 167.84 ± 32.19 and 160.28 ± 18.51 nm, respectively; p-value > 0.99), SEC particles showed larger size (194.1 ± 16.4 nm) (p-value $= 0.0026$) (Fig. 1B).

The ratio between the number of particles/mL and the µg of proteins/mL, as an estimation of the purity of the sample, was calculated the highest ratio being for UC samples ($5.97 \pm 6.24 \times 10^{10}$), followed by SEC ($2.01 \pm 0.97 \times 10^{10}$) and Exolute® ($0.44 \pm 0.28 \times 10^{10}$), respectively (Fig. 1C).

Non-significant differences between PCa patients and HDs were observed. EVs isolated from UC and SEC showed a similar pattern, with higher particle and protein concentration in samples derived from PCa patients, which was inverted in Exolute®-EVs samples (Fig. 1D and Additional file 1: Figure S1B).

Characterization of isolated EVs by transmission electron microscopy

To obtain an accurate determination of the size of the isolated EVs by the different isolation methods, and to confirm previous data obtained by NTA, a TEM analysis was performed. Membrane-limited vesicles were easily detected by TEM (Fig. 2A). Interestingly, whereas UC and SEC-isolated EVs preparations showed a clear background in most preparations, the presence of a "dense background smudge" was noted in Exolute® samples, consistent with the presence of protein aggregates, as it has been previously described by Karimi et al. [32]. TEM analysis showed that EVs displayed similar sizes between the three isolation methods, with a median size around 90 nm [ranged between 80.2 and 86.3; 84–91.5 and 78.7–105.7 for Exolute®, UC and SEC, respectively (p-value $= 0.65$)] (Fig. 2B). Differences in EVs size distribution were detected, where vesicles in the range of 60 to 90 nm represented the main isolated population (around 40% of total). Nevertheless, SEC-isolated EVs had a broader size distribution than those isolated with Exolute® and UC. In fact, Exolute® seemed to favor the isolation of medium size EVs (60–120 nm) in comparison with SEC and UC (Fig. 2C).

Comparative marker analyses by AlphaScreen™ Technology

Human EVs commonly present tetraspanin proteins at their surface, such as CD63, CD81 and CD9 [22, 33], which have been also detected in EVs from urine [32].

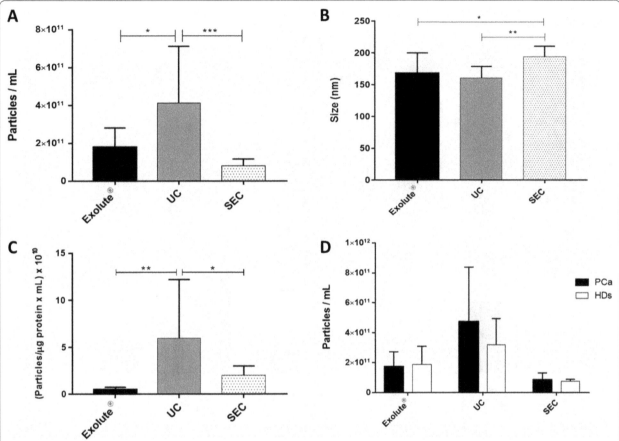

Fig. 1 Characterization of EVs by NTA. **A** Concentration and **B** size of the EVs. **C** Purity of sample calculated by ratio between the number of particles per mL and µg of proteins/mL. **D** The concentration of EVs is similar between PCa and HDs with the three isolation methods employed, with the number of EVs being higher in UC, followed by Exolute® and SEC. (*p-value < 0.05; **p-value < 0.001; ***p-value < 0.0001)

An adaptation of the amplified luminescent proximity homogeneous assay (ALPHA) technology [34] was used to detect two of these tetraspanins, CD9 and CD63, in EVs smaller than 200 nm. Our data showed that CD9 and CD63 were highly enriched in EVs from almost all the samples (with the exception of sample ID 129, which provided very low signals) when compared to total urine (TUr), confirming that the three methods were useful to isolate CD9 and CD63 positive EVs. As shown in Fig. 3A, SEC is the most efficient method in providing a reliable concentration of CD9 and CD63 positive EVs $(9.7 \times 10^5 \pm 9.1 \times 10^5)$, followed by UC $(6.7 \times 10^5 \pm 8.9 \times 10^5)$ and Exolute® $(1.1 \times 10^5 \pm 1.3 \times 10^5)$, respectively $(p$-value $= 0.0233)$. Interestingly, when luminescent data are disaggregated per sample and isolation method (Fig. 3B) it can be observed that SEC provides sufficient signal in almost every sample, whereas there is a broad variability in CD9 and CD63 combined signals in UC-EVs. Thus, whereas UC-EVs had the higher mean signal in four samples, EVs isolated from the rest provided low signals (below

200,000), SEC-EVs showed the higher mean signal in 6 out of 10 patients, but only 2 patients provided signals below 200,000. On the other hand, no differences were detected between PCa and HDs (Additional file 1: Figure S2).

Evaluation of the isolation method by HTG EdgeSeq miRNA whole transcriptome assay

A whole miRNA transcriptomic assay was performed on the isolated EVs using the WTA panel on an HTG EdgeSeq Sytem (HTG Molecular Diagnostics). miRNA expression levels were quantified by NGS. Median of the sum of the normalized miRNA counts was higher in EVs isolated from SEC [16814 (range: 15,650–17,121)], followed by UC [16260 (range: 15,796–16874], and Exolute® [16137 (range: 15,575–16,710)] $(p$-value $= 0.046)$ (Fig. 4).

Heatmap and PCA plots show that cases were not aggregated based on their miRNA expression profiles as would be expected, but they were classified more dependent of the EVs isolation method (Additional file 1: Figure S3). Despite this, correlations of miRNA

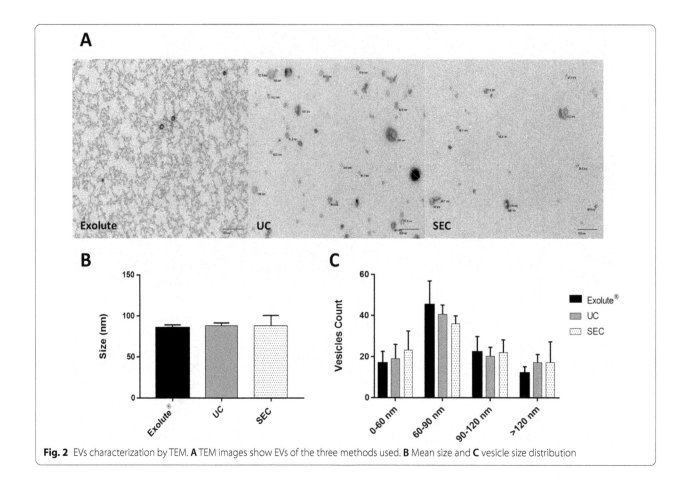

Fig. 2 EVs characterization by TEM. **A** TEM images show EVs of the three methods used. **B** Mean size and **C** vesicle size distribution

expression levels in each case between the three EVs isolation methods were statistically significant (Table 2, Additional file 1: Figures S4–S13). However, in global, the correlation was better between UC and SEC [Median $R^2 = 0.8$ (range: 0.62–0.91)] than any of these methods with Exolute® (Table 2).

The differential expression analysis (DEA) between PCa cases and HDs for each EVs isolation method showed that a total of 21 and 3 miRNAs were differentially expressed (p-adjusted < 0.1) between groups for SEC and UC, respectively. However, no miRNAs were discriminated in the case of Exolute®. Remarkably, only miR-8052 matched between the SEC and UC miRNA sets (Additional file 1: Figure S14).

Interestingly, the evaluation of two sets of RNAs (housekeeping genes and *Let-7* miRNA family) from different EVs isolation methods showed significant differences between UC and SEC with Exolute® (Fig. 5), suggesting that Exolute® method offers the lowest performance from the biological point of view.

Lastly, the overall miRNA expression was divided into different quartiles (q1 < q2 < q3 < q4), and a correlation with the EVs isolation method used was performed for

each quartile, indicating that those miRNAs with lower expression levels would be compromised depending on the type of isolation method used, as can be subtracted from the R^2 values of the different quartiles (Additional file 1: Figure S15).

Discussion

EVs have been postulated as a valuable source of potential biomarkers in PCa that at some point would complement or replace the routine diagnostic procedures [15, 35]. Urinary EVs take special relevance since their cargo reflect changes in the cellular biology of the tumour during progression and can be isolated by non-invasive procedures. However, translation of these biomarkers into the clinical setting is not exempt of limitations, including the irreproducibility of results as one of the most important [36]. In this regard, EVs isolation and characterization approaches still constitute a scientific challenge [23]. Hence, with the aim of deepening in the knowledge of EVs isolation methods, we evaluated three different methodologies including the classical UC and SEC, as well as a commercial eVs isolation kit (Exolute®). EVs characterization was performed using NTA, TEM,

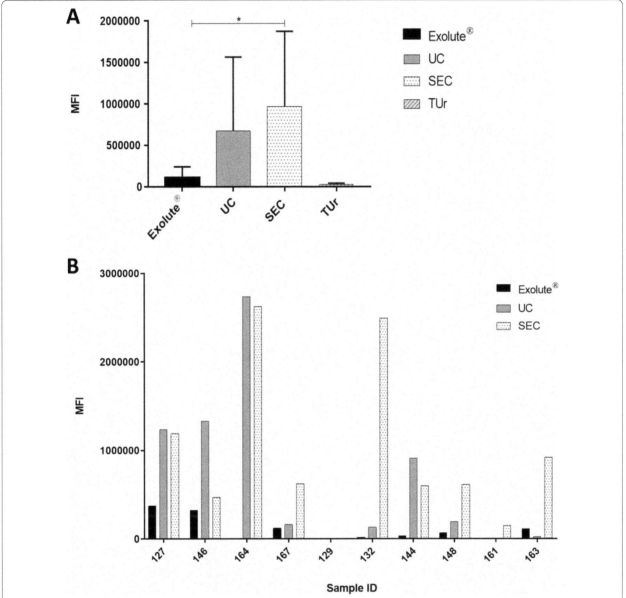

Fig. 3 AlphaScreen™ Technology analysis. **A** CD9 and CD 63 tretaspanins have been used to label EVs. A higher performance has been obtained by the three isolation methods of EVs compared to total urine (TUr), being SEC the method with the highest performance followed by UC and Exolute®. (*p-value < 0.05). **B** Luminiscent levels shows variability in CD9 and CD63 EVs signal in each sample

spectrophotometry (Nanodrop), AlphaScreen™ Technology and whole miRNA transcriptome expression analysis with the EdgeSeq System (HTG Molecular Diagnostics). For this purpose, a series of urines collected from 10 individuals (6 PCa patients and 4 HDs) were analysed with each isolation method.

Absorbance measurements showed similar protein concentrations in UC and SEC; however, a significant increase was noticed in Exolute® samples (Additional file 1: Figure S1A). This effect can be explained by TEM analysis, in which preparations from EVs obtained with Exolute® showed a background of precipitated proteins (Fig. 2A) consistent with the presence of protein aggregates, as it has been previously described [37]. NTA evaluation showed that UC provided the highest number of particles per mL and particles per µg protein ratio, in comparison with SEC and Exolute®, suggesting a higher EV yield obtained by this technique (Fig. 1A, C). Besides that, a significant increase in size of particles obtained by SEC was noticed (~ 190 nm),

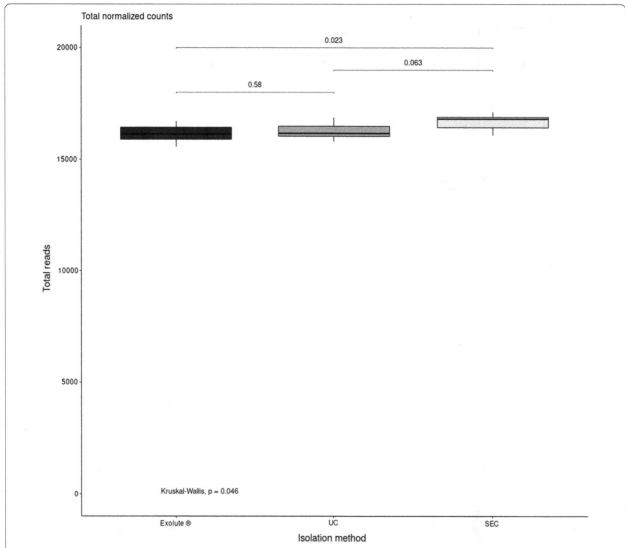

Fig. 4 Box plot of the sum of the normalized miRNA counts per EVs isolation methods. SEC reported a higher count reads in comparison to UC (*p*-value = 0.063) and Exolute® (*p*-value = 0.023)

when compared to the other EVs isolation procedures (~165 nm) (Fig. 1B). However, no differences in size were appreciated when EVs were analyzed by TEM with a median in size of around 90 nm (range: 30–200 nm). Interestingly, approximately 95% of EVs were ranged from 30 to 120 nm, and around 40% were between 60 and 90 nm of diameter (Fig. 2C). These findings correlate with previous reports showing that the size of urine EVs varies from 30 to 100 nm [38–41]. Discordances between NTA and TEM herein reported may be due to different aspects including: the difficulty of NTA to resolve EVs aggregates (a correct dilution of the sample is crucial to avoid this) [42]; the limitation of NTA in detecting particles which dimeter is lower than 100 nm

[43] and finally, the size overestimation of NTA [44, 45]. Additionally, and as mentioned above, TEM analyses revealed high variability in EVs yield obtained by Exolute®, with some samples showing the presence of protein aggregates that would explain the highest protein content of the spectrophotometric analysis (Fig. 2A). Interestingly, SEC-isolated EVs had a broader size distribution than those isolated with Exolute® and UC, which could be due to the growing evidence that SEC minimally alters the physical properties of EVs, whereas UC might cause vesicle rupture or fusion with proteins because of the high speed used in centrifugations [46]. No significant differences in particle concentration and size (measured by both NTA or TEM) were detected

Table 2 Coefficient correlation values (R^2) between the three EVs-isolation procedures

Sample ID	Type of sample	UC-SEC	SEC-Exolute®	UC-Exolute®
127	PCa patient	0.77	0.66	0.73
129	PCa patient	0.65	0.64	0.70
132	PCa patient	0.82	0.57	0.67
144	PCa patient	0.84	0.77	0.75
146	PCa patient	0.91	0.76	0.75
148	PCa patient	0.72	0.79	0.71
161	HDs	0.62	0.67	0.77
163	HDs	0.78	0.81	0.69
164	HDs	0.83	0.63	0.64
167	HDs	0.82	0.63	0.69
Median (range)		0.8 (0.62–0.91)	0.67 (0.57–0.81)	0.71 (0.64–0.77)
Average (SD)		0.78 (0.09)	0.69 (0.08)	0.71 (0.04)

SD, standard deviation; HDs, healthy donors; PCa, prostate cancer

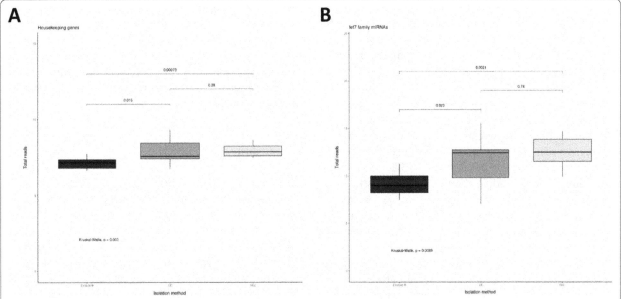

Fig. 5 Box plots showing the median expression values for different EVs isolation methods of: **A** Twelve housekeeping genes included in the WTA panel (probes for the following genes are included: *B2M, GAPDH, PPIA, RNU47, RNU75, RNY3, RPL19, RPL27, RPS12, RPS20, SNORA66 YWHAZ*); **B** Let-7 family of miRNAs (n = 15). In both cases, clear differences between UC and SEC with Exolute® were appreciated

between PCa samples and HDs (Fig. 1D) which is in accordance with previous studies [38].

Once characterized through NTA and TEM, EVs were analysed with AlphaScreen™ Technology, a strategy lately used to improve the typical immunoassays [34] through the simultaneous detection for two specific EV-tetraspanins, CD9 and CD63 [22, 33] and designed to specifically detect EVs lower than 200 nm. Our AlphaScreen data revealed that all three isolation methods obtained CD9 and CD63 positive EVs, as can be appreciated in Fig. 3A where luminescent signal was higher in purified EVs

compared to crude urine. Furthermore, SEC provided the highest luminescent intensity followed by UC and Exolute®, which luminescent intensity was significantly lower. Interestingly, a high signal variation was noted among the analysed cases, especially in Exolute® and UC isolated EVs, for which in some cases the luminescent signal was low or null, whereas SEC isolated EVs provided a measurable signal in most of the cases (Fig. 3B). These differences would be related to those herein noticed with regards EVs size distribution, or as suggested by some reports, as consequence of differences in the membrane proteomic content of small and large EVs [47]. Moreover, EVs rupture due to UC high-speed centrifugations [46] or the reported variability on EVs yield depending on the equipment and operator technical variability could have affected the results [48]. Hence, and according to the AlphaScreen™ Technology, our results highlight SEC as the most efficient method to isolate CD9 and CD63 positive microvesicles, followed by UC and Exolute®, respectively. Like the other characterization methods, no differences of luminescent signal were appreciated between EVs isolated from PCa patients and HDs for any of the isolation methods tested.

Forward characterization of EVs was carried through a whole miRNA transcriptomic analysis by using one of the newest and most reproducible RNA quantification platforms, the EdgeSeq Technology (HTG Molecular Diagnostics), currently used in many studies [49, 50]. Among the advantages of this system are that it does not require an RNA-extraction step which, reduces the extraction-associated data bias and sample loss; and the low input of sample necessary for being analysed [51]. Our results have shown that the sum of the normalized miRNA counts was higher in EVs isolated from SEC, followed by UC and Exolute® (Fig. 4), suggesting that the isolation methods influence on the yield of the transcriptomic analysis. Many -omic studies have been found to be highly dependent on the EVs isolation procedures, so that different methods produce EVs and EV sub-fractions of variable homogeneity, which makes difficult to extrapolate findings between different studies of EVs [7]. This is in line with the results we have obtained, in which samples were classified based more on the EVs isolation method than on their origin (PCa patients or HDs) (Additional file 1: Figure S3). Despite this, correlation of miRNA profiles between the different isolation approaches was high in all cases, being better between UC and SEC (Table 2). Interestingly, when miRNA expression was divided into quartiles, the best correlation coefficients (R^2) were obtained in q4 (higher number of miRNAs) with a $R^2 = 0.97$ between SEC and UC, the correlation in q2 and q1 being lower (Additional file 1: Figure S15). To demonstrate that the isolation procedures influence at biological level, two sets of RNA were evaluated: the housekeeping genes provided by the assay and the *Let-7* family of miRNAs. This approach showed significant differences with regards number of reads for any of the two RNA sets of UC and SEC with Exolute® (Fig. 5), indicating that Exolute® provides the lowest performance from the biological point of view.

DEA between PCa cases and HDs for each EVs isolation method showed that a total of 21 and 3 miRNAs were differentially expressed between groups for SEC and UC respectively, and none for Exolute®. The only miRNA that was differentially expressed in both methods was miR-8052 [52], a miRNA not previously described in PCa but in serum from sepsis patients with different outcomes [53]. Remarkably, two of the 3 miRNAs differentially expressed in EVs isolated by UC from urine of PCa patients were miR-142-5p and miR-223-3p, two miRNA that have been recently described in EVs from urine isolated also by UC as non-invasive PCa diagnostic biomarkers [54].

Although our study sample is limited, and further studies need to be addressed, our results point out to what other authors have suggested, the need of methodological standardization of EVs isolation and characterization to guaranty the success and reproducibility of the subsequent analysis, especially for clinical settings, where a large number of samples should be analysed [55–57]. In this line, we suggest developing a codification system focused on the EV isolation and characterization variables like the SPREC codification system for pre-analytical conditions [25] that we have introduce with our samples (Table 1) and that provides information on the handling of biological specimens before analysis, another critical point that not always comprehensively considered [58, 59].

Conclusion

Definitively, our study highlights the impact that the EV isolation method may have on the analytical results, as differences in the yield, purity, and status of the obtained EVs might have a great influence in the clinical setting. For this reason, methodological standardization in the isolation and subsequent analysis of EV is crucial to guaranty the reproducibility necessary for their implementation in different clinical scenarios.

Abbreviations

CREC: Clinical Research Ethics Committee; DEA: Differential expression analysis; DRE: Digital rectal examination; EVs: Extracellular vesicles; FIVO: Fundación Instituto Valenciano de Oncología; HDs: Healthy donors; miRNA: MicroRNA; NTA: Nanoparticle tracking analysis; PBS: Phosphate-Buffered Saline; PCa: Prostate cancer; PCR: Polymerase chain reaction; PSA: Prostate-specific antigen; qPCR: Quantitative PCR; RNA: Ribonucleic acid; RT: Room temperature; SCSIE: Central Service for Experimental Research; SEC: Size exclusion chromatography; SPREC: Sample PREanalytical Code; TEM: Transmission electron microscopy; UC: Ultracentrifugation; WTA: Whole Transcriptome Assay.

Supplementary Information

Additional file 1. Supplementary material.

Acknowledgements

Authors thank Patricia Carretero Hinojosa and Tania Mazcuñán Vitiello for technical assistance. We also thank the Biobank of the Fundación Instituto Valenciano de Oncología for providing the biological samples for the analysis.

Authors' contributions

MG-F: Methodology, formal analysis, investigation, data curation, writing-original draft preparation, visualization. CMS-L: Methodology, software, formal analysis, investigation, data curation, writing-original draft preparation, visualization. MR-C: Methodology, formal analysis, investigation, data curation. AF-S: Software, investigation, data curation, visualization. AM: Conceptualization, investigation, resources, writing—review and editing, supervision, funding acquisition. JAL-G: Conceptualization, investigation, resources, writing—review and editing, supervision, project administration, funding acquisition. All authors have read and agreed to the published version of the manuscript.

Author details

[1]Laboratory of Molecular Biology, Fundación Instituto Valenciano de Oncología, 46009 Valencia, Spain. [2]IVO-CIPF Joint Research Unit of Cancer, Príncipe Felipe Research Center (CIPF), 46012 Valencia, Spain. [3]Àrea de Parasitologia, Departament de Farmàcia i Tecnologia Farmacèutica i Parasitologia, Universitat de València, 46000 Burjassot, Valencia, Spain. [4]Joint Research Unit on Endocrinology, Nutrition and Clinical Dietetics, Health Research Institute La Fe, Universitat de Valencia, 46100 Valencia, Spain. [5]Department of Pathology, School of Medicine, Catholic University of Valencia "San Vicente Mártir", 46001 Valencia, Spain.

References

1. Bunting PS. Screening for prostate cancer with prostate-specific antigen: beware the biases. Clin Chim Acta. 2002;315:71–97.
2. Freedland SJ, Partin AW. Prostate-specific antigen: update 2006. Urology. 2006;67:458–60.
3. Thompson IM, Ankerst DP, Chi C, Lucia MS, Goodman PJ, Crowley JJ, Parnes HL, Coltman CA. Operating characteristics of prostate-specific antigen in men with an initial PSA level of 3.0 Ng/ml or lower. JAMA. 2005;294:66–70.
4. Thurtle DR, Greenberg DC, Lee LS, Huang HH, Pharoah PD, Gnanapragasam VJ. Individual prognosis at diagnosis in nonmetastatic prostate cancer: development and external validation of the PREDICT prostate multivariable model. PLoS Med. 2019;16:e1002758.
5. Filella X, Foj L. Prostate cancer detection and prognosis: from prostate specific antigen (PSA) to exosomal biomarkers. Int J Mol Sci. 2016;17:1784.
6. Lawson C, Vicencio JM, Yellon DM, Davidson SM. Microvesicles and exosomes: new players in metabolic and cardiovascular disease. J Endocrinol. 2016;228:R57–71.
7. Yáñez-mó M, Siljander PR, Andreu Z, Bedina A, Borràs FE, Buzas EI, Buzas K, Casal E, Cappello F, Carvalho J, et al. Biological properties of extracellular vesicles and their physiological functions. J Extracell Vesicles. 2015;4:27066.
8. Andreu Z, Rivas E, Sanguino-pascual A, Lamana A, Marazuela M, González-Alvaro I, Sánchez-Madrid F, de la Fuente H, Yáñez-Mó M. Comparative analysis of EV isolation procedures for miRNAs detection in serum samples. J Extracell Vesicles. 2016;5:31655.
9. Nilsson RJA, Skog J, Nordstrand A, Baranov V, Mincheva-Nilsson L, Breakefield XO, Widmark A. Prostate cancer-derived urine exosomes: a novel approach to biomarkers for prostate cancer. Br J Cancer. 2009;100:1603–7.
10. Emanueli C, Shearn AIU, Angelini GD, Sahoo S. Exosomes and exosomal miRNAs in cardiovascular protection and repair. Vasc Pharmacol. 2015;71:24–33.
11. Pol EVD, Böing AN, Harrison P, Sturk A, Nieuwland R. Classification, functions, and clinical relevance of extracellular vesicles. Pharmacol Rev. 2012;64:676–705.
12. Vader P, Breakefield XO, Wood MJA. Extracellular vesicles: emerging targets for cancer therapy. Trends Mol Med. 2015;20:385–93.
13. Patel GK, Khan MA, Bhardwaj A, Srivastava SK, Zubair H, Patton MC, Singh S, Khushman M, Singh AP. Exosomes confer chemoresistance to pancreatic cancer cells by promoting ROS detoxification and miR-155-mediated suppression of key gemcitabine-metabolising enzyme, DCK. Br J Cancer. 2017;116:609–19.
14. Kalluri R. The biology and function of exosomes in cancer. J Clin Investig. 2016;126:1208–15.
15. Tai Y, Lin C, Li T, Shen T, Hsieh J, Chen BPC. The role of extracellular vesicles in prostate cancer with clinical applications. Endocr Relat Cancer. 2020;27:R133–44.
16. Vlaeminck-Guillem V. Extracellular vesicles in prostate cancer carcinogenesis, diagnosis, and management. Front Oncol. 2018;8:222.
17. Greening DW, Xu R, Ji H, Tauro BJ, Simpson RJ. A protocol for exosome isolation and characterization: evaluation of ultracentrifugation, density-gradient separation, and immunoaffinity capture methods. Methods Mol Biol. 2015;1295:179–209.
18. Gould SJ, Raposo G. As we wait: coping with an imperfect nomenclature for extracellular vesicles. J Extracell Vesicles. 2013;2:10.
19. Helwa I, Cai J, Drewry MD, Zimmerman A, Dinkins B, Khaled ML, Seremwe M, Dismuke WM, Bieberich E, Stamer WD, et al. A Comparative study of serum exosome isolation using differential ultracentrifugation and three commercial reagents. PLoS ONE. 2017;22:e0170628.
20. Lee J, Kwon MH, Kim JA, Rhee WJ. Detection of exosome miRNAs using molecular beacons for diagnosing prostate cancer. Artif Cells Nanomed Biotechnol. 2018;46(sup3):S52–63.
21. Royo F, Zun P, Egia A, Perez A, Loizaga A, Arceo R, Lacasa I, Rabade A, Arrieta E, Bilbao R, et al. Different EV enrichment methods suitable for clinical settings yield different subpopulations of urinary extracellular vesicles from human samples. J Extracell Vesicles. 2016;1:1–11.
22. Lötvall J, Hill AF, Hochberg F, Buzás EI, Di D, Gardiner C, Gho YS, Kurochkin IV, Quesenberry P, Sahoo S, et al. Minimal experimental requirements for definition of extracellular vesicles and their functions: a position statement from the international society for extracellular vesicles. J Extracell Vesicles. 2014;3:26913.
23. Szatanek R, Baran J, Siedlar M, Baj-krzyworzeka M. Isolation of extracellular vesicles: determining the correct approach (review). Int J Mol Med. 2015;36:11–7.
24. Zhou H, Yuen PST, Pisitkun T, Gonzales PA, Yasuda H, Dear JW, Gross P, Knepper MA, Star RA. Collection, storage, preservation, and normalization of human urinary exosomes for biomarker discovery. Kidney Int. 2006;69:1471–6.
25. Betsou F, Bilbao R, Case J, Chuaqui R, Clements JA, De Souza Y, De Wilde A, Geiger J, Grizzle W, Guadagni F, et al. Standard PREanalytical code version 3.0. Biopreserv Biobank. 2018;16:9–12.
26. Betsou F, Lehmann S, Ashton G, Barnes M, Benson EE, Coppola D, DeSouza Y, Eliason J, Glazer B, Guadagni F, et al. Standard preanalytical coding for biospecimens: defining the sample PREanalytical code. Cancer Epidemiol Biomark Prev. 2010;19:1004–11.
27. Lehmann S, Guadagni F, Moore H, Ashton G, Barnes M, Benson E, Clements J, Koppandi I, Coppola D, Demiroglu SY, et al. Standard preanalytical coding for biospecimens: review and implementation of the Sample PREanalytical Code (SPREC). Biopreserv Biobank. 2012;10:366–74.
28. Kosanovic M, Jankovi M. Isolation of urinary extracellular vesicles from tamm- horsfall protein-depleted urine and their application in the development of a lectin-exosome-binding assay. Biotechniques. 2014;57:143–9.
29. Böing AN, van der Pol E, Grootemaat AE, Coumans FAW, Sturk A, Nieuwland R. Single-step isolation of extracellular vesicles by size-exclusion chromatography. J Extracell Vesicles. 2014;3:23430–511.
30. Théry C, Clayton A, Amigorena S, Raposo G, editors. Isolation and characterization of exosomes from cell culture supernatants and biological fluids. Hoboken: Wiley; 2006. p. 3221–32229.
31. Love MI, Huber W, Anders S. Moderated estimation of fold change and-dispersion for RNA-Seq data with DESeq2. Genome Biol. 2014;15:550.
32. Campos-Silva C, Suarez H, Jara-Acevedo R, Linares-Espinos E, Martinez-Pineiro L, Yanez-Mo M, Vales-Gomez M. High sensitivity detection of extracellular vesicles immune-captured from urine by conventional flow cytometry. Sci Rep. 2019;9:2042–8.
33. Mathivanan S, Ji H, Simpson RJ. Exosomes: extracellular organelles important in intercellular communication. J Proteom. 2010;73:1907–20.

34. Yoshioka Y, Kosaka N, Konishi Y, Ohta H, Okamoto H, Sonoda H, Nonaka R, Yamamoto H, Ishii H, Mori M, et al. Ultra-sensitive liquid biopsy of circulating extracellular vesicles using ExoScreen. Nat Commun. 2014;5:3591.

35. Braun F, Müller R. Urinary extracellular vesicles as a source of biomarkers reflecting renal cellular biology in human disease. Methods Cell Biol. 2019;154:43–65.

36. Scherer A. Reproducibility in biomarker research and clinical development: a global challenge. Biomark Med. 2017;11:309–12.

37. Karimi N, Cvjetkovic A, Jang SC, Crescitelli R, Hosseinpour Feizi MA, Nieuwland R, Lötvall J, Lässer C. Detailed analysis of the plasma extracellular vesicle proteome after separation from lipoproteins. Cell Mol Life Sci. 2018;75:2873–86.

38. Bryzgunova OE, Zaripov MM, Skvortsova TE, Lekchnov EA, Grigor'eva AE, Zaporozhchenko IA, Morozkin ES, Ryabchikova EI, Yurchenko YB, Voitsitskiy VE, et al. Comparative study of extracellular vesicles from the urine of healthy individuals and prostate cancer patients. PLoS ONE. 2016;11:e0157566.

39. Fang DY, King HW, Li JY, Gleadle JM. Exosomes and the kidney: blaming the messenger. Nephrology (Carlton). 2013;18:1–10.

40. Murakami T, Oakes M, Ogura M, Tovar V, Yamamoto C, Mitsuhashi M. Development of glomerulus-, tubule-, and collecting duct-specific mRNA assay in human urinary exosomes and microvesicles. PLoS ONE. 2014;9:e109074.

41. Singhto N, Vinaiphat A, Thongboonkerd V. Discrimination of urinary exosomes from microvesicles by lipidomics using thin layer liquid chromatography (TLC) coupled with MALDI-TOF mass spectrometry. Sci Rep. 2019;9:13834–911.

42. Lozano-Ramos I, Bancu I, Oliveira-Tercero A, Armengol MP, Menezes-Neto A, Portillo HAD, Lauzurica-Valdemoros R, Borràs FE. Size-exclusion chromatography-based enrichment of extracellular vesicles from urine samples. J Extracell Vesicles. 2015;4:27369.

43. Van der Pol E, Coumans FAW, Grootemaat AE, Gardiner C, Sargent IL, Harrison P, Sturk A, van Leeuwen TG, Nieuwland R. Particle size distribution of exosomes and microvesicles determined by transmission electron microscopy, flow cytometry, nanoparticle tracking analysis, and resistive pulse sensing. J Thromb Haemost. 2014;12:1182–92.

44. Bachurski D, Schuldner M, Nguyen P, Malz A, Reiners KS, Grenzi PC, Babatz F, Schauss AC, Hansen HP, Hallek M, et al. Extracellular vesicle measurements with nanoparticle tracking analysis: an accuracy and repeatability comparison between NanoSight NS300 and ZetaView. J Extracell Vesicles. 2019;8:1596016.

45. Serrano-Pertierra E, Oliveira-Rodríguez M, Matos M, Gutiérrez G, Moyano A, Salvador M, Rivas M, Blanco-López MC. Extracellular vesicles: current analytical techniques for detection and quantification. Biomolecules (Basel, Switzerland). 2020;10:824.

46. Monguió-Tortajada M, Gálvez-Montón C, Bayes-Genis A, Roura S, Borràs FE. Extracellular vesicle isolation methods: rising impact of size-exclusion chromatography. Cell Mol Life Sci. 2019;76:2369–82.

47. Mariscal J, Vagner T, Kim M, Zhou B, Chin A, Zandian M, Freeman MR, You S, Zijlstra A, Yang W, et al. Comprehensive palmitoyl-proteomic analysis identifies distinct protein signatures for large and small cancer-derived extracellular vesicles. J Extracell Vesicles. 2020;9:1764192.

48. Torres Crigna A, Fricke F, Nitschke K, Worst T, Erb U, Karremann M, Buschmann D, Elvers-Hornung S, Tucher C, Schiller M, et al. Inter-laboratory comparison of extracellular vesicle isolation based on ultracentrifugation. Transfus Med Hemother. 2020;48:48–59.

49. Bustos MA, Tran KD, Rahimzadeh N, Gross R, Lin SY, Shoji Y, Murakami T, Boley CL, Tran LT, Cole H, et al. Integrated assessment of circulating cell-free microRNA signatures in plasma of patients with melanoma brain metastasis. Cancers. 2020;12:1692.

50. Nziza N, Jeziorski E, Delpont M, Cren M, Chevassus H, Carbasse A, Mahe P, Abassi H, Joly-Monrigal P, Schordan E, et al. Synovial-fluid miRNA signature for diagnosis of juvenile idiopathic arthritis. Cells (Basel). 2019;8:1521.

51. Godoy PM, Barczak AJ, DeHoff P, Srinivasan S, Etheridge A, Galas D, Das S, Erle DJ, Laurent LC. Comparison of reproducibility, accuracy, sensitivity, and specificity of miRNA quantification platforms. Cell Rep. 2019;29:4212-4222.e5.

52. Griffiths-Jones S. miRBase: microRNA sequences, targets and gene nomenclature. Nucleic Acids Res. 2006;34:D140–4.

53. Wang H, Zhang P, Chen W, Jie D, Dan F, Jia Y, Xie L. Characterization and identification of novel serum microRNAs in sepsis patients with different outcomes. Shock. 2013;39:480–7.

54. Barceló M, Castells M, Bassas L, Vigués F, Larriba S. Semen miRNAs contained in exosomes as non-invasive biomarkers for prostate cancer diagnosis. Sci Rep. 2019;9:13772–816.

55. Gurunathan S, Kang M, Jeyaraj M, Qasim M, Kim J. Review of the isolation, characterization, biological function, and multifarious therapeutic approaches of exosomes. Cells. 2019;8:307.

56. Ma C, Jiang F, Ma Y, Wang J, Li H, Zhang J. Isolation and detection technologies of extracellular vesicles and application on cancer diagnostic. Nanotechnol Microtechnol Drug Deliv Syst. 2019;17:155932581989100–1559325818991004.

57. Xu R, Greening DW, Zhu H, Takahashi N, Simpson RJ. Extracellular vesicle isolation and characterization: toward clinical application. J Clin Invest. 2016;126:1152–62.

58. Carraro P, Zago T, Plebani M. Exploring the initial steps of the testing process: frequency and nature of pre-preanalytic errors. Clin Chem. 2012;58:638–42.

59. Moore HM, Compton CC, Lim MD, Vaught J, Christiansen KN, Alper J. 2009 Biospecimen research network symposium: advancing cancer research through biospecimen science. Cancer Res. 2009;69:6770–2.

19

Evaluation of a rapid one-step PSA test for primary prostate cancer screening

Shingo Ashida[1*], Ichiro Yamasaki[2], Chiaki Kawada[1], Hideo Fukuhara[1], Satoshi Fukata[1], Kenji Tamura[1], Takashi Karashima[1], Keiji Inoue[1] and Taro Shuin[3]

Abstract

Background: To enhance the convenience and reduce the cost of prostate cancer (PC) screening, a one-step prostate-specific antigen (PSA) test was evaluated in a large population. The PSA SPOT test kit enables rapid detection of human PSA in serum or plasma at or above a cutoff level of 4 ng/mL to aid in the diagnosis of PC.

Methods: PC screening using the PSA SPOT test was offered to male participants in educational public lectures that we conducted in various cities. Test results were reported to participants at the end of the lectures. Blood samples from 1429 men were evaluated. Two independent observers interpreted the tests at 15 and 30 min. The remaining serum samples were subsequently tested using a conventional quantitative assay.

Results: The sensitivity, specificity, positive predictive value, negative predictive value, and accuracy of the test were 79.9, 93.0, 65.4, 96.6, and 91.2%, respectively. The sensitivity and specificity of the test changed with variations in the reading time. Quantitative assessment of the intensity of the band was correlated with the PSA value.

Conclusions: PSA testing using this kit can be easily performed. The low cost and speed of the test make it a useful and convenient tool for primary PC screening.

Keywords: Prostate cancer, Screening, Prostate-specific antigen, Rapid test

Background

Prostate cancer (PC) is one of the most common malignancies and causes of cancer death among men worldwide [1], with an estimated 78,500 new cases in 2019 in Japan. The widespread use of the prostate-specific antigen (PSA) test is thought to be responsible for the rapid increase in PC diagnoses between 1988 and 1992 in the United States [2, 3].

Both the high prevalence of PC and availability of PSA tests capable of detecting PC at an early stage are important criteria required to support mass screening. The significant increase in the diagnosis of organ-confined PC—which means a reduction in metastatic disease—justifies PC screening [4–6]. Moreover, recent randomized clinical trials (RCTs) demonstrated a 21 to 44% decline in PC mortality rates due to PSA screening [7, 8], which could represent one of the most persuasive arguments in support of PC screening.

However, PC screening is still controversial, as the potential benefits and harms continue to be debated among health professionals. Major controversies regarding PC screening center on the possibilities of over-diagnosis and over-treatment. Some patients might suffer from complications associated with the treatment of clinically insignificant PCs that would probably never lead to death. Another issue involves the economics of PC screening, including the costs associated with detection, treatment, and treatment-related complications. Optenberg and Thompson estimated that the cost of screening could be as high as $25 billion annually if all men

*Correspondence: ashidas@kochi-u.ac.jp
[1] Department of Urology, Kochi Medical School, Nankoku, Kochi 783-8505, Japan
Full list of author information is available at the end of the article

50–70 years of age in the United States participated in a screening program [9].

In this study, we evaluated a rapid, one-step, qualitative PSA test, called the PSA SPOT test, as a possible way to enhance the convenience and reduce the cost of PC screening in a large population.

Methods
PSA SPOT test
The PSA SPOT test was performed according to the instructions provided by Prof. Rajvir Dahiya, PhD, Department of Urology, Veterans Affairs Medical Center and University of California, San Francisco, California. The format of the PSA SPOT test is a double-antibody sandwich. Antibodies specific to PSA are conjugated to colloidal gold and incorporated into a strip pad, and these antibodies capture any PSA after the sample is added to the test strip. The antigen-antibody-gold complexes migrate along the nitrocellulose membrane via capillary action and are then captured by marker-specific antibodies immobilized on the membrane. A red-colored band will appear in the test zone (T) if PSA protein is present in the specimen (Fig. 1). Antibody-gold complexes are captured in the control zone (C), where goat anti-mouse IgG is immobilized. To serve as an internal process control, a red-colored control band was designed to appear as an indication that the test was performed properly and should always be seen after the test is completed. The absence of a red control band in the control region is an indication of an invalid result.

The PSA SPOT test kit is designed for the rapid detection of human PSA in serum or plasma at or above a cutoff level of 4 ng/mL. In the present study, two independent observers interpreted the test results at 15 and 30 min. The remaining serum samples were subsequently tested using a conventional quantitative assay (Access Hybritech PSA, Beckman Coulter, Inc.). The tests were interpreted as negative if no band appeared in the test

region; if a band developed, the test was judged as either weakly positive (+) or strongly positive (++) according to the intensity of the color reaction.

Validation of the PSA SPOT test
To validate the PSA SPOT test, serum samples obtained from 53 consecutive patients suspected of having or followed up for PC were tested using the PSA SPOT test and quantitative PSA test (Access Hybritech PSA). The sensitivity and specificity of the PSA SPOT test were determined using the cut-off value of 4.0 ng/mL.

PC screening using the PSA SPOT test
PC screening using the PSA SPOT test kit was offered to male participants in educational public lectures that we conducted in various cities from June 2005 to July 2016. Blood samples from 1429 men (mean age, 70.8 years; range, 30–93 years) were evaluated. The blood samples were obtained before the lectures, serum was separated from blood by centrifugation, and the PSA SPOT test was immediately performed. The results of the tests were reported to the participants at the end of the lectures. We then enclosed and passed referral letters if the results were judged as positive.

This study was approved by the ethical review board of Kochi Medical School (ethical approval no. 16–12). Written informed consent was obtained regarding PC screening using the PSA SPOT test. All methods were carried out in accordance with relevant guidelines and regulations.

Statistical analysis
All statistical analyses were performed using JMP® software (SAS Institute Inc., Cary, NC, USA). A P value < 0.05 was considered to indicate a statistically significant difference. The sensitivity, specificity, positive predictive value (PPV), negative predictive value (NPV), and accuracy of the PSA SPOT test were calculated. A box-and-whisker plot was used to show the correlation between the PSA quantitative value and intensity of the color reaction band on the PSA SPOT test. Pearson's correlation test was used to correlate the two variables described above.

Results
In the validation series using serum samples from 54 patients suspected of having or followed up for PC, the sensitivity and specificity of the PSA SPOT test were 9.1 and 96.8%, respectively, at a reading time of 15 min and 90.9 and 93.5%, respectively, at 30 min.

Of 1429 participants, 1223 (85.6%) had a PSA value of less than 4 ng/mL (median PSA, 1.270 ng/mL; range, 0.001–3.972 ng/mL), and 206 (14.4%) presented a PSA value higher than 4 ng/mL (median PSA, 6.304 ng/mL;

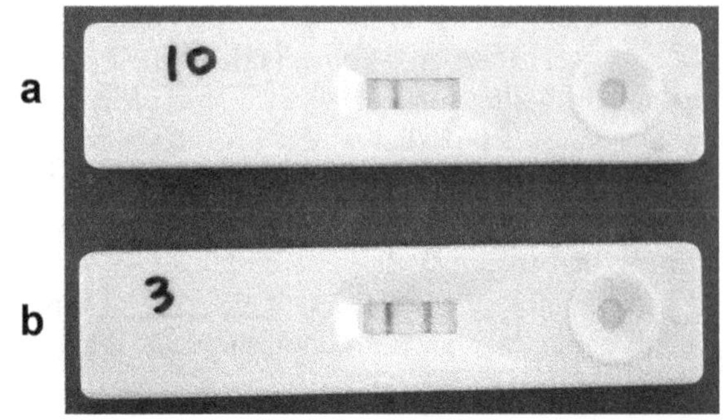

Fig. 1 PSA SPOT test. **a** No band appears in the test zone (negative). **b** A red-colored band appears in the test zone (positive)

range, 4.018–237.518 ng/mL). A total of 164 (11.5%) participants had a PSA value between 4 and 10 ng/mL.

The results of the test were affected by variations in the reading time. The sensitivity was very low at a reading time of 15 min (41.7%) but increased at a reading time of 30 min (79.9%), whereas the specificity of the test was similar (98.7% at 15 min, 93.0% at 30 min). Thus, we chose 30 min as the optimal reading time for further analyses.

The sensitivity, specificity, PPV, NPV, and accuracy of the test were 79.9, 93.0, 65.4, 96.6, and 91.2%, respectively. Among the 1151 participants with a PSA value < 4 ng/mL, 1071 were correctly interpreted as negative using the PSA SPOT test, whereas 80 were interpreted as positive, resulting in a test specificity of 93.0%. Of the 80 false-positive results, 39 (48.8%) were in the PSA range of 3–4 ng/mL (Table 1). The specificity of the test in the PSA range of 3–4 ng/mL was 63.9% (69/108).

Of 151 true positive results, 112 exhibited a PSA value between 4 and 10 ng/mL; 34/112 (30.4%) were interpreted as weakly positive by the PSA SPOT test, whereas 78/112 (69.6%) were judged as strongly positive (Table 1). A total of 40 participants presented a PSA value > 10 ng/mL; 1/40 (2.5%) was judged as weakly positive, whereas 38/40 (95.0%) were judged as strongly positive. As shown in Fig. 2, the intensity of the color reaction was correlated with the PSA quantitative value (Pearson's correlation test: $r = 0.39$, $P < 0.0001$).

Discussion

Since Catalona et al. first demonstrated in 1991 that determination of PSA could be used as a first-line screening test for PC in men without suspicious digital rectal examination findings [10], PSA testing has been widely applied. This has resulted in a spike in PC incidence rates, as previously undetectable cases of PC were unmasked.

Although mass screening for PC remains one of the most controversial issues in oncology, two large,

Table 1 Correlation of PSA SPOT test interpretations with PSA quantitative values

PSA (ng/mL)	n*	PSA SPOT test			Accuracy (%)
		−	+	++	
< 3	1043	1002	32	9	96.1
3–4	108	69	23	16	63.9
4–5	52	23	12	17	55.8
5–10	97	14	22	61	85.6
10–20	23	0	1	22	100.0
> 20	17	1	0	16	94.1

*Some samples not included due to invalid results

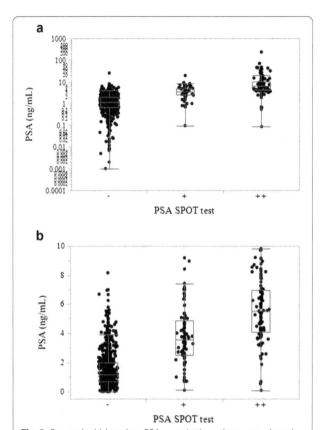

Fig. 2 Box-and-whisker plots. PSA quantitative values were plotted according to the intensity of the red bands in PSA SPOT tests among all samples (**a**) and samples in which the PSA value was between 0 and 10 ng/mL (**b**). The horizontal line within each box represents the median, the ends of the box represent the 25th and 75th percentiles, the whiskers extend from the ends of the box to the minimum and maximum, and the individual dots beyond the whiskers represent outliers

high-quality RCTs were carried out to evaluate PSA screening. The Swedish Göteborg trial demonstrated a 44% lower PC mortality rate in the screening arm among men aged 55 to 69 years over approximately 14 years [7]. The European Randomized Study of Screening for Prostate Cancer (ERSPC) reported a 21% reduction in PC mortality in the screening arm during 13 years of follow-up [8].

The controversy over PSA screening includes the possibilities of detecting insignificant PCs that would never lead to death (over-diagnosis) and then treating these PCs (over-treatment). Other issues include cost and convenience, which are possible reasons why the rate of PSA screening is low in Japan. To overcome these issues, we conducted educational public lectures in Japanese cities and offered a one-step PSA test for free.

Several reports have described rapid, one-step, qualitative PSA tests, as summarized in Table 2 [11–16]. However, the sample sizes of these studies have been limited,

Table 2 One-step PSA tests reported in the literature

Author	n	PSA test	Sensitivity (%)	Specificity (%)
Madersbacher et al.	238	Oncoscreen	93	93
Jung et al.	99	Chembio	67	87
Jung et al.	99	Medpro	87	88
Jung et al.	99	Seratec	80	97
Jung et al.	99	Syntron	93	93
Dok An et al.	147	One Step PSA	100	90
Berg et al.	2322	Uralen	91	81
Miano et al.	188	PSA RapidScreen	97.6	90.4
Shigeno et al.	614	PSA Rapid Test	89.5	94.2

with the exception of the study of Berg et al., which reported a specificity (81%) that appears to be unacceptable. Therefore, we evaluated a one-step PSA test in a large population of Japanese males to potentially enhance the convenience and reduce the cost of PC screening. The one-step PSA test we describe is very easy to administer and can be performed without costly additional equipment, although centrifuge is needed to separate serum from blood. The low cost and speed of the test make it useful and convenient as a tool for primary PC screening, even in general practitioner or urologist office settings. The economic drawbacks to PSA mass screening could be overcome using this one-step PSA test. In general, a rapid test can be priced much lower because it utilizes a simple method [16]. Therefore, the use of this test could spare a significant number of costly quantitative PSA determinations in screening populations due to the high percentage of negative PSA results in PC mass screening, although we could not show expected cost savings because the PSA SPOT test kit is not commercially available and not priced.

Although the overall specificity was 93.0% in our study, it was lower in the PSA range 3–4 ng/mL, within which false-positive results were quite common (36.1%). The results of the PSA SPOT test were comparable to those of other one-step PSA tests described in the literature (Table 2). The primary limitations of this test appear to be poor accuracy in the PSA range 3–4 ng/mL. As such, greater precision is needed to minimize the number of false-positive results. The secondary limitations might be poor accuracy in the PSA range 4–5 ng/mL. The overall sensitivity will increase to 89.1% if the PSA cut-off value of 5.0 ng/mL is used. Nonetheless, the one-step PSA SPOT test could be useful in the general practitioner or urologist office setting as well as in mass screening. If the test could be modified to allow administration at home, PSA testing might be reassessed as a means of mass screening for PC.

Conclusions

The PSA SPOT test is a simple, feasible, and reproducible tool for PC screening. The lower cost, ease of handling, and rapid procedure could make this test useful in the general practitioner or urologist office setting as well as for mass primary PC screening.

Abbreviations

PC: Prostate cancer; PSA: Prostate-specific antigen; RCTs: Randomized clinical trials; PPV: Positive predictive value; NPV: Negative predictive value; ERSPC: European Randomized Study of Screening for Prostate Cancer.

Acknowledgements

The PSA SPOT test was obtained from Prof. Rajvir Dahiya, PhD, Department of Urology, Veterans Affairs Medical Center and University of California, San Francisco, California. We sincerely thank Prof. Dahiya for his kind and essential support.

Authors' contributions

SA and IY contributed to the writing of the manuscript. KI and TS were involved in the design of the study. CK performed the PSA SPOT test. SA, IY, and CK analyzed and interpreted the data. HF, SF, KT, and TK were study investigators. All authors read and approved the final manuscript.

Author details

[1]Department of Urology, Kochi Medical School, Nankoku, Kochi 783-8505, Japan. [2]Department of Urology, Kubokawa Hospital, Takaoka-gun, Kochi 786-0002, Japan. [3]Kochi Medical School Hospital, Nankoku, Kochi 783-8505, Japan.

References

1. Kimura T, Egawa S. Epidemiology of prostate cancer in Asian countries. Int J Urol Off J Jpn Urol Assoc. 2018;25(6):524–31.
2. Potosky AL, Miller BA, Albertsen PC, Kramer BS. The role of increasing detection in the rising incidence of prostate cancer. JAMA. 1995;273(7):548–52.
3. Siegel RL, Miller KD, Jemal A. Cancer statistics, 2019. CA Cancer J Clin. 2019;69(1):7–34.
4. Catalona WJ, Richie JP, Ahmann FR, Hudson MA, Scardino PT, Flanigan RC, DeKernion JB, Ratliff TL, Kavoussi LR, Dalkin BL, et al. Comparison of digital rectal examination and serum prostate specific antigen in the early detection of prostate cancer: results of a multicenter clinical trial of 6630 men. J Urol. 1994;151(5):1283–90.

5. Crawford ED. Prostate cancer awareness week: September 22 to 28, 1997. CA Cancer J Clin. 1997;47(5):288–96.

6. Stephenson RA, Stanford JL. Population-based prostate cancer trends in the United States: patterns of change in the era of prostate-specific antigen. World J Urol. 1997;15(6):331–5.

7. Hugosson J, Carlsson S, Aus G, Bergdahl S, Khatami A, Lodding P, Pihl CG, Stranne J, Holmberg E, Lilja H. Mortality results from the Göteborg randomised population-based prostate-cancer screening trial. Lancet Oncol. 2010;11(8):725–32.

8. Schröder FH, Hugosson J, Roobol MJ, Tammela TL, Zappa M, Nelen V, Kwiatkowski M, Lujan M, Määttänen L, Lilja H, et al. Screening and prostate cancer mortality: results of the European Randomised Study of Screening for Prostate Cancer (ERSPC) at 13 years of follow-up. Lancet (Lond, Engl). 2014;384(9959):2027–35.

9. Optenberg SA, Thompson IM. Economics of screening for carcinoma of the prostate. Urol Clin N Am. 1990;17(4):719–37.

10. Catalona WJ, Smith DS, Ratliff TL, Dodds KM, Coplen DE, Yuan JJ, Petros JA, Andriole GL. Measurement of prostate-specific antigen in serum as a screening test for prostate cancer. N Engl J Med. 1991;324(17):1156–61.

11. Berg W, Linder C, Eschholz G, Schubert J. Pilot study of the practical relevance of a one-step test for prostate-specific antigen in capillary blood to improve the acceptance rate in the early detection program of prostate carcinoma. Int Urol Nephrol. 2001;32(3):381–8.

12. Dok An C, Yoshiki T, Lee G, Okada Y. Evaluation of a rapid qualitative prostate specific antigen assay, the One Step PSA(TM) test. Cancer Lett. 2001;162(2):135–9.

13. Jung K, Zachow J, Lein M, Brux B, Sinha P, Lenk S, Schnorr D, Loening SA. Rapid detection of elevated prostate-specific antigen levels in blood: performance of various membrane strip tests compared. Urology. 1999;53(1):155–60.

14. Madersbacher S, Mian C, Maier U, Simak R. Validation of a 10-minute dipstick test for serum prostate-specific antigen. Eur Urol. 1996;30(4):446–50.

15. Miano R, Mele GO, Germani S, Bove P, Sansalone S, Pugliese PF, Micali F. Evaluation of a new, rapid, qualitative, one-step PSA Test for prostate cancer screening: the PSA RapidScreen test. Prostate Cancer Prostatic Dis. 2005;8(3):219–23.

16. Shigeno K, Arichi N, Yoneda T, Kishi H, Shiina H, Igawa M. Usefulness of an immunochromatographical assay, PSA Rapid Test as a primary screening test for prostate cancer. Int Urol Nephrol. 2006;38(3–4):565–9.

20

Combining prostate health index and multiparametric magnetic resonance imaging in estimating the histological diameter of prostate cancer

Po-Fan Hsieh[1,2,3†], Tzung-Ruei Li[1†], Wei-Ching Lin[2,4], Han Chang[5], Chi-Ping Huang[1,2], Chao-Hsiang Chang[1], Chi-Rei Yang[1], Chin-Chung Yeh[1], Wen-Chin Huang[3] and Hsi-Chin Wu[1,2,6*]

Abstract

Background: Although multiparametric magnetic resonance imaging (mpMRI) is widely used to assess the volume of prostate cancer, it often underestimates the histological tumor boundary. The aim of this study was to evaluate the feasibility of combining prostate health index (PHI) and mpMRI to estimate the histological tumor diameter and determine the safety margin during treatment of prostate cancer.

Methods: We retrospectively enrolled 72 prostate cancer patients who underwent radical prostatectomy and had received PHI tests and mpMRI before surgery. We compared the discrepancy between histological and radiological tumor diameter stratified by Prostate Imaging-Reporting and Data System (PI-RADS) score, and then assessed the influence of PHI on the discrepancy between low PI-RADS (2 or 3) and high PI-RADS (4 or 5) groups.

Results: The mean radiological and histological tumor diameters were 1.60 cm and 2.13 cm, respectively. The median discrepancy between radiological and histological tumor diameter of PI-RADS 4 or 5 lesions was significantly greater than that of PI-RADS 2 or 3 lesions (0.50 cm, IQR (0.00–0.90) vs. 0.00 cm, IQR (−0.10–0.20), $p = 0.02$). In the low PI-RADS group, the upper limit of the discrepancy was 0.2 cm; so the safety margin could be set at 0.1 cm. In the high PI-RADS group, the upper limits of the discrepancy were 1.2, 1.6, and 2.2 cm in men with PHI < 30, 30–60, and > 60; so the safety margin could be set at 0.6, 0.8, and 1.1 cm, respectively.

Conclusions: Radiological tumor diameter on mpMRI often underestimated the histological tumor diameter, especially for PI-RADS 4 or 5 lesions. Combining mpMRI and PHI may help to better estimate the histological tumor diameter.

Keywords: Multiparametric magnetic resonance imaging, Prostate cancer, Prostate health index, Tumor diameter

Introduction

Prostate cancer is the second most common cancer in men and the fifth leading cause of death worldwide [1]. With increasingly popular screening protocols and the adoption of multiparametric magnetic resonance imaging (mpMRI) in the diagnostic pathway, an increasing number of prostate cancer cases can be diagnosed at an early stage [2]. Radical prostatectomy has long been the

*Correspondence: wuhc4746@gmail.com
†Po-Fan Hsieh and Tzung-Ruei Li have contributed equally to this article.
[1] Department of Urology, China Medical University Hospital, No. 2, Yu-Der Rd, Taichung 40447, Taiwan
Full list of author information is available at the end of the article

standard of care for clinically localized prostate cancer, and focal therapy is an emerging treatment modality which may also achieve oncological control and result in lower rates of urinary incontinence and erectile dysfunction [3, 4]. The importance of the preoperative delineation of tumor boundaries cannot be underestimated, because it may help preserve neurovascular bundles during radical prostatectomy as well as determine the safety margin during focal therapy. Specifically, the purpose of determining the safety margin for focal therapy is to safely achieve the trifecta, i.e. destruction of sufficient tissue for oncological control, whilst preserving enough normal prostatic tissue to retain both continence and potency, and carefully balance these three elements.

Based on the high sensitivity and specificity for clinically significant prostate cancer, mpMRI is widely used to assess the tumor location and volume [5]. The tumor diameter on mpMRI has been correlated with extraprostatic extension, seminal vesicle invasion, and positive margin after radical prostatectomy [6]. Nevertheless, mpMRI is limited by a low positive predictive value for Prostate Imaging-Reporting and Data System (PI-RADS) 3 or 4 lesions and high inter-reader variability [7, 8]. The staging accuracy of mpMRI has also been reported to vary across risk groups [9]. Moreover, mpMRI often underestimates the histological tumor boundary [10, 11]. Although a safety margin of at least 5–10 mm has been suggested for focal therapy of prostate cancer, how to individualize the safety margin for each patient remains unknown [10, 12–14]. Recently, a pilot study suggested performing intraoperative digital analysis of ablation margins using fluorescent confocal microscopy given the relevance of MRI targeting errors and the presence of MRI invisible cancer [15]. On the other hand, prostate health index (PHI) is a serum biomarker which has a higher specificity compared with prostate specific antigen (PSA) [16]. Some studies have reported that PHI is significantly correlated with tumor volume and adverse pathological outcomes [17–22].

Our previous work showed that the combination of PHI and mpMRI had a higher accuracy for detecting clinically significant prostate cancer compared with PHI or mpMRI alone [23]. Therefore, the aim of the present study was to evaluate the feasibility of combining PHI and mpMRI to estimate the histological tumor diameter and determine the safety margin during treatment of prostate cancer.

Materials and methods

We retrospectively collected patients with biopsy-proven prostate cancer who underwent robot-assisted laparoscopic radical prostatectomy (RALRP) from January 2016 to December 2020 and had received preoperative

PHI tests and mpMRI at a tertiary referral center. The exclusion criteria were metastatic prostate cancer (N1 or M1), PHI tested during an episode of urinary tract infection, defined as pyuria (3 or more white blood cells per high power field of unspun, voided mid-stream urine), or poor quality of mpMRI, which included inadequate field of view, inadequate in-plane resolution, inadequate slice thickness, lack of multiple and high b values, unclear delineation of anatomical landmarks, or the presence of artifacts. This study was approved by the Research Ethics Committee of China Medical University and Hospital, Taichung, Taiwan (Protocol Number: CMUH110-REC3-048). The need for informed consent was waived by the Research Ethics Committee because all clinical practice in this study was routine work for prostate cancer patients and carried out in accordance with EAU guidelines [3]. In addition, the retrospective analysis did not influence any clinical decision making or violate the patients' rights.

PHI and mpMRI
PSA parameters including total PSA, free PSA, and p2PSA were tested using a Beckman Coulter DxI 800 Immunoassay System (Beckman Coulter, Taiwan Inc.) to obtain PHI (PHI = (p2PSA/free PSA) × √PSA) before prostate biopsy.

Prostate mpMRI examinations were done using a 3-T scanner (Signa HDxt, GE Healthcare, Milwaukee, WI) with a four-channel high definition (HD) cardiac array coil before prostate biopsy or at least 6 weeks after prostate biopsy. The mpMRI protocol included T2-weighted imaging (T2WI), dynamic contrast enhanced (DCE) imaging, diffusion-weighted imaging (DWI) with b values of 0 and 1000–1400 s/mm^2, and apparent diffusion coefficient (ADC) mapping. All mpMRI scans were interpreted by an experienced radiologist (W. C. L.) who had 12 years of prostate MRI experience with > 500 scans per year, and reported according to PI-RADS version 2 [24]. The index lesion was defined as the single lesion with the highest PI-RADS score. If there were two or more lesions with the same PI-RADS score, the index lesion was defined as the largest one. We measured the maximal diameter of the index lesion on the axial, coronal, or sagittal view of T2WI to determine the radiological tumor diameter.

Prostate biopsy
For men who underwent mpMRI before biopsy, we performed targeted biopsies for at least 2 cores and systematic biopsies for at least 12 cores. Initially, we performed transrectal cognitive biopsies based on lesions revealed on mpMRI. In April 2019, we introduced the MRI/ultrasound fusion platform, BioJet® (D&K Technologies GmbH, Barum, Germany), and thereafter we exclusively

performed transperineal software fusion biopsies. For men who did not undergo mpMRI before biopsy, we performed systematic biopsies for at least 12 cores.

Histology

RALRP was performed by urologists who were specialists in the procedure. The prostatectomy specimens were fixed with 10% neutral buffered formalin for 24 h, and subsequently each entire prostate specimen was sectioned. The proximal (bladder neck) margins were thinly shaved. We amputated the distal 1 cm of the apex, and then sectioned this apical cone at right angles to the cut edge in thin parallel slices to accurately assess the distal margin. After the margins had been measured, we serially sectioned the prostate at 3-mm intervals from the apex to base. Individual slices were sectioned carefully to maintain the orientation. To fit into standard tissue cassettes, a median section was made through the urethra to divide the slice into right and left sides, and a coronal section was made through the urethra to further divide the slice into anterior and posterior quadrants. All slices were performed using routine tissue processing and embedding in paraffin, and 4 μ thick slices were cut from these paraffin blocks and stained by hematoxylin and eosin (H&E). A uropathologist (H. C.) who had 22 years of experience with > 100 cases per year reviewed all of the specimens. The grading of prostate cancer was in accordance with the 2014 International Society of Urological Pathology Consensus Conference guidelines [25]. All of the cases were reviewed in a multidisciplinary team meeting by urologists, radiologists and pathologists to confirm the concordance of the index tumor on histology and mpMRI. The histological tumor diameter was defined as the maximal diameter of the index tumor on histology.

Statistical analysis

Continuous variables were reported as median (interquartile range, IQR) or mean (standard deviation, SD) and 95% confidence interval (CI), and categorical variables were reported as proportions. The normality of data was tested using the Kolmogorov–Smirnov test. We performed Pearson correlation analysis between histological tumor diameter and clinical parameters including age, PSA, PHI, radiological tumor diameter, biopsy/histology grade group, and histology T stage. We then compared the median discrepancy between radiological and histological tumor diameter stratified by different PI-RADS score, PSA, biopsy grade group, and PHI using the Mann–Whitney U test or Kruskal–Wallis test. Finally, we separated the study population into low PI-RADS (2 or 3) and high PI-RADS (4 or 5) groups and assessed the influence of PHI on the discrepancy in each group. All statistical analyses were conducted using SPSS version 22 (IBM

Corp, Armonk, NY, USA), assuming a two-sided test with an alpha of 5% for statistical significance.

Results

Overall, 572 patients received RALRP, of whom 564 patients underwent mpMRI before surgery. Of these patients, 76 (13.5%) had PHI tests. Four patients were excluded; one had a concurrent urinary tract infection during PHI test, one had lymph node involvement on pathology, one had prostate cancer diagnosed by transurethral resection of the prostate, and one had poor quality mpMRI due to motion artifacts. Finally, a total of 72 men were enrolled in this study, and their clinical characteristics are shown in Table 1. The median age was 66 (IQR 60–69) years old. The median PSA level was 9.03 (IQR 5.95–13.36) ng/mL, and the median PHI was 54.97 (IQR 42.41–78.04). Forty-two men underwent mpMRI before the prostate biopsy, including a transrectal cognitive biopsy in 29, and a transperineal software fusion biopsy in 13. Thirty men underwent mpMRI after a systematic biopsy, and the mean duration between biopsy and mpMRI was 58.6 (SD 40.4, range 42–252) days. The PI-RADS scores of the index tumor were 2, 3, 4, and 5 in 4, 3, 29, and 36 men, respectively. The mean radiological and histological tumor diameters were 1.6 (SD 0.89, 95% CI [1.39, 1.81]) cm, and 2.13 (SD 1.11, 95% CI [1.86, 2.39]) cm, respectively. The mean discrepancy between radiological and histological tumor diameter was 0.53 (SD 0.67, 95% CI [0.37, 0.68]) cm. The Kolmogorov–Smirnov test revealed that the histological tumor diameters were normally distributed, while the radiological tumor diameters and their discrepancy were not normally distributed.

Table 2 shows the Pearson correlation analysis between the histological tumor diameter and clinical parameters. The histological tumor diameter was highly correlated with radiological tumor diameter ($r = 0.80$, $p < 0.01$). In addition, the histological tumor diameter was also correlated with PHI ($r = 0.52$, $p < 0.01$), histology grade group ($r = 0.37$, $p < 0.01$), biopsy grade group ($r = 0.32$, $p = 0.01$), histology T stage ($r = 0.32$, $p = 0.01$), and PSA ($r = 0.30$, $p = 0.01$).

The median discrepancy between radiological and histological tumor diameter of PI-RADS 4 or 5 lesions was significantly greater than that of PI-RADS 2 or 3 lesions (0.5 cm vs. 0 cm, $p = 0.02$). On the other hand, the median discrepancy between radiological and histological tumor diameter was not significantly correlated with PSA ($p = 0.36$), biopsy grade group ($p = 0.07$), or PHI ($p = 0.55$).

Finally, in the low PI-RADS group, the upper limit of the discrepancy between radiological and histological tumor diameter was 0.2 cm. In the high PI-RADS group,

Table 1 Patient characteristics

Parameters	Overall population (n = 72)
Age (years), median (IQR)	66 (60–69)
PSA (ng/mL), median (IQR)	9.03 (5.95–13.36)
Free PSA/PSA (%), median (IQR)	12.76 (9.38–17.39)
PSA density (ng/mL), median (IQR)	0.26 (0.16–0.37)
%p2PSA, median (IQR)	2.04 (1.4–2.5)
PHI, median (IQR)	54.97 (42.41–78.04)
PI-RADS score, n (%)	
2	4 (5.6)
3	3 (4.2)
4	29 (40.3)
5	36 (50)
Radiological tumor diameter (cm), mean ± SD (95% CI)	1.6 ± 0.89 (1.39–1.81)
Biopsy cores, median (IQR)	
Targeted biopsy + systematic biopsy	4 (2–8) + 15 (12–18)
Systematic biopsy alone	14 (12–16)
Biopsy grade group, n (%)	
1	25 (34.7)
2	19 (26.4)
3	13 (18.1)
4	12 (16.7)
5	3 (4.2)
Histology grade group, n (%)	
1	10 (13.89)
2	28 (38.89)
3	28 (38.89)
4	1 (1.39)
5	5 (6.94)
Histology T stage, n (%)	
2	52 (72.2)
3a	16 (22.2)
3b	3 (4.2)
4	1 (1.4)
Histological tumor diameter (cm), mean ± SD (95% CI)	2.13 ± 1.11 (1.86–2.39)
Discrepancy between histological and radiological tumor diameter (cm), mean ± SD (95% CI)	0.53 ± 0.67 (0.37–0.68)

PHI: Prostate Health Index; PI-RADS: Prostate Imaging Reporting and Data System; PSA: prostate specific antigen; %p2PSA: percentage of p2PSA to free PSA

the upper limits of the discrepancy between radiological and histological tumor diameter were 1.2 cm, 1.6 cm, and 2.2 cm in men with PHI < 30, 30–60, and > 60, respectively. Assuming that the tumor had a spherical shape, the safety margin could be set at 0.1 cm for PI-RADS 2 or 3 lesions. For PI-RADS 4 or 5 lesions, the safety margins could be set at 0.6 cm, 0.8 cm, and 1.1 cm when the PHI was < 30, 30–60, and > 60, respectively (Fig. 1).

Discussion

In this study, we found that the radiological tumor diameter on mpMRI underestimated the histological tumor diameter by a mean of 0.53 cm. In addition, the discrepancy between radiological and histological tumor diameter of PI-RADS 4 or 5 lesions was greater than that of PI-RADS 2 or 3 lesions. For PI-RADS 2 or 3 lesions, a safety margin of 0.1 cm may be sufficient. For PI-RADS 4

Table 2 Pearson correlation between histological tumor diameter and clinical parameters

Parameters	r	p value
Age	0.11	0.38
PSA	0.30	0.01
Free/total PSA	−0.20	0.10
PSA density	0.22	0.06
%p2PSA	0.21	0.08
PHI	0.52	< 0.01
Radiological tumor diameter	0.80	< 0.01
Biopsy grade group	0.32	0.01
Histology grade group	0.37	< 0.01
Histology T stage	0.32	0.01

PHI: Prostate Health Index; PSA: prostate specific antigen; %p2PSA: percentage of p2PSA to free PSA

or 5 lesions, the safety margins should be 0.6 cm, 0.8 cm, and 1.1 cm when the PHI is < 30, 30–60, and > 60, respectively. To the best of our knowledge, this is the first study

to estimate histological tumor diameter and safety margin using a combination of PHI and mpMRI.

Accurately estimating the tumor boundary is key to successful focal therapy, and it can also decrease the positive margin rate after radical prostatectomy. Although mpMRI is the most commonly used tool to estimate tumor volume [5], underestimation of the histological tumor volume has frequently been reported [10, 11]. This may be because at the periphery of the index tumor the cancer may be low grade or intermixed with normal prostatic tissue, making the tumor inconspicuous on mpMRI [26]. In this study, we found that mpMRI underestimated the histological tumor diameter by a mean of 0.53 cm. Consistent with Le Nobin's study [10], the discrepancy between radiological and histological tumor diameter was greater in PI-RADS 4 or 5 lesions compared with PI-RADS 2 or 3 lesions. To achieve oncological control, a safety margin beyond the index lesion is necessary during any treatment of localized prostate cancer. However, there is currently no consensus on how to determine the safety margin. Practically, the best strategy currently

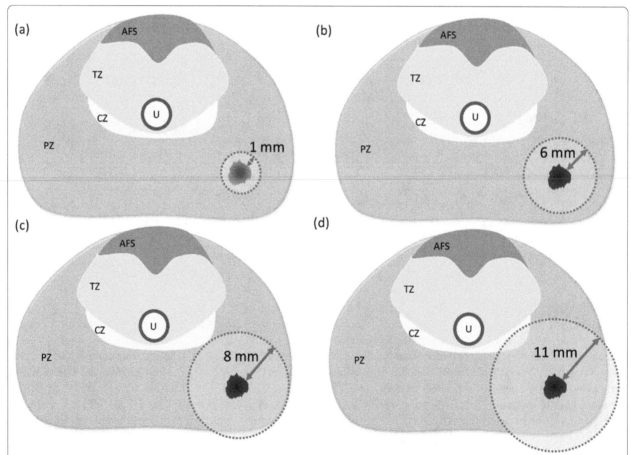

Fig. 1 The schematic diagram the safety margin of PI-RADS 2 or 3 lesions (**a**), and safety margin of PI-RADS 4 or 5 lesions stratified by PHI < 30 (**b**), 30 ≤ PHI ≤ 60 (**c**), PHI > 60 (**d**). AFS: anterior fibromuscular stroma; CZ: central zone; PHI: Prostate Health Index; PI-RADS: Prostate Imaging Reporting and Data System; PZ: peripheral zone; TZ: transition zone; U: urethra

available to estimate tumor volume is to combine biopsy results and MRI information. Specially directed biopsies around the lesion may assist in margin determination. In addition, several nomograms incorporating 4 K score, clinical and imaging parameters have been developed to predict the presence of cancer outside the index lesion and the added value of systematic biopsies [27, 28].

PHI is a serum biomarker for prostate cancer, and it has been associated with cancer detection, stage, grade, surgical margin status, and tumor volume [21, 22, 29]. Previous studies have reported area under the curve values of PHI to predict a tumor volume greater than $0.5cm^3$ ranging from 0.72 to 0.94 [18–20]. Friedersdorff et al. reported that PHI had a significantly higher correlation with tumor volume than Gleason score (Pearson's $r = 0.588$ vs. 0.385, $p = 0.008$) [20]. In our study, PHI was significantly correlated with histological tumor diameter ($r = 0.52$, $p < 0.001$). The correlation coefficient of PHI was superior to that of PSA ($r = 0.30$) and biopsy grade group ($r = 0.32$), and just inferior to radiological tumor diameter ($r = 0.80$).

Importantly, we used PHI to calibrate tumor diameter on mpMRI. For PI-RADS 2 or 3 lesions, the discrepancy between radiological and histological tumor diameter was 0.2 cm, which means that extending of the radius of the index lesion by 0.1 cm may be sufficient to cover the tumor boundary. On the other hand, for PI-RADS 4 or 5 lesions, the safety margins should be extended to 0.6 cm, 0.8 cm, and 1.1 cm when the PHI is < 30, 30–60, and > 60, respectively. In other words, combining PHI and mpMRI may be able to estimate the histological tumor diameter more accurately than using mpMRI alone. Individualized treatment margins can help to decide whether neurovascular bundles can be preserved and how wide the bladder neck or urethra should be resected. It may also be possible to achieve complete tumor destruction during focal therapy, and preserve more normal prostatic parenchyma to lower the risk of injury to neurovascular bundles, external sphincter, bladder neck and urethra. Namely, the combination of imaging and serological biomarkers has the potential to achieve the best oncological outcomes whilst preserving functional outcomes including continence and sexual function. Future interventional studies on PHI and mpMRI are warranted to clarify whether these endpoints can be achieved.

In this study, we used the maximal tumor diameter as a surrogate of tumor volume. In fact, there is still no robust evidence for how best to measure tumor volume on mpMRI [30]. Tumor volume can also be estimated using planimetric maps or three-dimensional quantification, which require time for segmentation and lesion contouring [10, 31]. In contrast, measuring the maximal tumor diameter on mpMRI is a relatively simple

and practically feasible method. Mizuno et al. reported that the maximal tumor diameter on mpMRI had a higher correlation with extraprostatic disease than maximal tumor area or total tumor volume [32]. In our study, the histological tumor diameter was significantly correlated with radiological tumor diameter ($r = 0.80$, $p < 0.01$), pathological T stage ($r = 0.32$, $p = 0.01$) and grade group ($r = 0.37$, $p < 0.01$). That is, the tumor diameter may help to predict cancer aggressiveness and prognosis. Research on prostate MRI radiomics and machine learning may lead to automatic lesion localization, volumetry, and assessment of tumor biology in the future [33, 34].

There are several limitations to this study. First, only 7 men were enrolled in the low PI-RADS group. This is because biopsies are not routinely suggested for PI-RADS 2 or 3 lesions unless the patient has a high clinical suspicion of prostate cancer. The limited number of cases may have reduced the power of comparisons between the high PI-RADS and low PI-RADS groups. The overall small sample size also precluded us from adding a validation cohort. However, our preliminary study addresses an important issue. Prospective large-scale studies, either in a real-world or in silico setting, are needed to assess the combined value of PHI and mpMRI in estimating tumor volume. Second, there was selection bias associated with the RALRP-only population. Other modalities of radical prostatectomy, including open or laparoscopic procedures, are needed to validate our results. Third, patients with mpMRI scheduled before or after a prostate biopsy were enrolled. Awareness of the biopsy outcomes may have affected the radiologist's interpretation of post-biopsy mpMRI. Nevertheless, the mean duration between biopsy and mpMRI was up to 58.6 days, and the small amount of residual hemorrhage did not influence identification of the index lesion. Fourth, the prostate biopsy protocol was not uniform. Systematic biopsy alone was performed in the men without pre-biopsy mpMRI, and the lack of targeted biopsy may have resulted in undergrading of the biopsy outcome. Fifth, this study was conducted among an Asian population. Although a recent study showed similar staging accuracy of mpMRI in African Americans and Caucasian Americans, the application of combining PHI and mpMRI needs to be validated in different races [35]. Finally, we assessed the diameter of the index tumor based on the hypothesis that the index tumor drives the natural course of prostate cancer and determines the prognosis [36]. However, prostate cancer is usually a multifocal disease. The prognostic roles of satellite lesions are variable and remain to be investigated, and the combination of mpMRI, biomarkers, and genetic signatures may help in decision making for the treatment of prostate cancer [37].

Conclusions

In conclusion, the radiological tumor diameter on prostate mpMRI often underestimated the histological tumor diameter, especially for PI-RADS 4 or 5 lesions. The combination of mpMRI and PHI may help to better estimate the boundary of prostate cancer and refine the procedures of radical prostatectomy and focal therapy. Prospective, large-scale studies are needed to validate our results.

Acknowledgements

The authors would like to thank the editors and reviewers for constructive criticisms.

Authors' contributions

P.-F.H., T.-R.L., and H.-C.W. designed the study. P.-F.H., T.-R.L., W.-C.L., H.C., C.-P.H., C.-H.C., C.-R.Y., C.-C.Y., W.-C.H., H.-C.W. helped acquisition of data. P.-F.H., T.-R.L., and H.-C.W. performed data and statistical analysis. P.-F.H., T.-R.L., and H.-C.W. edited the manuscript. All authors read and approved the final manuscript.

Author details

[1]Department of Urology, China Medical University Hospital, No. 2, Yu-Der Rd, Taichung 40447, Taiwan. [2]School of Medicine, China Medical University, Taichung 40402, Taiwan. [3]Graduate Institute of Biomedical Sciences, School of Medicine, China Medical University, Taichung 40402, Taiwan. [4]Department of Radiology, China Medical University Hospital, Taichung 40447, Taiwan. [5]Department of Pathology, China Medical University Hospital, Taichung 40447, Taiwan. [6]Department of Urology, China Medical University Beigang Hospital, Beigang, Yunlin 651012, Taiwan.

References

1. Rawla P. Epidemiology of prostate cancer. World J Oncol. 2019;10:63–89.
2. Litwin MS, Tan HJ. The diagnosis and treatment of prostate cancer: a review. JAMA. 2017;317:2532–42.
3. Mottet N, van den Bergh RC, Briers E, Van den Broeck T, Cumberbatch MG, De Santis M, et al. EAU-EANM-ESTRO-ESUR-SIOG guidelines on prostate cancer—2020 update. part 1: screening, diagnosis, and local treatment with curative intent. Eur Urol. 2021;79:243–62.
4. Valerio M, Ahmed HU, Emberton M, Lawrentschuk N, Lazzeri M, Montironi R, et al. The role of focal therapy in the management of localised prostate cancer: a systematic review. Eur Urol. 2014;66:732–51.
5. Eldred-Evans D, Tam H, Smith AP, Winkler M, Ahmed HU. Use of imaging to optimise prostate cancer tumour volume assessment for focal therapy planning. Curr Urol Rep. 2020;21:1–10.
6. Tonttila PP, Kuisma M, Pääkkö E, Hirvikoski P, Vaarala MH. Lesion size on prostate magnetic resonance imaging predicts adverse radical prostatectomy pathology. Scand J Urol. 2018;52:111–5.
7. Falagario UG, Jambor I, Lantz A, Ettala O, Stabile A, Taimen P, et al. Combined use of prostate-specific antigen density and magnetic resonance imaging for prostate biopsy decision planning: a retrospective multi-institutional study using the prostate magnetic resonance imaging outcome database (PROMOD). Eur Urol Oncol. 2020;S2588–9311(20):30142–5.
8. Wajswol E, Winoker JS, Anastos H, Falagario UG, Okhawere K, Martini A, et al. A cohort of transperineal electromagnetically tracked magnetic resonance imaging/ultrasonography fusion-guided biopsy: assessing the impact of inter-reader variability on cancer detection. BJU Int. 2020;125:531–40.
9. Falagario UG, Jambor I, Ratnani P, Martini A, Treacy PJ, et al. Performance of prostate multiparametric MRI for prediction of prostate cancer extraprostatic extension according to NCCN risk categories: implication for surgical planning. Minerva Urol Nefrol. 2020;72:746–54.
10. Le Nobin J, Rosenkrantz AB, Villers A, Orczyk C, Deng FM, Melamed J, et al. Image guided focal therapy for magnetic resonance imaging visible prostate cancer: defining a 3-dimensional treatment margin based on magnetic resonance imaging histology co-registration analysis. J Urol. 2015;194:364–70.
11. Cornud F, Khoury G, Bouazza N, Beuvon F, Peyromaure M, Flam T, et al. Tumor target volume for focal therapy of prostate cancer—does multiparametric magnetic resonance imaging allow for a reliable estimation? J Urol. 2014;191:1272–9.
12. Donaldson IA, Alonzi R, Barratt D, Barret E, Berge V, Bott S, et al. Focal therapy: patients, interventions, and outcomes—a report from a consensus meeting. Eur Urol. 2015;67:771–7.
13. Karagiannis A, Varkarakis J. Irreversible electroporation for the ablation of prostate cancer. Curr Urol Rep. 2019;20:1–8.
14. Van den Bos W, Scheltema MJ, Siriwardana AR, Kalsbeek AM, Thompson JE, Ting F, et al. Focal irreversible electroporation as primary treatment for localized prostate cancer. BJU Int. 2018;121:716–24.
15. Selvaggio O, Falagario UG, Bruno SM, Recchia M, Sighinolfi MC, Sanguedolce F, et al. Intraoperative digital analysis of ablation margins (DAAM) by fluorescent confocal microscopy to improve partial prostate gland cryoablation outcomes. Cancers. 2021;13:4382.
16. De La Calle C, Patil D, Wei JT, Scherr DS, Sokoll L, Chan DW, et al. Multicenter evaluation of the prostate health index to detect aggressive prostate cancer in biopsy naive men. J Urol. 2015;194:65–72.
17. Ferro M, Lucarelli G, Bruzzese D, Perdonà S, Mazzarella C, Perruolo G, et al. Improving the prediction of pathologic outcomes in patients undergoing radical prostatectomy: the value of prostate cancer antigen 3 (PCA3), prostate health index (phi) and sarcosine. Anticancer Res. 2015;35:1017–23.
18. Chiu PK-F, Lai FM-M, Teoh JY-C, Lee WM, Yee CH, Chan ES-Y, et al. Prostate health index and %p2PSA predict aggressive prostate cancer pathology in Chinese patients undergoing radical prostatectomy. Ann Surg Oncol. 2016;23:2707–14.
19. Tallon L, Luangphakdy D, Ruffion A, Colombel M, Devonec M, Champetier D, et al. Comparative evaluation of urinary PCA3 and TMPRSS2: ERG scores and serum PHI in predicting prostate cancer aggressiveness. Int J Mol Sci. 2014;15:13299–316.
20. Friedersdorff F, Groß B, Maxeiner A, Jung K, Miller K, Stephan C, et al. Does the prostate health index depend on tumor volume? A study on 196 patients after radical prostatectomy. Int J Mol Sci. 2017;18:488.
21. Cheng YT, Huang CY, Chen CH, Chiu ST, Hong JH, Pu YS, et al. Preoperative% p2PSA and prostate health index predict pathological outcomes in patients with prostate cancer undergoing radical prostatectomy. Sci Rep. 2020;10:1–7.
22. Huang YP, Lin TP, Cheng WM, Wei TC, Huang IS, Fan YH, et al. Prostate health index density predicts aggressive pathological outcomes after radical prostatectomy in Taiwanese patients. J Chin Med Assoc. 2019;82:835–9.
23. Hsieh PF, Li WJ, Lin WC, Chang H, Chang CH, Huang CP, et al. Combining prostate health index and multiparametric magnetic resonance imaging in the diagnosis of clinically significant prostate cancer in an Asian population. World J Urol. 2020;38:1207–14.
24. Weinreb JC, Barentsz JO, Choyke PL, Cornud F, Haider MA, Macura KJ, et al. PI-RADS prostate imaging–reporting and data system: 2015, version 2. Eur Urol. 2016;69:16–40.
25. Epstein JI, Egevad L, Amin MB, Delahunt B, Srigley JR, Humphrey PA. The 2014 International Society of Urological Pathology (ISUP) consensus conference on Gleason grading of prostatic carcinoma. Am J Surg Pathol. 2016;40:244–52.
26. Langer DL, van der Kwast TH, Evans AJ, Sun L, Yaffe MJ, Trachtenberg J, et al. Intermixed normal tissue within prostate cancer: effect on MR imaging measurements of apparent diffusion coefficient and T2—sparse versus dense cancers. Radiology. 2008;249:900–8.
27. Falagario UG, Lantz A, Jambor I, Martini A, Ratnani P, Wagaskar V, et al. Using biomarkers in patients with positive multiparametric magnetic resonance imaging: 4Kscore predicts the presence of cancer outside the index lesion. Int J Urol. 2021;28:47–52.
28. Falagario UG, Jambor I, Taimen P, Syvänen KT, Kähkönen E, Merisaari H, et al. Added value of systematic biopsy in men with a clinical suspicion of prostate cancer undergoing biparametric MRI-targeted biopsy: multi-institutional external validation study. World J Urol. 2021;39:1879–87.

29. Ferro M, De Cobelli O, Lucarelli G, Porreca A, Busetto GM, Cantiello F, et al. Beyond PSA: the role of prostate health index (phi). Int J Mol Sci. 2020;21:1184.

30. Moore CM, Giganti F, Albertsen P, Allen C, Bangma C, Briganti A, et al. Reporting magnetic resonance imaging in men on active surveillance for prostate cancer: the PRECISE recommendations: a report of a European School of Oncology Task Force. Eur Urol. 2017;71:648–55.

31. Harvey H, Orton MR, Morgan VA, Parker C, Dearnaley D, Fisher C, et al. Volumetry of the dominant intraprostatic tumour lesion: intersequence and interobserver differences on multiparametric MRI. Br J Radiol. 2017;90:20160416.

32. Mizuno R, Nakashima J, Mukai M, Ookita H, Nakagawa K, Oya M, et al. Maximum tumor diameter is a simple and valuable index associated with the local extent of disease in clinically localized prostate cancer. Int J Urol. 2006;13:951–5.

33. Sun Y, Reynolds H, Wraith D, Williams S, Finnegan ME, Mitchell C, et al. Predicting prostate tumour location from multiparametric MRI using Gaussian kernel support vector machines: a preliminary study. Australas Phys Eng Sci Med. 2017;40:39–49.

34. Sun Y, Reynolds HM, Parameswaran B, Wraith D, Finnegan ME, Williams S, et al. Multiparametric MRI and radiomics in prostate cancer: a review. Australas Phys Eng Sci Med. 2019;42:3–25.

35. Falagario UG, Ratnani P, Lantz A, Jambor I, Dovey Z, Verma A, et al. Staging accuracy of multiparametric magnetic resonance imaging in Caucasian and African American men undergoing radical prostatectomy. J Urol. 2020;204:82–90.

36. Ahmed HU. The index lesion and the origin of prostate cancer. N Engl J Med. 2009;361:1704–6.

37. Tourinho-Barbosa RR, de la Rosette J, Sanchez-Salas R. Prostate cancer multifocality, the index lesion, and the microenvironment. Curr Opin Urol. 2018;28:499–505.

21

The urologist's learning curve of "in-bore" magnetic resonance-guided prostate biopsy

Barak Rosenzweig[1,2,3*], Tomer Drori[1,2], Orit Raz[4], Gil Goldinger[1,2], Gadi Shlomai[2,3,5], Dorit E. Zilberman[1,2], Moshe Shechtman[2,6], Jacob Ramon[1,2], Zohar A. Dotan[1,2†] and Orith Portnoy[2,7†]

Abstract

Background: The combination of multi-parametric MRI to locate and define suspected lesions together with their being targeted by an MRI-guided prostate biopsy has succeeded in increasing the detection rate of clinically significant disease and lowering the detection rate of non-significant prostate cancer. In this work we investigate the urologist's learning curve of in-bore MRI-guided prostate biopsy which is considered to be a superior biopsy technique.

Materials and methods: Following Helsinki approval by The Chaim Sheba Medical Center ethics committee in accordance with The Sheba Medical Center institutional guidelines (5366-28-SMC) we retrospectively reviewed 110 IB-MRGpBs performed from 6/2016 to 1/2019 in a single tertiary center. All patients had a prostate multi-parametric MRI finding of at least 1 target lesion (prostate imaging reporting and data system [PI-RADS] score $\geq$ 3). We analyzed biopsy duration and clinically significant prostate cancer detection of targeted sampling in 2 groups of 55 patients each, once by a urologist highly trained in IB-MRGpBs and again by a urologist untrained in IB-MRGpBs. These two parameters were compared according to operating urologist and chronologic order.

Results: The patients' median age was 68 years (interquartile range 62–72). The mean prostate-specific antigen level and prostate size were 8.6 $\pm$ 9.1 ng/d and 53 $\pm$ 27 cc, respectively. The mean number of target lesions was 1.47 $\pm$ 0.6. Baseline parameters did not differ significantly between the 2 urologists' cohorts. Overall detection rates of clinically significant prostate cancer were 19%, 55%, and 69% for PI-RADS 3, 4 and 5, respectively. Clinically significant cancer detection rates did not differ significantly along the timeline or between the 2 urologists. The average duration of IB-MRGpB targeted sampling was 28 $\pm$ 15.8 min, correlating with the number of target lesions ($p < 0.0001$), and independent of the urologist's expertise. Eighteen cases defined the cutoff for the procedure duration learning curve ($p < 0.05$).

Conclusions: Our data suggest a very short learning curve for IB-MRGpB-targeted sampling duration, and that clinically significant cancer detection rates are not influenced by the learning curve of this technique.

Keywords: Prostate MRI, In-bore MRI, Prostate biopsy, Learning curve

*Correspondence: Barak.rosenzweig@sheba.health.gov.il; barak22@gmail.com
†Zohar A. Dotan and Orith Portnoy have contributed equally to this work.
[1] Department of Urology, Chaim Sheba Medical Center, 5262080 Ramat Gan, Israel
Full list of author information is available at the end of the article

Introduction

Magnetic resonance-guided prostate biopsy (MRGpB) is considered superior to transrectal ultrasound (TRUS)-guided biopsy, and multi-parametric magnetic resonance imaging (mpMRI) is now regarded as a leading tool in diagnosing clinically significant prostate cancer [1–3]. The combination of mpMRI to locate and define suspected lesions together with their being targeted by an MRI-guided prostate biopsy (MRGpB) has succeeded in increasing the detection rate of clinically significant disease and lowering the detection rate of non-significant prostate cancer [1]. Incorporating MRI data with the biopsy technique can be accomplished by means of several methods. The "MR/TRUS fusion" approach uses software-based registration platforms which overlay the TRUS images with the MRI, allowing the physician to target lesions seen only on the mpMRI at the corresponding location in real-time sonographic imaging. In the "in-bore" approach, following an initial diagnostic mpMRI, the patient undergoes a biopsy within the bore of the magnet at a later date [4, 5]. These high-end technologies incorporate multidisciplinary efforts, and may therefore suggest a long learning curve and possible slow adaptation of biopsy techniques whose applications are limited by the number of trained personnel. Indeed, prostate MRI reading itself has been associated with a significant learning curve [6–8]. Similarly, a TRUS biopsy is also reportedly subject to some learning curve, and that its operator serves as an independent predictor of prostate cancer detection [9, 10]. The MR/TRUS fusion approach also bears a significant learning curve on both the individual physician as well as on the institution [11–13].

The in-bore MRI-guided prostate biopsy (IB-MRGpB) is considered by some to be a superior biopsy technique [14]. To the best of our knowledge, the learning curve for IB-MRGpB has not been reported before, and that is the aim of the current study.

Materials and methods

Methods and study population

Following Helsinki approval by The Chaim Sheba Medical Center ethics committee in accordance with The Sheba Medical Center institutional guidelines (5366-28-SMC) and waiver of informed consent, we retrospectively reviewed 110 consecutive IB-MRGpBs performed from June 2016 to January 2019 in a single tertiary center. The patients had been referred to our institution by their urologist or general practitioner due to elevated PSA serum levels and/or abnormal digital rectal examination, and following an mpMRI finding of at least one target lesion, which is defined as a score ≥ 3 on the prostate imaging reporting and data system (PI-RADS v.2).

MRI analysis and biopsy technique

The referring institutions had carried out the mpMRI studies by means of 1.5 T or 3 T MRI scanners, and some of them had applied an endorectal coil and a variety of imaging protocols. All of those studies included multiplanar high-resolution T2, diffusion-weighted and dynamic contrast enhancement series. All of the scans and original readings were reviewed by a single expert radiologist who

had more than 8 years' experience in prostate mpMRI reading. Only patients with lesions suspected as clinically significant cancer (i.e., PI-RADS score ≥ 3) were sent to IB-MRGpB. The same radiologist attended all subsequent biopsy procedures, and reviewed the previous diagnostic and MRI images taken real-time during guided biopsy. The IB-MRGpBs were carried out with 3 T MRI scanners and external coil application.

The IB-MRGpB patients were placed in a prone position and administered general anesthesia. A transrectal probe (DynaTRIM; Philips, USA) containing an MR "visible" gel was positioned against the apex of the prostate and attached externally to a manual biopsy device (DynaTRIM; Philips, USA). Axial and sagittal T2-weighted images were obtained to visualize the prostate and identify the target lesion. Diffusion-weighted series were used at the radiologist's discretion. A dedicated software package was used for device tracking and target localization (DynaCAD; Philips, USA) as described elsewhere [15]. Suspected clinically significant target lesions that were detected by MRI were sampled first, followed by 12-core template systematic prostate sampling when applicable.

The biopsies were performed by 2 senior urologists. The first urologist was trained and highly experienced in IB-MRGpBs (> 250 cases). The second urologist had no prior experience in performing IB-MRGpBs. Following training comprised of observation and a stepwise-guided hands-on approach with 8 cases, the second urologist performed the subsequent biopsies independently. All of the IB-MRGpBs sessions included in this study were then performed by one of these 2 urologists. With the exception of the urologist, the same team that was comprised of a radiologist, anesthesiologist, nurse, and technicians participated in the procedures. The patients were monitored in the recovery room for 1–2 h post-biopsy and discharged home following the anesthesiologist's evaluation.

Biopsy specimens were processed by routine pathologic fixation with formalin solution and evaluated by a single dedicated uropathologist with > 20 years of experience. Cancer cells retrieved in the IB-MRGpB specimens were used as the reference standard to determine the biopsy result. Clinically significant disease was defined as a biopsy Gleason score of ≥ 7 (International Society of Urological Pathology, ISUP ≥ 2).

Learning curve evaluation

Evaluation of the IB-MRGpB learning curve consisted of assessing biopsy duration and histology results according to the precision of the PI-RADS score (a "hit"). Procedure duration was defined as the time that elapsed from the first MRI scan at the time of performing the IB-MRGpB until the last target lesion sampling. We analyzed target lesion characteristics on the MRI, and assessed their effect on procedure duration according to number of lesions, lesion size, and use of diffusion MRI studies at the time of biopsy (as a surrogate for difficulty in identifying the target lesion). We divided the cohort into thirds per chronological order, and evaluated the duration of time needed to sample target lesions accordingly, i.e., comparing target sampling time at the first, second, and last thirds of patients, controlling for lesion characteristics. We then compared procedure time between the expert and novice urologists.

Since all of the MRIs before and during biopsies were read by a single radiologist, we used percentage of clinical significant disease diagnosis (ISUP ≥ 2) per PI-RADS score as surrogate for IB-MRGpB precision ("hit"). We also analyzed the effect of chronological order, lesion size as well as the urologist's background (trained vs. untrained) on IB-MRGpB precision.

Statistical analysis

We applied 2-sample t tests, Levene's test, and ANOVA to compare the "trained" and the "untrained" urologists' performances. A p value < 0.05 was considered statistically significant. Time analysis was by logarithmic conversion, and multiple comparison testing

by Benjamini–Hochberg correction. All tests were calculated using SPSS (version 25.0, IBM Corporation).

Results

In total, 110 biopsies were evaluated, comprised of 55 for each of the 2 participating urologists. Table 1 lists the patient characteristics and MRI findings. The average time for sampling IB-MRGpB target lesions and per-lesion sampling was 28 ± 15 and 20 ± 10 min, respectively, and there was a gradual decrease in time to completion (per chronological order) (Fig. 1). The number of target lesions correlated with IB-MRGpB-targeted sampling time, showing a significant difference for sampling a single lesion compared to sampling 2 or 3 lesions ($p < 0.0001$) (Fig. 2). Targeted sampling time between 2 and 3 lesions did not differ significantly. Dividing the entire cohort into thirds and evaluating the change in sampling time per lesion needed in the first 18 cases to cases 19–55 revealed a decrease from 37 ± 19 to 24 ± 10 min ($p < 0.05$).

We evaluated targeted sampling duration per chronological order (i.e., first third of patients vs. second third vs. last third) for each of the urologists separately, controlling for the number of target lesions on MRI (Fig. 3), and then compared their results. The less experienced

Table 1 Patient characteristics and MRI imaging findings

Variable		All		Untrained		Trained		p value
Age	Median, IQR	68	62–72	68	62–72	67	62.5–72.5	0.68
PSA (ng/dL)	Mean, STD	8.6	9.1	8.6	9.9	8.7	8.3	0.95
Prostate size (cc)	Mean, STD	53	27	53	27	56	52	0.72
PSA density (ng/dL/cc)	Mean, STD	0.20	0.30	0.22	0.37	0.15	0.10	0.31
Previous biopsy	Number, %	76	70	34	63[*]	42	76	0.13
Number of target lesions on MRI	Mean, STD	1.47	0.6	1.44	0.6	1.51	0.6	0.54
MRI target lesions' characteristics								
PI-RADS 3	Number, %	84	51.9	38	48.1	46	55.4	0.43
PI-RADS 4	Number, %	62	38.3	34	43.0	28	33.7	0.26
PI-RADS 5	Number, %	16	9.9	7	8.9	9	10.8	0.79
Lesion size (mm)	Median, IQR	7	5–11	7.5	6–11	7	4–12	0.4
Large lesion size (mm)	Mean, STD	10	6	10	6	9	6	0.63
Small lesion size (mm)	Mean, STD	8	6	9	6	7	4	0.095
Lesion location—Base[#]	Number, %	27	17	10	13	17	20	0.2
Lesion location—Mid-gland[#]	Number, %	91	56	39	49	52	63	0.11
Lesion location—Apex[#]	Number, %	56	35	30	38	26	31	0.4
Number of targeted cores/lesion	Mean, STD	3.3	1.6	3.0	1.1	3.6	1.9	0.07

Untrained urologist with no experience in performing IB-MRGpBs, *Trained* urologist highly trained in performing IB-MRGpBs, *Large lesion size* represents the size of the larger lesion when more than 1 target lesion was identified on pre-biopsy imaging, *Small lesion size* represents the size of the smaller lesion when more than 1 target lesion was identified on pre-biopsy imaging, *PSA* prostate-specific antigen, *STD* standard deviation, *IQR* interquartile range, *PI-RADS* prostate imaging reporting and data system v.2, *MRI* magnetic resonance imaging

*One patient had no available data regarding former biopsy

[#] Percentages calculated per total number of lesions. Numbers may not add up due to overlap with some lesions located in more than one anatomical section (e.g. base-mid etc.)

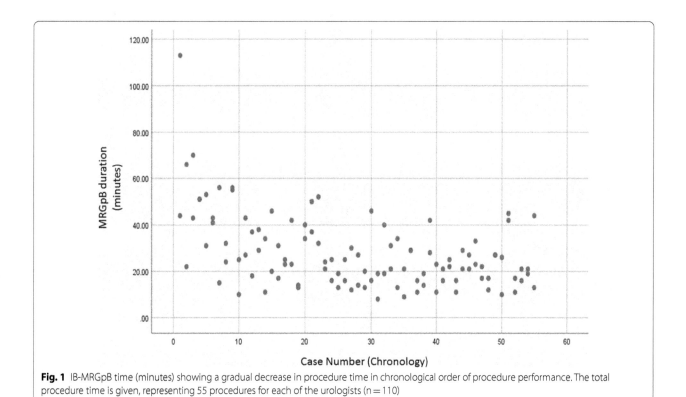

Fig. 1 IB-MRGpB time (minutes) showing a gradual decrease in procedure time in chronological order of procedure performance. The total procedure time is given, representing 55 procedures for each of the urologists (n = 110)

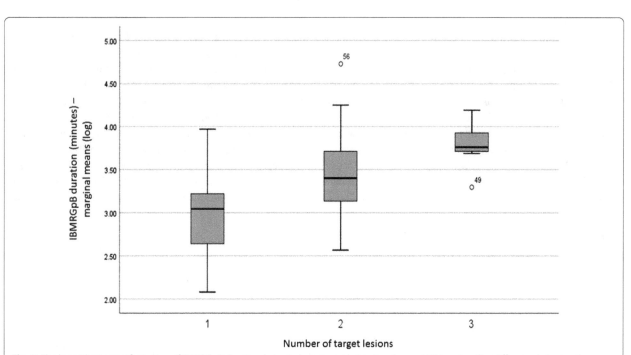

Fig. 2 The logarithmic transformation of IB-MRGpB duration (minutes) per target lesion number on MRI imaging. The difference between the sampling time of a single-target lesion compared to that of 2 or 3 target lesions was significant ($p < 0.0001$)

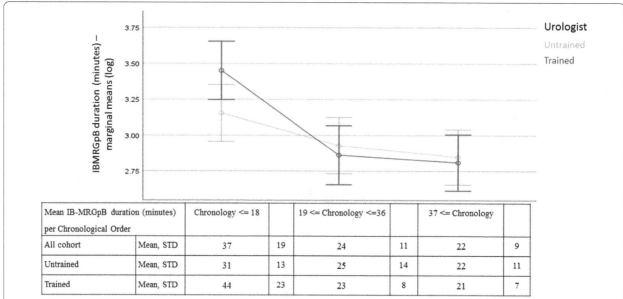

Mean IB-MRGpB duration (minutes) per Chronological Order		Chronology <= 18		19 <= Chronology <=36		37 <= Chronology	
All cohort	Mean, STD	37	19	24	11	22	9
Untrained	Mean, STD	31	13	25	14	22	11
Trained	Mean, STD	44	23	23	8	21	7

Fig. 3 Estimated marginal means of IB-MRGpB time (logarithmic transformation) showing a gradual decrease in procedure time in chronological order of the procedures performed for a single target lesion on MRI. The first 18 cases took longer than the subsequent ones. The table presents the average IB-MRGpB time per single lesion sampling, the procedure time for the entire cohort and the procedure time for the highly trained vs. the untrained urologist. There was no significant difference between the 2 urologists

urologist's IB-MRGpB targeted sampling time for the first 18 cases (i.e., the first third) showed a trend toward shorter duration ($p = 0.05$). No difference in the IB-MRGpB targeted sampling duration was found between the two urologists for the subsequent two-thirds of patients (from patient number 19 onward). Similar results were found in the analysis of the per urologist IB-MRGpB targeted sampling duration for multiple target lesions (i.e., 2 and 3 lesions) for the first 18 patients compared to the subsequent two-thirds (data not shown).

Neither prostate size, target lesion size (average, maximal, or minimal) nor the usage of diffusion studies during the MRI protocol of IB-MRGpB correlated with the time needed to sample target lesions for the cohort as a whole nor for each urologist's caseload on separate analyses.

Table 2 lists the correlation between the PI-RADS score with clinically significant disease. A multivariate analysis demonstrated no correlation between positive "hits"

(i.e., the finding of clinically significant prostate cancer in correlation with the PI-RADS score) and the following covariates: number of lesions, chronological order of biopsy (i.e., biopsy taken at the first, second, or last third of the cohort) and the operating urologist.

Discussion

Multiple techniques are available for performing a biopsy of suspicious prostatic MRI lesions, and we evaluated the urologist's learning curve of the high-end technique of IB-MRGpB, considered by some to be the leading tool in the diagnosis of clinically significant prostate cancer [1–3, 16]. Our reported correlation between IB-MRGpB targeted sampling and clinically significant disease diagnosis is in agreement with current literature [1, 17]. We achieved a similar level of precision of clinically significant disease diagnosis for smaller lesions as well. For example, the median lesion size was 12 mm (interquartile

Table 2 PI-RADS score correlation with clinically significant disease ("hit")

PI-RADS score	Clinical significant disease (ISUP ≥ 2)						*p* value
	All	%	Untrained	%	Trained	%	
3	16 (of 84)	19	7 (of 38)	18	9 (of 46)	20	0.89
4	34 (of 62)	55	20 (of 34)	59	14 (of 28)	50	0.49
5	11 (of 16)	69	7 (of 7)	100	4 (of 9)	44	0.74*

PI-RADS prostate imaging reporting and data system v.2, *ISUP* International Society of Urological Pathology, *Untrained* urologist with no experience in performing IB-MRGpBs, *Trained* urologist highly trained in performing IB-MRGpBs

*A preliminary *p* value of 0.034 was calculated for PIRADS5 lesions. This value was later corrected following Benjamini–Hochberg correction

range [IQR] 8–15) in the PRECISION trial [1], while it was 7 mm (IQR 5–11) in the current work. We believe that the ability to achieve a similar level of biopsy precision for the more challenging smaller lesions represents a real advantage of the IB-MRGpB technique. Our finding is supported by Pokorny et al. [17] who showed that a lesion's diameter had no impact on cancer diagnosis when using IB-MRGpB.

The most important outcome of prostate biopsy is the ability to detect clinically significant cancer. There was no difference between an experienced urologist's clinically significant cancer detection rate with that of the less experienced urologist in the present analysis (Table 2). Furthermore, the chronological order of biopsy did not affect the detection rate of clinically significant disease in the entire cohort or in either of the urologists' cohorts analyzed separately. These data suggest that a urologist's experience has no effect on the cancer detection rate. El Fegoun et al. and Karam et al. reported similar results for TRUS prostate biopsy and cancer detection rate, supporting the lack of a learning curve regarding cancer detection rates [9, 18]. Lawrentschuk et al. even suggested that it was the operator, rather than the operator's experience, that influenced the TRUS biopsy cancer detection rate [10]. Acknowledging the aforementioned advantage of MRI-guided prostate biopsy, multiple papers looked at the learning curve of MR/TRUS fusion biopsy and reported that an operator's learning curve affected sampling accuracy, suggesting that this represents the learning curves of both radiologists and urologists, and that it further affects procedural costs [8, 12, 13]. Similarly, Mager et al. reported that the MR/TRUS fusion biopsy detection rate for the initial 42 cases to be lower compared to the subsequent 42 cases, suggesting that accumulating experience influenced the ability to detect cancer. Of note is the fact that all of the cases reported by those authors were reviewed by a skilled radiologist and with the same supporting team (MRI technician, nurse, and anesthesiologist), suggesting that this learning curve represented the urologist's improvement rather than that of the rest of the biopsy team members [11].

Despite the application of high-end technology, the IB-MRGpB interface itself is rather simple. The ability to visualize a target lesion traversed by the sampling needle in real time together with a simple operator interface can explain such ease and precision, even at the very early phases of adopting this technology [15]. Our findings of a short learning curve for clinically significant cancer detection suggests an important advantage of the IB-MRGpB over the MR/TRUS fusion biopsy. It should be noted that a comparison of the significant cancer detection rates of PI-RADS 5 lesions between our two urologists' cohorts might have appeared to reveal a difference

in favor of the untrained urologist. Since only very few patients included in this study were diagnosed with PI-RADS 5, however, small diversions can translate into a difference, but this difference did not remain valid after statistical correction.

We perform IB-MRGpB with the patients under general anesthesia. The team consists of technicians, a nurse, radiologist, anesthesiologist, and urologist for ensuring a high standard of care, although it translates into a high procedure cost. As such, the length of a procedure plays a role in preserving resources. The reported procedure time for a transrectal MR-guided biopsy varies from 30 to 68 min [19]. Pokorny et al. [17] estimated the IB-MRGpB execution time to range between 24 and 63 min, and that their own experience averaged 20 min per single target. In line with those figures, our average IB-MRGpB time for sampling of all of the targeted lesions was 28 ± 15 min and the per-lesion sampling duration was 20 ± 15 min, with an average of 3.3 cores sampled per lesion. Importantly, 2 parameters significantly correlated with IB-MRGPB duration, the number of lesions (Fig. 2) and the urologists' accumulated experience (i.e., chronology) (Fig. 3), representing the procedure's learning curve. Our findings suggest that the 18th biopsy represents the cut-off point after which procedure time does not improve significantly. Compared to MR/TRUS fusion biopsy, for which the proposed learning curve was 98 cases for targeted biopsy and 84 cases for systematic biopsies in 1 series [13] and 42 cases in another [11], a learning curve of only 18 cases is clearly indicative of a quick and easy-to-adopt technique.

The procedure's duration plateaued after 18 cases for both urologists. While this may be interpreted as the learning curve of the untrained urologist, shortening the procedure duration over time for the highly trained urologist suggests an alternative explanation. Considering the high level of expertise of all team members to begin with, alongside the fact that they were putting this service together for the first time in our hospital, we believe this to represents the team's learning curve adopting a synchronized biopsy routine rather than the trained urologists further improvement of skills.

The utilization of MRGpB may be influenced by resource availability and costs, a consideration even suggested by some to specifically limit IB-MRGpB widespread use [20]. While IB-MRGpB indeed necessitates designated team as well as longer MR machine occupancy time, we believe its advantages may overcome these limitations [17, 21]. In the current work we describe how using the IB-MRGpB device and applying high-end technology together with a very simple interface compensates for much of the learning curve needed with other MRI-guided prostate biopsies and allows quick and easy mastering of this technique. In an era in which MRGpB plays such a critical role in prostate cancer diagnosis, such an easy learning curve is an important consideration for choosing a biopsy technique at both the institutional as well as the practicing urologist's level.

We recognize that our study has several limitations that bear mention. First, we used the PI-RADS correlation with the significant cancer pathology result as surrogate to a positive lesion "hit". The fact that all MRI reads and IB-MRGpBs were done with the same trained uroradiologist, and that all specimens were evaluated by a single dedicated expert uropathologist, we believe such consistency and level of expertise translates into true representation of a lesion's traversing rates. Second, our evaluation of procedure duration included the contribution of multiple personnel, and we extrapolated the urologist's learning curve from these findings. The fact that all other team members were highly experienced to begin with supports this approach. Lastly, our data is limited by the small cohort size, however, we believe the significant findings we show can serve the urologic-radiologic community.

In conclusion, these data suggest a very short learning curve for IB-MRGpB-targeted sampling duration, and that clinically significant cancer detection rates are not influenced by the learning curve of this technique.

Abbreviations

mpMRI: Multi-parametric magnetic resonance imaging; MRGpB: MRI-guided prostate biopsy; IB-MRGpB: In-bore MRI-guided prostate biopsy; TRUS: Transrectal ultrasound; PI-RADS: Prostate imaging reporting and data system.

Acknowledgements

The authors wish to thank the dedicated team of IB-MRGpBs for their constant help and professionalism.

Authors' contributions

BR: Conceptualization, Methodology, Formal analysis, Visualization, Writing—Original Draft, Project administration. TD: Investigation, Data curation, Formal analysis. OR: Investigation, Data curation. GG: Investigation, Data curation, Visualization. GS: Formal analysis, Writing—Original Draft. DEZ—Investigation, Writing—Original Draft. MS: Investigation, Data curation. JR: Methodology, Writing—Review and Editing. ZAD: Writing—Review and Editing, Supervision. OP: Writing—Review and Editing, Supervision. All authors read and approved the final manuscript.

Author details

[1]Department of Urology, Chaim Sheba Medical Center, 5262080 Ramat Gan, Israel. [2]The Sackler Faculty of Medicine, Tel Aviv University, Tel Aviv, Israel. [3]The Talpiot Medical Leadership Program, Chaim Sheba Medical Center, Tel Hashomer, Ramat Gan, Israel. [4]Assuta Ashdod University Hospital, Ashdod, Israel. [5]Department of Internal Medicine D and the Hypertension Unit, Chaim Sheba Medical Center, Tel Hashomer, Ramat Gan, Israel. [6]Department of Anesthesiology, Chaim Sheba Medical Center, Ramat Gan, Israel. [7]Department of Diagnostic Imaging, Chaim Sheba Medical Center, Ramat Gan, Israel.

References

1. Kasivisvanathan V, Rannikko AS, Borghi M, Panebianco V, Mynderse LA, Vaarala MH, et al. MRI-targeted or standard biopsy for prostate-cancer diagnosis. N Engl J Med [Internet]. 2018;378(19):1767–77.

2. Schoots IG, Roobol MJ, Nieboer D, Bangma CH, Steyerberg EW, Hunink MGM. Magnetic resonance imaging–targeted biopsy may enhance the diagnostic accuracy of significant prostate cancer detection compared to standard transrectal ultrasound-guided biopsy: a systematic review and meta-analysis. Eur Urol [Internet]. 2015;68(3):438–50.

3. Ahmed HU, El-Shater Bosaily A, Brown LC, Gabe R, Kaplan R, Parmar MK, et al. Diagnostic accuracy of multi-parametric MRI and TRUS biopsy in prostate cancer (PROMIS): a paired validating confirmatory study. Lancet [Internet]. 2017;389(10071):815–22.

4. Rothwax JT, George AK, Wood BJ, Pinto PA. Multiparametric MRI in biopsy guidance for prostate cancer: fusion-guided. Biomed Res Int [Internet]. 2014;2014:439171.

5. Wegelin O, van Melick HHE, Hooft L, Bosch JLHR, Reitsma HB, Barentsz JO, et al. Comparing three different techniques for magnetic resonance imaging-targeted prostate biopsies: a systematic review of in-bore versus magnetic resonance imaging-transrectal ultrasound fusion versus cognitive registration. Is there a preferred technique? Eur Urol [Internet]. 2017;71(4):517–31.

6. Rosenkrantz AB, Ayoola A, Hoffman D, Khasgiwala A, Prabhu V, Smereka P, et al. The learning curve in prostate MRI interpretation: self-directed learning versus continual reader feedback. AJR Am J Roentgenol [Internet]. 2017;208(3):W92–100. https://doi.org/10.2214/AJR.16.16876.

7. Akin O, Riedl CC, Ishill NM, Moskowitz CS, Zhang J, Hricak H. Interactive dedicated training curriculum improves accuracy in the interpretation of MR imaging of prostate cancer. Eur Radiol [Internet]. 2010;20(4):995–1002. https://doi.org/10.1007/s00330-009-1625-x.

8. Gaziev G, Wadhwa K, Barrett T, Koo BC, Gallagher FA, Serrao E, et al. Defining the learning curve for multiparametric magnetic resonance imaging (MRI) of the prostate using MRI-transrectal ultrasonography (TRUS) fusion-guided transperineal prostate biopsies as a validation tool. BJU Int [Internet]. 2016;117(1):80–6. https://doi.org/10.1111/bju.12892.

9. Benchikh El Fegoun A, El Atat R, Choudat L, El Helou E, Hermieu J-F, Dominique S, et al. The learning curve of transrectal ultrasound-guided prostate biopsies: implications for training programs. Urology [Internet]. 2013;81(1):12–5.

10. Lawrentschuk N, Toi A, Lockwood GA, Evans A, Finelli A, O'Malley M, et al. Operator is an independent predictor of detecting prostate cancer at transrectal ultrasound guided prostate biopsy. J Urol [Internet]. 2009;182(6):2659–63.

11. Mager R, Brandt MP, Borgmann H, Gust KM, Haferkamp A, Kurosch M. From novice to expert: analyzing the learning curve for MRI-transrectal ultrasonography fusion-guided transrectal prostate biopsy. Int Urol Nephrol [Internet]. 2017;49(9):1537–44. https://doi.org/10.1007/s11255-017-1642-7.

12. Meng X, Rosenkrantz AB, Huang R, Deng F-M, Wysock JS, Bjurlin MA, et al. The institutional learning curve of magnetic resonance imaging-ultrasound fusion targeted prostate biopsy: temporal improvements in cancer detection in 4 years. J Urol [Internet]. 2018;200(5):1022–9. https://doi.org/10.1016/j.juro.2018.06.012.

13. Kasabwala K, Patel N, Cricco-Lizza E, Shimpi AA, Weng S, Buchmann RM, et al. The learning curve for magnetic resonance imaging/ultrasound fusion-guided prostate biopsy. Eur Urol Oncol [Internet]. 2019;2(2):135–40.

14. Costa DN, Goldberg K, de Leon AD, Lotan Y, Xi Y, Aziz M, et al. Magnetic resonance imaging-guided in-bore and magnetic resonance imaging-transrectal ultrasound fusion targeted prostate biopsies: an adjusted comparison of clinically significant prostate cancer detection rate. Eur Urol Oncol [Internet]. 2019;2(4):397–404.

15. Schiavina R, Vagnoni V, D'Agostino D, Borghesi M, Salvaggio A, Giampaoli M, et al. "In-bore" MRI-guided prostate biopsy using an endorectal nonmagnetic device: a prospective study of 70 consecutive patients. Clin Genitourin Cancer [Internet]. 2017;15(3):417–27.

16. Kasivisvanathan V, Stabile A, Neves JB, Giganti F, Valerio M, Shanmugabavan Y, et al. Magnetic resonance imaging-targeted biopsy versus systematic biopsy in the detection of prostate cancer: a systematic review and meta-analysis. Eur Urol [Internet]. 2019;76(3):284–303.

17. Pokorny M, Kua B, Esler R, Yaxley J, Samaratunga H, Dunglison N, et al. MRI-guided in-bore biopsy for prostate cancer: what does the evidence say? A case series of 554 patients and a review of the current literature. World J Urol [Internet]. 2019;37(7):1263–79.

18. Karam JA, Shulman MJ, Benaim EA. Impact of training level of urology residents on the detection of prostate cancer on TRUS biopsy. Prostate Cancer Prostatic Dis [Internet]. 2004;7(1):38–40.

19. Overduin CG, Fütterer JJ, Barentsz JO. MRI-guided biopsy for prostate cancer detection: a systematic review of current clinical results. Curr Urol Rep [Internet]. 2013;14(3):209–13.

20. Hutchinson R, Lotan Y. Cost consideration in utilization of multiparametric magnetic resonance imaging in prostate cancer. Transl Androl Urol [Internet]. 2017;6(3):345.

21. Hosseiny M, Shakeri S, Felker ER, Lu D, Sayre J, Ahuja P, Raman SS, et al. 3-T multiparametric MRI followed by in-bore MR-guided biopsy for detecting clinically significant prostate cancer after prior negative transrectal ultrasound-guided biopsy. AJR Am J Roentgenol [Internet]. 2020;215(3):660–6.

22

Clinically significant prostate cancer (csPCa) detection with various prostate sampling schemes based on different csPCa definitions

Fei Wang[1], Tong Chen[1], Meng Wang[1], Hanbing Chen[1], Caishan Wang[1], Peiqing Liu[1], Songtao Liu[1], Jing Luo[1], Qi Ma[1*] and Lijun Xu[2*]

Abstract

Background: Combining targeted biopsy (TB) with systematic biopsy (SB) is currently recommended as the first-line biopsy method by the European Association of Urology (EAU) guidelines in patients diagnosed with prostate cancer (PCa) with an abnormal magnetic resonance imaging (MRI). The combined SB and TB indeed detected an additional number of patients with clinically significant prostate cancer (csPCa); however, it did so at the expense of a concomitant increase in biopsy cores. Our study aimed to evaluate if ipsilateral SB (ipsi-SB) + TB or contralateral SB (contra-SB) + TB could achieve almost equal csPCa detection rates as SB + TB using fewer cores based on a different csPCa definition.

Methods: Patients with at least one positive prostate lesion were prospectively diagnosed by MRI. The combination of TB and SB was conducted in all patients. We compared the csPCa detection rates of the following four hypothetical biopsy sampling schemes with those of SB + TB: SB, TB, ipsi-SB + TB, and contra-SB + TB.

Results: The study enrolled 279 men. The median core of SB, TB, ipsi-SB + TB, and contra-SB + TB was 10, 2, 7 and 7, respectively (P < 0.001). ipsi-SB + TB detected significantly more patients with csPCa than contra-SB + TB based on the EAU guidelines (P = 0.042). They were almost equal on the basis of the Epstein criteria (P = 1.000). Compared with SB + TB, each remaining method detected significantly fewer patients with csPCa regardless of the definition (P < 0.001) except ipsi-SB + TB on the grounds of D1 (P = 0.066). Ten additional subjects were identified with a higher Gleason score (GS) on contra-SB + TB, and only one was considered as significantly upgraded (GS = 6 on ipsi-SB + TB to a GS of 8 on contra-SB + TB).

Conclusions: Ipsi-SB + TB could acquire an almost equivalent csPCa detection value to SB + TB using significantly fewer cores when csPCa was defined according to the EAU guidelines. Given that there was only one significantly upgrading patient on contra-SB, our results suggested that contra-SB could be avoided.

Keywords: Clinically significant prostate cancer, Contralateral, Ipsilateral, Systematic biopsy, Targeted biopsy

Background

The number of patients with prostate cancer (PCa) has increased in the last decades in the USA. An estimated 174,650 and 191,930 men were diagnosed with PCa in 2019 and 2020, respectively, and the number of related deaths was 31,620 and 33,330, respectively [1, 2]. PCa is the only tumor diagnosed by blindly puncturing the

*Correspondence: maqisz@126.com; xulijun7313079@163.com
[1] Department of Ultrasound, The Second Affiliated Hospital of Soochow University, 1055 Sanxiang Road, Suzhou, Jiangsu, China
[2] Department of Urology, The Second Affiliated Hospital of Soochow University, 1055 Sanxiang Road, Suzhou, Jiangsu, China

entire organ rather than just the identified lesion by imaging due to the considerable overlap between benign and malignant lesion appearances in the imaging [3]. Despite its relatively low sensitivity (39–75%) [4] and specificity (40–82%) [5], routine transrectal ultrasound (TRUS)-guided systematic biopsy (SB) remains the diagnostic standard for PCa [6].

The ability to precisely detect PCa using magnetic resonance imaging (MRI) has led to the development of software-assisted MRI–ultrasound fusion guided targeted biopsy (TB). The European Association of Urology (EAU) guidelines currently recommend the combination of TB and SB as the first-line biopsy method for patients with suspected PCa with an abnormal MRI [7]. SB + TB indeed captures an additional number of PCa, but it does so at the expense of a concomitant increase in biopsy cores and overdetection of clinically insignificant prostate cancer (ciPCa) [8, 9]. The more the biopsy cores, the higher the complication rates, such as hematuria and urinary retention [10]. Besides, overdiagnosis and the following unnecessary treatment of low-grade PCa bear heavily on patients [9]. Thus, exploring a new biopsy method that could achieve an acceptable clinically significant prostate cancer (csPCa) detection rate with fewer cores is important.

A previous study has demonstrated that ipsilateral SB (ipsi-SB) + TB could detect more patients with csPCa than contralateral SB (contra-SB) + TB [11]. However, the study was performed on a single definition of csPCa. At present, no universally accepted definition of csPCa exists [12]. Therefore, we performed this study to evaluate the csPCa detection rate of various prostate sampling schemes and verify whether ipsi-SB + TB or contra-SB + TB could achieve almost equal csPCa detection rates to SB + TB using fewer cores based on different csPCa definitions.

Methods

Patient selection

Men with increased serum prostate-specific antigen (PSA) levels (PSA > 4 ng/mL) or an abnormal digital rectal examination (DRE) underwent 3.0-T prostate MRI. We included patients whose MRI was positive [with at least one lesion with a Prostate Imaging Reporting and Data System (PI-RADS) score of 3 or greater]. Patients with clinical stage T > 3 or metastases, prior treatment for PCa, and under active surveillance were excluded from the study (Fig. 1).

Multiparametric MRI

Multiparametric MRI was performed using a 3.0-T scanner with a 32-channel surface coil (Ingenia, Philips, Netherlands). In a nutshell, the study involved triplanar

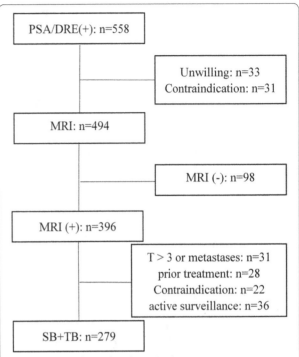

Fig. 1 Flowchart for study inclusion/exclusion. PSA = prostate-specific antigen; DRE = digital rectal examination; MRI = magnetic resonance imaging; SB = systematic biopsy; TB = targeted biopsy

T2-weighted imaging, diffusion-weighted imaging with a b value of 0–100–1000–2000 s/mm^2, apparent diffusion coefficient maps (calculated by the b value of 100–1000 s/mm^2 automatically), and dynamic contrast (gadolinium, 2.5 mL/s, 0.1 mmol/kg)-enhanced imaging sequences according to the minimum standards set by consensus guidelines [10]. One genitourinary radiologist interpreted all the lesions visible in MRI according to the PI-RADS version 2 on a scale from 1 (no suspicion) to 5 (high suspicion).

Biopsy procedure

A fluoroquinolone antibiotic was prescribed 3 days before biopsy to prevent postoperative infection, and an enema was generally performed. A MyLab Twice ultrasound system was used with an EC-123 7.5-MHz transrectal end-fire probe (EsaoteSpA, Genova, Italy) accompanied by an automatic biopsy gun with an 18-G needle for sampling.

TB procedure

MRI-TRUS registration (i.e., matching of the previously obtained suspicious MRI lesions with the real-time image of the prostate during TRUS biopsy) was performed by software-assisted rigid registration Virtual Navigator

(Esaote, Genoa, Italy). Each MRI suspicious lesion was biopsied with at least two cores.

SB procedure

The MRI overlay TB was then removed, and a second physician performed an SB with ultrasonographic guidance alone. The standard 10-core biopsy was obtained from the lateral and medial aspects of the base and midgland, and the apical prostate of the left and right sides [13] (Fig. 2).

Hypothetical biopsy sampling schemes and different definitions of csPCa

We hypothesized four biopsy sampling schemes in this study: SB only, TB only, ipsi-SB + TB, and contra-SB + TB. Among these, SB + TB was regarded as the reference. csPCa was defined according to the EAU guidelines [International Society for Urological Pathology (ISUP) 2 or higher, definition 1 (D1)] [14] or the Epstein criteria [Gleason score (GS) > 6 or GS 6 with ≥ 50% of cancer per core involvement or > 2 cores with cancer, definition 2 (D2)] [15].

Outcomes of interest

A comparison of the csPCa detection rate of the four hypothetical biopsy sampling schemes based on different csPCa definitions was our primary endpoint. The secondary endpoint was to assess the diagnostic concordance and upgrading between the aforementioned sampling schemes and SB + TB.

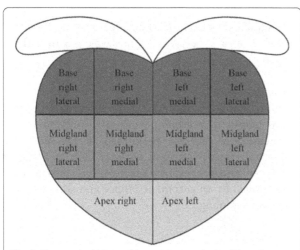

Fig. 2 The standard 10-core biopsy. 10 cores obtained from the lateral and medial aspects of the base and midgland and apical prostate of the left and right side. (Reprinted with the kind permission from Ma et al., 2017 [13])

Statistical analysis

Data were prospectively collected according to the Standards of Reporting for MRI-targeted Biopsy Studies database [16]. Descriptive statistics were used to describe the patient characteristics. The difference in the needed cores of different biopsy methods was compared by employing the Wilcoxon signed-rank test. We compared the csPCa detection rate of different biopsy strategies head-to-head using the McNemar test. A Cochran's Q test was used for comparing the pathological concordance and upgrading between different biopsy methods. We evaluated the potential predictors of biopsy result upgrading using multivariable logistic regression. All statistical analyses were conducted using SPSS, version 22.0, and a statistical significance level of 5% was used.

Results

Baseline characteristics of patients

In this prospective single-center diagnostic study, 279 subjects with a median age of 71 years [interquartile range (IQR): 62–80] and median PSA of 10.04 ng/mL (IQR: 6.38–18.00) were enrolled from January 2017 to December 2020 irrespective of the biopsy history. Abnormal DRE was found in 74 men (26.52%). The patients' demographics are given in Table 1.

Table 1 Patients' baseline characteristics, TRUS findings and MRI findings

Men, no	279
Age, year (IQR)	71 (65–77)
PSA, ng/mL (IQR)	10.04 (6.38–18.00)
Suspicious DRE findings, n (%)	74 (26.52)
TRUS prostate volume, mL (IQR)	57.00 (41.00–82.30)
Men with prior biopsy, n (%)	89 (31.90)
Men without biopsy history, n(%)	190 (68.10)
Abnormal TRUS findings, n (%)	139 (49.82)
Urologists' biopsy experience, year (IQR)	4 (4–5)
MRI suspicious lesions per patient, no. (IQR)	1 (1–1)
Total lesions, no	353
PIRADS v2 score, n (%)	
3	113 (32.01)
4	169 (47.88)
5	71 (20.11)
Location	
Peripheral zone, n (%)	232 (65.72)
Transitional zone, n (%)	121 (34.28)

Values are presented as median (interquartile range [IQR]). Statistically significant at P < 0.05. TRUS, transrectal ultrasound; MRI, magnetic resonance imaging; PSA, prostate-specific antigen; DRE, digital rectal examination; PIRADS, prostate imaging reporting and data system

Biopsy cores

The median core of SB, TB, ipsi-SB+TB, and contra-SB+TB was 10, 2, 7, and 7, respectively; they all differed significantly from SB+TB (12, P < 0.001) (Table 2). Obviously, TB showed the best detection of csPCa for the total number of cores regardless of the definition (P < 0.001) and SB performed the worst (P < 0.001). A comparison of the csPCa positive core rates of ipsi-SB+TB and contra-SB+TB revealed that the former performed better irrespective of the definition of csPCa (P < 0.001) (Table 2).

PCa detection rates

On the basis of D1, 104 and 90 patients with csPCa were detected by ipsi-SB+TB and contra-SB+TB, respectively (P = 0.042). And on the basis of D2, both ipsi-SB+TB and contra-SB+TB detected 146 patients with csPCa (P = 1.000). SB could detect more patients with csPCa than TB when used alone; however, the difference was insignificant on the grounds of D1 (D1: 82 vs. 80, P = 0.302; D2: 143 vs. 118, P = 0.002). Compared with SB+TB, each remaining method detected significantly fewer patients with csPCa regardless of the definition of csPCa (P < 0.001) except ipsi-SB+TB, which achieved almost the same csPCa detection rate as that of SB+TB based on D1 (P = 0.066) (Table 3). SB, TB, ipsi-SB+TB, and contra-SB+TB detected 61, 38, 42, and 56 patients with PCa, respectively, which were clinically insignificant when csPCa was defined as D1. It was obvious that TB

(P = 0.018) and ipsi-SB+TB (P = 0.021) detected significantly fewer patients with ciPCa compared with SB+TB (55).

GS distribution, concordance, and upgrading

The distribution of the GS on each biopsy method could be seen in Fig. 3. It is worth noting that the number of PCa with a GS of 6 detected by SB was more than that by TB (P < 0.001), but the number of PCa with a GS of ≥ 7 detected by both of them was almost equal (P = 0.311). ipsi-SB+TB identified the same number of PCa as that of contra-SB+TB (P = 1.000) but higher number of patients with a GS of ≥ 7 (P < 0.001) and fewer patients with a GS of 6 (P < 0.001).

ipsi-SB detected 92 patients with a higher GS, and 38 patients were still detected after combining with TB. Of the 38 patients, 9 had a GS of 6, 14 had a GS of ≤ 6 on contra-SB+TB to $\geq 3+4$ on ipsi-SB+TB, and the remaining 15 were concordant patients (Fig. 4a). The upgrading of a patient from a GS of ≤ 6 in one biopsy method to higher than a GS of ≤ 6 in another was considered as insignificantly upgraded. A patient upgrading from a GS of ≤ 6 in one biopsy method to a GS of $\geq 3+4$ in another was considered as significantly upgraded. A patient upgrading from a GS of $\geq 3+4$ in one biopsy method to higher than a GS of $\geq 3+4$ in another was considered concordant. Details of the 38 upgrading patients on ipsi-SB are summarized in Additional file 1: Table S1.

Table 2 Summary of biopsy cores

	SB	TB	ipsi-SB+TB	contra-SB+TB	SB+TB
Biopsy cores, no	10 (10–10)	2 (2–2)	7 (7–7)	7 (7–7)	12 (12–12)
Positive biopsy cores, no	1 (0–4)	0 (0–2)	2 (0–5)	2 (0–3)	2 (0–6)
D1 positive core rate, n (%)	373 (10.69)	230 (29.72)	509 (20.21)	324 (12.86)	603 (14.14)
P	< 0.001	< 0.001	< 0.001	0.017	–
D2 positive core rate, n (%)	678 (19.43)	357 (46.12)	817 (32.43)	575 (22.83)	1035 (24.27)
P	< 0.001	< 0.001	< 0.001	0.051	–

Values are presented as median (interquartile range). Statistically significant at P < 0.05. SB, systematic biopsy; TB, targeted biopsy; ipsi-SB, ipsilateral SB; contra-SB, contralateral SB; D1, definition 1 (EAU guidelines); csPCa, clinically significant prostate cancer; D2, definition 2 (Epstein criteria)

Table 3 Detection rates of csPCa

	SB	TB	ipsi-SB+TB	contra-SB+TB	SB+TB
Detected D1 csPCa cases, n (%)	82 (29.39)	80 (28.67)	104 (37.28)	90 (32.26)	106 (37.99)
P	< 0.001	< 0.001	0.066	< 0.001	-
Detected D2 csPCa cases, n (%)	143 (51.25)	118 (42.29)	146 (52.33)	146 (52.33)	161 (57.71)
P	< 0.001	< 0.001	< 0.001	< 0.001	-

Statistically significant at P < 0.05. csPCa, clinically significant prostate cancer; SB, systematic biopsy; TB, targeted biopsy; ipsi-SB, ipsilateral SB; contra-SB, contralateral SB; D1, definition 1 (EAU guidelines); D2, definition 2 (Epstein criteria); GS, Gleason score

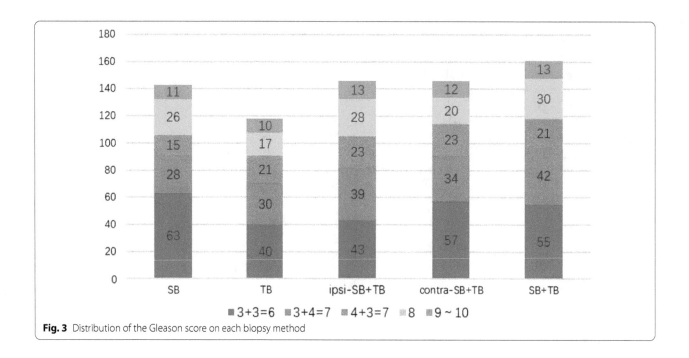

Fig. 3 Distribution of the Gleason score on each biopsy method

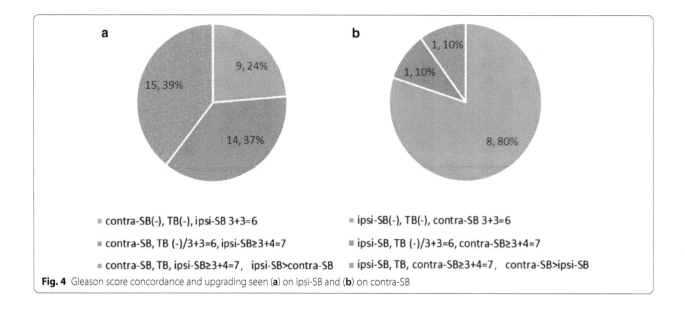

Fig. 4 Gleason score concordance and upgrading seen (**a**) on ipsi-SB and (**b**) on contra-SB

In contrast, 17 subjects were identified with a higher GS on contra-SB compared with ipsi-SB, and only 10 additional upgrades occurred after combining with TB. Among them, eight patients had a GS of 6, one had a GS of 6 on ipsi-SB + TB to a GS of 8 on contra-SB + TB, and one had a GS of 9 on ipsi-SB + TB to a GS of 10 on contra-SB + TB (Fig. 4b). Details of the 10 upgrading patients on contra-SB are summarized in Additional file 2: Table S2.

Potential predictors of GS upgrading on ipsi-SB + TB and contra-SB + TB

We evaluated the potential predictors of GS upgrading on ipsi-SB + TB and contra-SB + TB. For all 38 patients with a higher GS on ipsi-SB + TB, decreased TRUS prostate volume, prior biopsy history, lesion located in the peripheral zone (PZ), and higher PSA level were associated with GS upgrading. Among them, prior biopsy history had the strongest association with GS upgrading

Table.4 Associated predictors of Gleason score upgrading on ipsi-SB + TB

	38 upgrading			14 significantly upgrading		
	OR	95% CI	P value	OR	95% CI	P value
TRUS prostate volume (per 10 volume)	0.970	0.950–0.990	0.004	0.980	0.950–1.012	0.022
Biopsy history (yes or no)	2.365	0.903–6.192	0.008	–	–	–
Location (PZ or TZ)	1.949	0.713–5.324	0.019	8.424	1.201–59.065	0.032
PSA (per ng/mL)	1.001	0.999–1.004	0.028	–	–	–

Statistically significant at $P < 0.05$. SB, systematic biopsy; TB, targeted biopsy; ipsi-SB, ipsilateral SB; OR, odds ratio; CI, confidence interval; TRUS, transrectal ultrasound; PZ, peripheral zone; TZ, transitional zone; PSA, prostate-specific antigen

Table.5 Associated predictors of 10 Gleason score upgrading on contra-SB + TB

	OR	95% CI	P value
Biopsy history (yes or no)	3.148	0.527–18.802	0.021
Urologists' biopsy experience (per year)	0.701	0.349–1.409	0.032

Statistically significant at $P < 0.05$. SB, systematic biopsy; TB, targeted biopsy; contra-SB, contralateral SB; OR, odds ratio; CI, confidence interval

[odds ratio (OR): 2.365; P = 0.008] (Table 4). In the 14 significantly upgrading patients on ipsi-SB + TB, decreased TRUS prostate volume and lesion located in the PZ remained significant (Table 4).

Prior biopsy history (OR: 3.148; P = 0.021) and inadequate biopsy experience (OR: 0.701; P = 0.032) were associated with a GS of 10 upgrading on contra-SB + TB (Table 5).The basic characteristics of the only patient with significant upgrading on contra-SB + TB were as follows: age 82 years, PSA 30.24 ng/mL, DRE (+), TRUS prostate volume 66.9 mL, prior biopsy history, abnormal TRUS findings, urologists' biopsy experience 5, MRI suspicious lesions 1, maximum PI-RADS 5, and lesion position PZ.

Discussion

SB is a relatively cost-effective and nonoperator-dependent method of detecting PCa and does not need specialized equipment. However, the method suffers from relatively lower diagnostic accuracy and more biopsy cores. Despite several limitations, systematic sampling of the prostate with different core numbers (commonly 10–12 cores) still represents an integral aspect of diagnosing or excluding PCa [17]. The MRI pathway (MRI with or without TB) has been increasingly used for the detection and risk stratification of csPCa [18, 19]. Van der Leest M et al. [20] concluded that MRI-TB had an identical detection rate of csPCa and significantly fewer ciPCa using fewer needles compared with SB.

In this study, TB indeed had a significantly higher csPCa positive core rate than SB; however, SB still could detect significantly more patients with csPCa than TB at least based on D2. Similar results were reported by Hakozaki et al. [21] with a higher csPCa detection rate in the SB group; they defined csPCa according to D2 in this context. More patients with csPCa were also detected by SB than by TB on the grounds of D1, although the difference was insignificant in this article. This finding was compatible with that of a previous similar study (Radtke et al. [22]), which reported that the csPCa (in line with D1 in our study) detection rate was higher using SB alone than using TB alone. Compared with D1, D2 of csPCa is more inclusive. For example, cancer with a GS of 6 and three cores would be considered ciPCa on the grounds of D1 but csPCa based on D2. In the series by Filson et al. [23], TB offered the potential to identify more higher-risk patients with PCa. As a consequence, although SB still detected more patients with csPCa than TB, the difference was insignificant when using the stricter D1 of csPCa. Therefore, TB was nonsuperior to SB in terms of detecting csPCa at least in the current study.

Recently, many different modified sampling schemes have emerged to increase the detection of aggressive tumors and decrease biopsy cores and concomitant complications [24]. A regional TB strategy (10.58 cores) proposed by Raman et al. [25] detected a similar number of patients with csPCa to SB + TB. And many other studies [26, 27] also focused on optimizing the number of cores sampled from the targeted area and reached the conclusion that saturation TB (10–20 cores) detected as many patients with csPCa as 20- to 26-core SB + TB. However, omitting SB or not was still in dispute, and the scheme of saturation TB was not unified. In an early study, Ploussard et al. [28] evaluated the added value of concomitant SB for predicting the final grade group in patients with positive MRI findings who underwent TB. The results showed that SB reclassified a non-negligible proportion of patients in a higher-risk category and modified the final treatment decision-making. As a consequence, SB should not be omitted at least in MRI-positive cases, just identical to the EAU guidelines [7]. Although SB + TB indeed led to the detection of more PCa and csPCa among patients with MRI-visible lesions, the cores were also increased [8].

Bryk et al. [9] enrolled a cohort of 211 men with a single unilateral suspicious lesion on MRI and recommended ipsi-SB + TB, as the detection of csPCa increased with only a modest increase in ciPCa detection. Our findings were consistent with those of Bryk et al. when we used nearly the same definition of csPCa (D1). ipsi-SB + TB also performed better in terms of a positive core rate than contra-SB + TB irrespective of the definition of csPCa. However, the two methods had an equivalent detection of csPCa based on D2 in this study. Thus, no matter which csPCa definition was chosen in this study, ipsi-SB + TB did not perform worse than contra-SB + TB in the detection of patients with csPCa.

In this study, both ipsi-SB + TB and contra-SB + TB detected fewer patients with csPCa regardless of the definition of csPCa when compared with SB + TB. The aforementioned findings were identical with those of Freifeld et al. [11], who found that patients were more or less missed or misclassified by TB alone, TB + ipsi-SB, and TB + contra-SB. However, slightly different from the previous study, ipsi-SB + TB detected an almost equal number of patients with csPCa as SB + TB based on D1 in this study. This provided us a novel biopsy scheme that could acquire an equivalent csPCa detection value to SB + TB using significantly fewer cores.

Further, we analyzed the specific GS of each biopsy method. Also, we found that ipsi-SB + TB identified the same number of PCa as contra-SB + TB did but with a higher number of patients with a GS of ≥ 7 and fewer patients with a GS of 6. With respect to the upgrading condition, combining ipsi-SB and contra-SB + TB led to 38 GS upgrading; however, combining contra-SB and ipsi-SB + TB only resulted in 10 GS upgrading. Also, a large number of the 38 patients upgraded from GS ≤ 6 to GS ≥ 7; conversely, 80% of the 10 cases with no cancer on ipsi-SB + TB were diagnosed with PCa with a GS of 6 when combined with contra-SB. Recently, as a result of the widespread use of PSA testing, the incidence of PCa has increased (including ciPCa) [29]. Also, after many years of aggressive treatment of PCa, the reduced overdiagnosis and overtreatment of ciPCa have caught the attention of the urology community [30]. According to the EAU guidelines [14], active surveillance should be discussed for patients at low risk of PCa (PSA < 10 ng/mL and GS < 7 and cT1-2a). Patients at intermediate risk (PSA 10–20 ng/mL or GS 7 or cT2b) and those at high risk of PCa (PSA > 20 ng/mL or GS > 7 or cT2c) are strongly recommended to undergo radical prostatectomy. As a result, additional contra-SB results in the overdetection of low-risk PCa, while additional ipsi-SB is more likely to change the patients' recommended treatment strategy.

This study has some limitations. First, the inclusion criteria of this study are confined to patients with abnormal MRI; thus, no statement of cancer missed in the initial MRI could be made. Siddiqui et al. [31] reported that MRI showed a negative predictive value of 98% for PCa with a GS of 7 or greater; hence, further studies are needed to explore the negative predictive value of MRI. Second, whole-mount histopathology was not the reference specimen when the cancer detection rate was compared. Third, the rigid registration system did not allow us to make adjustments; even deformations happened to the prostate by the TRUS probe, although some anatomical landmarks can be used to make cognitive fusion at that time in our study [32]. Finally, the same patient was tested with SB and TB, and biopsy complications, such as hemorrhage and swelling of the first conducted one-TB procedure might have negatively affected the SB.

Conclusions

Ipsi-SB + TB could acquire an almost equivalent csPCa detection value to SB + TB using significantly fewer cores when csPCa was defined according to the EAU guidelines. Given that there was only one significantly upgrading patient on contra-SB, our results suggested that contra-SB could be avoided.

Abbreviations

PCa: Prostate cancer; TRUS: Transrectal ultrasound; SB: Systematic biopsy; MRI: Magnetic resonance imaging; TB: Targeted biopsy; EAU: European Association of Urology; ciPCa: Clinically insignificant prostate cancer; csPCa: Clinically significant prostate cancer; ipsi-SB: Ipsilateral SB; contra-SB: Contralateral SB; PSA: Prostate-specific antigen; DRE: Digital rectal examination; PI-RADS: Prostate Imaging Reporting and Data System; ISUP: International Society for Urological Pathology; GS: Gleason score; IQR: Interquartile range; PZ: Peripheral zone; TZ: Transitional zone; OR: Odds ratio.

Supplementary Information

Additional file 1. Table S1 Detail of the 38 upgrading patients on ipsi-SB.

Additional file 2. Table S2 Detail of the 10 upgrading patients on contra-SB.

Acknowledgements

Not applicable.

Authors' contributions

FW and QM conceived and designed the study, participated in the collection of data and data analysis, and drafted the manuscript. LJ X assisted in the design of this research and project development. TC, MW, HB C, CS W, PQ L, ST L, JL participated in the collection of data. All authors read and approved the final manuscript.

References

1. Sterling J, Smith K, Farber N, et al. Fourteen-core systematic biopsy that includes two anterior cores in men with PI-RADS lesion >/= 3 is comparable with magnetic resonance imaging-ultrasound fusion biopsy in detecting clinically significant prostate cancer: a single-institution experience. Clin Genitourin Cancer. 2020. https://doi.org/10.1016/j.clgc.2020.09.006.

2. Morris DC, Chan DY, Lye TH, et al. Multiparametric ultrasound for targeting prostate cancer: combining ARFI, SWEI, QUS and B-mode. Ultrasound Med Biol. 2020;46(12):3426–39. https://doi.org/10.1016/j.ultrasmedbio.2020.08.022.

3. Gunzel K, Cash H, Buckendahl J, et al. The addition of a sagittal image fusion improves the prostate cancer detection in a sensor-based MRI/ultrasound fusion guided targeted biopsy. BMC Urol. 2017;17(1):7. https://doi.org/10.1186/s12894-016-0196-9.

4. Postema A, Mischi M, de la Rosette J, Wijkstra H. Multiparametric ultrasound in the detection of prostate cancer: a systematic review. World J Urol. 2015;33(11):1651–9. https://doi.org/10.1007/s00345-015-1523-6.

5. Heijmink SW, Futterer JJ, Strum SS, et al. State-of-the-art uroradiologic imaging in the diagnosis of prostate cancer. Acta Oncol. 2011;50(Suppl 1):25–38. https://doi.org/10.3109/0284186X.2010.578369.

6. Pinto PA, Chung PH, Rastinehad AR, et al. Magnetic resonance imaging/ultrasound fusion guided prostate biopsy improves cancer detection following transrectal ultrasound biopsy and correlates with multiparametric magnetic resonance imaging. J Urol. 2011;186(4):1281–5. https://doi.org/10.1016/j.juro.2011.05.078.

7. Guideline. Secondary Guideline. https://uroweb.org/guidelines/.

8. Ahdoot M, Wilbur AR, Reese SE, et al. MRI-targeted, systematic, and combined biopsy for prostate cancer diagnosis. N Engl J Med. 2020;382(10):917–28. https://doi.org/10.1056/NEJMoa1910038.

9. Bryk DJ, Llukani E, Taneja SS, et al. The role of ipsilateral and contralateral transrectal ultrasound-guided systematic prostate biopsy in men with unilateral magnetic resonance imaging lesion undergoing magnetic resonance imaging-ultrasound fusion-targeted prostate biopsy. Urology. 2017;102:178–82. https://doi.org/10.1016/j.urology.2016.11.017.

10. Borghesi M, Ahmed H, Nam R, et al. Complications after systematic, random, and image-guided prostate biopsy. Eur Urol. 2017;71(3):353–65. https://doi.org/10.1016/j.eururo.2016.08.004.

11. Freifeld Y, Xi Y, Passoni N, et al. Optimal sampling scheme in men with abnormal multiparametric MRI undergoing MRI-TRUS fusion prostate biopsy. Urol Oncol. 2019;37(1):57–62. https://doi.org/10.1016/j.urolonc.2018.10.009.

12. Shin T, Smyth TB, Ukimura O, et al. Diagnostic accuracy of a five-point Likert scoring system for magnetic resonance imaging (MRI) evaluated according to results of MRI/ultrasonography image-fusion targeted biopsy of the prostate. BJU Int. 2018;121(1):77–83. https://doi.org/10.1111/bju.13972.

13. Ma Q, Yang DR, Xue BX, et al. Transrectal real-time tissue elastography targeted biopsy coupled with peak strain index improves the detection of clinically important prostate cancer. Oncol Lett. 2017;14(1):210–6. https://doi.org/10.3892/ol.2017.6126.

14. Mottet N, van den Bergh RCN, Briers E, et al. EAU-EANM-ESTRO-ESUR-SIOG guidelines on prostate cancer-2020 update. Part 1: screening, diagnosis, and local treatment with curative intent. Eur Urol. 2021;79(2):243–62. https://doi.org/10.1016/j.eururo.2020.09.042.

15. Epstein JI, Walsh PC, Carmichael M, Brendler CB. Pathologic and clinical findings to predict tumor extent of nonpalpable (stage T1c) prostate cancer. JAMA. 1994;271(5):368–74.

16. Moore CM, Kasivisvanathan V, Eggener S, et al. Standards of reporting for MRI-targeted biopsy studies (START) of the prostate: recommendations from an International Working Group. Eur Urol. 2013;64(4):544–52. https://doi.org/10.1016/j.eururo.2013.03.030

17. Bjurlin MA, Taneja SS. Standards for prostate biopsy. Curr Opin Urol. 2014;24(2):155–61. https://doi.org/10.1097/mou.0000000000000031.

18. Weinreb JC, Barentsz JO, Choyke PL, et al. PI-RADS prostate imaging—reporting and data system: 2015, version 2. Eur Urol. 2016;69(1):16–40. https://doi.org/10.1016/j.eururo.2015.08.052.

19. Turkbey B, Rosenkrantz AB, Haider MA, et al. Prostate imaging reporting and data system version 2.1: 2019 update of prostate imaging reporting and data system version 2. Eur Urol. 2019;76(3):340–51. https://doi.org/10.1016/j.eururo.2019.02.033.

20. Van der Leest M, Cornel E, Israël B, et al. Head-to-head comparison of transrectal ultrasound-guided prostate biopsy versus multiparametric prostate resonance imaging with subsequent magnetic resonance-guided biopsy in biopsy-naïve men with elevated prostate-specific antigen: a large prospective multicenter clinical study. Eur Urol. 2019;75(4):570–8. https://doi.org/10.1016/j.eururo.2018.11.023.

21. Hakozaki Y, Matsushima H, Kumagai J, et al. A prospective study of magnetic resonance imaging and ultrasonography (MRI/US)-fusion targeted biopsy and concurrent systematic transperineal biopsy with the average of 18-cores to detect clinically significant prostate cancer. BMC Urol. 2017;17(1):117. https://doi.org/10.1186/s12894-017-0310-7.

22. Radtke JP, Schwab C, Wolf MB, et al. Multiparametric magnetic resonance imaging (MRI) and MRI-transrectal ultrasound fusion biopsy for index tumor detection: correlation with radical prostatectomy specimen. Eur Urol. 2016;70(5):846–53. https://doi.org/10.1016/j.eururo.2015.12.052.

23. Filson CP, Natarajan S, Margolis DJ, et al. Prostate cancer detection with magnetic resonance-ultrasound fusion biopsy: the role of systematic and targeted biopsies. Cancer. 2016;122(6):884–92. https://doi.org/10.1002/cncr.29874.

24. Loeb S, Vellekoop A, Ahmed HU, et al. Systematic review of complications of prostate biopsy. Eur Urol. 2013;64(6):876–92. https://doi.org/10.1016/j.eururo.2013.05.049.

25. Raman AG, Sarma KV, Raman SS, et al. Optimizing spatial biopsy sampling for the detection of prostate cancer. J Urol. 2021;206(3):595–603. https://doi.org/10.1097/JU.0000000000001832.

26. Hansen NL, Barrett T, Lloyd T, et al. Optimising the number of cores for magnetic resonance imaging-guided targeted and systematic transperineal prostate biopsy. BJU Int. 2020;125(2):260–9. https://doi.org/10.1111/bju.14865.

27. Tschirdewahn S, Wiesenfarth M, Bonekamp D, et al. Detection of significant prostate cancer using target saturation in transperineal magnetic resonance imaging/transrectal ultrasonography-fusion biopsy. Eur Urol Focus. 2020;20:30186–93. https://doi.org/10.1016/j.euf.

28. Ploussard G, Beauval JB, Lesourd M, et al. Added value of concomitant systematic and fusion targeted biopsies for grade group prediction based on radical prostatectomy final pathology on positive magnetic resonance imaging. J Urol. 2019;202(6):1182–7. https://doi.org/10.1097/ju.0000000000000418.

29. Borkowetz A, Platzek I, Toma M, et al. Comparison of systematic transrectal biopsy to transperineal magnetic resonance imaging/ultrasound-fusion biopsy for the diagnosis of prostate cancer. BJU Int. 2015;116(6):873–9. https://doi.org/10.1111/bju.13023.

30. Albisinni S, Aoun F, Noel A, et al. Are concurrent systematic cores needed at the time of targeted biopsy in patients with prior negative prostate biopsies? Prog Urol. 2018;28(1):18–24. https://doi.org/10.1016/j.purol.2017.10.001.

31. Siddiqui MM, Rais-Bahrami S, Turkbey B, et al. Comparison of MR/ultrasound fusion-guided biopsy with ultrasound-guided biopsy for the diagnosis of prostate cancer. JAMA. 2015;313(4):390–7. https://doi.org/10.1001/jama.2014.17942.

32. Venderink W, Bomers JG, Overduin CG, et al. Multiparametric magnetic resonance imaging for the detection of clinically significant prostate cancer: what urologists need to know. Part 3: targeted biopsy. Eur Urol. 2020;77(4):481–90. https://doi.org/10.1016/j.eururo.2019.10.009.

23

The risk factors related to the severity of pain in patients with Chronic Prostatitis/Chronic Pelvic Pain Syndrome

Jing Chen[1,2], Haomin Zhang[3], Di Niu[1,2], Hu Li[1,2], Kun Wei[1,2], Li Zhang[1,2], Shuiping Yin[1,2], Longfei Liu[5], Xiansheng Zhang[1,2,4], Meng Zhang[1,2,4,6]* and Chaozhao Liang[1,2,4]*

Abstract

Background: Chronic Prostatitis/Chronic Pelvic Pain Syndrome (CP/CPPS) is a disease with diverse clinical manifestations, such as pelvic pain or perineal pain. Although recent studies found several risk factors related to the pain severity of CP/CPPS patients, results were inconsistent. Here, we aimed to identify novel risk factors that are closely related to the severity of pain in patients with CP/CPPS.

Methods: We retrospectively collected the clinical records from patients with CP/CPPS from March 2019 to October 2019. The questionnaire was used to obtain related parameters, such as demographics, lifestyle, medical history, etc. To identify potential risk factors related to pain severity, we used the methods of univariate and multivariate logistic regression analyses. Further, to confirm the relationship between these confirmed risk factors and CP/CPPS, we randomly divided CP/CPPS patients into the training and the validation cohorts with a ratio of 7:3. According to the co-efficient result of each risk factor calculated by multivariate logistic regression analysis, a predicting model of pain severity was established. The receiver operating characteristic curve (ROC), discrimination plot, calibration plot, and decision curve analyses (DCA) were used to evaluate the clinical usage of the current model in both the training and validation cohorts.

Results: A total of 272 eligible patients were enrolled. The univariate and multivariate logistic regression analysis found that age [odds ratio (OR): 2.828, 95% confidence intervals (CI): 1.239–6.648, $P = 0.004$], holding back urine (OR: 2.413, 95% CI: 1.213–4.915, $P = 0.005$), anxiety or irritability (OR: 3.511, 95% CI: 2.034–6.186, $P < 0.001$), contraception (OR: 2.136, 95% CI:1.161–3.014, $P = 0.029$), and smoking status (OR: 1.453, 95% CI: 1.313–5.127, $P = 0.013$) were the risk factors of pain severity. We then established a nomogram model, to test whether these factors could be used to predict the pain severity of CP/CPPS patients in turn. Finally, ROC, DCA, and calibration analyses proved the significance and stability of this nomogram, further confirmed that these factors were closely related to the pain severity of CP/CPPS patients.

*Correspondence: zhangmeng1930@126.com; liang_chaozhao@ahmu.edu.cn
[4] Anhui Province Key Laboratory of Genitourinary Diseases, Anhui Medical University, Hefei, People's Republic of China
[6] Institute of Urology of Shenzhen University, The Third Affiliated Hospital of Shenzhen University, Shenzhen Luohu Hospital Group, Shenzhen, People's Republic of China
Full list of author information is available at the end of the article

Conclusions: We identify age, holding back urine, anxiety or irritability, contraception, and smoking are risk factors closely related to the pain severity in patients with CP/CPPS. Our results provide novel inspirations for clinicians to design the personalized treatment plan for individual CP/CPPS patient who has suffered different encounters.

Keywords: Chronic prostatitis, Risk factors, Pain, Nomogram, Personalized treatment

Background

Prostatitis is a common urologic disease [1, 2], with studies reporting that during their lifetime, approximately 35–50% of men will suffer from prostatitis. The morbidity of prostatitis is higher in men who are not over 50-year-old [3]. According to previous work, we know that the prevalence rate of chronic prostatitis in Chinese males is approximately 8.4% [4]. Based on a proposal from the National Institutes of Health (NIH) [5], prostatitis is divided into four categories; of them, Category III, which is defined as chronic prostatitis or chronic pelvic pain syndrome (CP/CPPS), accounts for most cases of prostatitis [6]. CP/CPPS has a variety of clinical manifestations, such as pelvic pain or perineal pain, irritative or obstructive voiding symptoms, sexual dysfunction, or psychological disorders, and is without any evidence of urinary tract infection [7, 8]. Commonly, chronic pelvic pain occurs with pelvic floor tenderness, thus the patients will feel pain at the time of palpation [9].

Clinically, doctors always apply NIH-CPSI to judge the severity of chronic prostatitis. According to the subscores for pain, the pain levels are graded as mild (0 to 7), moderate (8 to 13), and severe (14 to 21). A recent study showed that the relationship between pain with the quality of life (QoL) in CP/CPPS patients was more important than urinary symptoms and the pain severity was more important than pain localization/type [10]. So, studying the risk factors for pain severity and clarifying the pain severity are helpful in improving the strategy of individualized phenotypically guided treatment. Although recent studies had found several risk factors related to the pain of CP/CPPS patients, results were inconsistent. Some studies had shown that a sedentary lifestyle, smoking, and stress were potential risk factors for the pain in patients with CP/CPPS [11]. But other studies showed that cigarette smoking was not related to the pain in patients with CP/CPPS [12]. Therefore, studying the risk factors for the pain severity in patients with CP/CPPS is particularly important for designing the personalized treatment plan.

In this study, we recorded the NIH-CPSI scores and other parameters from the outpatients with CP/CPPS to explore the risk factors related to the pain severity in patients with CP/CPPS and establish a predicting model of it.

Methods

Population selection

From March 2019 to October 2019, approximately 322 patients were diagnosis of CP/CPPS according to physical examination, microbiologic localization cultures, laboratory testing of stamey test, urodynamic studies and the UPOINTs classification [13] in the clinic of the First Affiliated Hospital of Anhui Medical University; we recorded the information from those patients. This study was approved by the Institutional Review Board of the First Affiliated Hospital of Anhui Medical University. Each patient had signed informed consent. The inclusion criteria for CP/CPPS patients were as follows: (1) symptoms lasting for at least 3 months; (2) discomfort or pain in the pelvic area or perineum that participants were excluded from the study if they had the urologic disease, such as acute prostatitis or bacterial prostatitis, urinary tract infection, urinary tuberculosis, bladder stone, interstitial cystitis, urethritis [14], and (3) the score of NIH-CPSI ≥ 4 [15]. The patients whose age was older than 50 years underwent a test of serum PSA based on the cut point of less than 4.0 ng/ml to exclude prostate cancer [16]. The patients who had benign prostatic hyperplasia (BPH) that the prostate ultrasound showed the prostate volume greater than 2*3*4 cm with the post-void residual urine volume of 50 ml were ruled out. Of all 322 recorded patients, 50 were excluded because of missing baseline values for continuous variables.

Records of the variables

From the available records that we obtained from the CP/CPPS patients; according to some studies of the risk factors for CP/CPPS and the pain of CP/CPPS [11], the 11 variables were about basic information, lifestyle, and medical history were selected for further analysis. The sedentary lifestyle was defined as sitting or lying down when took part in an activity, such as reading, watching television, driving [17]. Holding back urine was defined as that waiting until the last second to go to the bathroom to pee [18]. In China, the main contraceptive method was the use of condoms, so in our study, the contraceptive method was set as the use of condoms. The questionnaire of the Self-Rating Anxiety Scale (SAS) was used to judge whether patients with CP/CPPS had the diagnosis of anxiety. When the scores of SAS was more than 50, the patients were diagnosed with anxiety [19]. 100 ml of beer per week differed significantly from 100 ml of liquor or spirits. To accurately assess the alcohol intake of patients, we uniformly defined the patient's alcohol intake as grams of alcohol intake per week. According to the number of cigarettes daily in Paul's study, we divided smokers into two groups: daily smoker of < 10 cigarettes and daily smoker of ≥ 10 cigarettes [20]. Skewed data were log-transformed or coded as categorical variables, and the detailed information was presented in Additional file 1: Table S1.

Statistical analysis

For the information of the patients, the normality was checked by the Shapiro–Wilk test and the demographic characteristics were compared by X^2-test. When the p-value was lower than 0.05, the difference of risk factors between mild pain and moderately to severely pain groups was considered statistically significant. Univariate logistic regression analysis and multivariate logistic regression analysis were used to estimate those potential factors. The variables were considered as odds ratios (ORs), 95% confidence intervals (CIs), and P-values. To confirm the relationship between these confirmed risk factors and CP/CPPS, we randomly divided CP/CPPS patients into the training and the validation cohorts at a ratio of 7:3 (Fig. 1) to establish a predicting model of pain severity in patients with CP/CPPS. Based on these results of multivariate logistic regression analysis, a predicting model was created by using the "rms" package in

R version 3.6.1. To assess the discrimination, calibration, and clinical usage of this predicting model, the methods of ROC, calibration plot, and DCA were executed. The validation cohort was used to confirm the significance and performance of this model.

Results

Risk factors for pain severity in patients with CP/CPPS

According to the NIH-CPSI's subscores for pain, all patients were divided into two groups: CP/CPPS patients with mild pain (less than eight scores) and patients with moderate to severe pain (higher than a score of eight). The variables included age, BMI, white cells in the urine, sedentary, holding back urine, anxiety or irritability, sex life, contraception, past medical history, alcohol consumption, and smoking. The distributions of variables among CP/CPPS patients and the P-value of variables between the two groups were shown in Table 1. According to the univariate logistic regression analysis, age ($P=0.041$), BMI ($P=0.007$), holding back urine ($P=0.004$), anxiety or irritability ($P<0.001$), contraception ($P=0.012$) and smoking ($P<0.001$) were potential risk factors for the pain severity in patients with CP/CPPS. Multivariate logistic regression analysis was used to measure the variables to exclude the internal effects of the participants. We found that age [OR: 2.828, 95% CI: 1.239–6.648, $P=0.004$], holding back urine (OR: 2.413, 95% CI: 1.213–4.915, $P=0.005$), anxiety or irritability (OR: 3.511, 95% CI: 2.034–6.186, $P<0.001$), contraception (OR: 2.136,

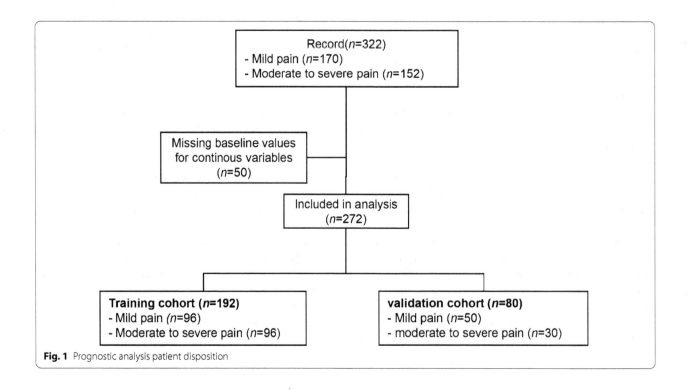

Fig. 1 Prognostic analysis patient disposition

Table 1 Comparison of risk factors in pain severity in patients of CP/CPPS

Characteristic	Mildly pain (n = 146)	Moderately to severely pain (n = 126)	P value
Age, years			
≤ 30 years	60 (41.10)	43 (34.13)	0.046*
30 to ≤ 40 years	52 (35.61)	36 (28.57)	
40 to ≤ 50 years	22 (15.07)	33 (26.19)	
> 50 years	12 (8.22)	14 (11.11)	
BMI (kg/m^2)			
< 18.5 kg/m^2	10 (6.85)	5 (3.97)	0.007**
18.5 to < 24 kg/m^2	84 (57.53)	50 (39.68)	
24 to < 27 kg/m^2	41 (28.08)	53 (42.06)	
≥ 27 kg/m^2	11 (7.54)	18 (14.29)	
White cell in urine, n (%)			
No	135 (92.46)	114 (90.48)	0.385
Yes	11 (7.54)	12 (9.52)	
Sedentary, n (%)			
No	77 (52.74)	54 (42.86)	0.066
Yes	69 (47.26)	72 (57.14)	
Holding back urine, n (%)			
No	123 (84.25)	88 (69.84)	0.004**
Yes	23 (15.75)	38 (30.16)	
Anxiety or irritability, n (%)			
No	88 (60.27)	43 (34.13)	< 0.001***
Yes	58 (39.73)	83 (65.87)	
Sex life, n (%)			
No	17 (11.64)	9 (7.12)	0.146
Yes	129 (88.36)	117 (92.88)	
Contraception, n (%)			
No	94 (64.38)	68 (53.97)	0.012*
Yes	52 (35.62)	58 (46.03)	
Past medical history, n (%)			
No	114 (78.08)	90 (71.43)	0.333
Urologic diseases	28 (19.18)	29 (23.02)	
Others	4 (2.74)	7 (5.55)	
Alcohol consumption, n (%)			
No	94 (64.38)	90 (71.43)	> 0.05
≤ 100 g/w	35 (23.97)	27 (21.43)	
> 100 g/w	17 (11.65)	9 (7.14)	
Smoking, n (%)			
No	110 (75.34)	8 (6.35)	< 0.001***
≤ 10 cigarettes/d	26 (17.81)	28 (22.22)	
> 10 cigarettes/d	10 (6.85)	90 (71.43)	

BMI Body Mass Index (obtained as weight divided by height squared)

95% CI: 1.161—3.014, $P = 0.029$) and smoking (OR: 1.453, 95% CI: 1.313–5.127, $P = 0.013$) were the risk factors. The OR, 95% CI, and P-value of each variable were presented in Table 2.

Table 2 Multivariate logistic regression analysis found out the factors related to pain severity prediction

Parameters	OR	95% CI	P value
Age	2.828	1.239–6.648	0.004**
Holding back urine	2.413	1.213–4.915	0.005**
Anxiety or irritability	3.511	2.034–6.186	< 0.001***
Contraception	2.136	1.161–3.014	0.029*
Smoking	1.453	1.313–5.127	0.013*

CI confidential interval, OR odd ratio

*$P < 0.05$, **$P < 0.01$ and ***$P < 0.001$

Establishment of the predictive nomogram

To confirm the relationship between these confirmed risk factors and CP/CPPS, a predicting model of pain severity in patients with CP/CPPS was established. The distributions of variables among CP/CPPS patients between mild pain and moderately to severely pain groups in the training and the validation cohorts were shown in Table 3. Based on the six variables derived from multivariate logistic regression analysis, we created a nomogram that could be used to predict the pain severity in patients with CP/CPPS. As shown in Fig. 2, the top bar indicated the scale for estimating the risk score of each variable, while the bottom bar corresponds to the pain severity in patients with CP/CPPS.

Apparent performance of the predictive nomogram in the cohort

To evaluate the calibration and discrimination of the nomogram, the calibration and ROC curves were applied. The calibration curve demonstrated a good agreement in the training cohort (Fig. 3a) and the ROC curve confirmed the predictive value of the nomogram, with the AUC value of 0.781 (Fig. 3b). Meanwhile, the DCA analysis was used to evaluate the clinical utility of this nomogram (Fig. 3c). We then used the validation cohort to verify the calibration, discrimination, and clinical utility of the nomogram. The calibration plot (Fig. 3d), AUC value (Fig. 3e), and DCA analysis (Fig. 3f) derived from the validation cohort showed similar results as the training cohort. These results reflected that the nomogram can precisely and steadily judge pain severity in patients with CP/CPPS.

Discussion

Prostatitis is a common outpatient disease in urology. Recent research has shown that the prevalence rates of prostatitis in Europe and the USA are 10% to 14% [21]. In the USA, this health problem motivates 8% of urology consultations [1]. Among all types of prostatitis, CP/CPPS accounts for most cases. As shown in previous studies, men of all ages and ethnic origins can suffer

Table 3 Baseline patient and disease characteristics of the training and validation cohorts

Characteristic	Training cohort (n = 192)		Validation cohort (n = 80)	
	Mildly pain (n = 96)	Moderately to severely Pain (n = 96)	Mildly pain (n = 50)	Moderately to severely pain (n = 30)
Age, years				
≤ 30 years	37 (38.54)	31 (32.29)	23 (46.00)	12 (40.00)
30 to ≤ 40 years	36 (37.50)	29 (30.21)	16 (32.00)	7 (23.33)
40 to ≤ 50 years	17 (17.71)	27 (28.125)	5 (10.00)	6 (20.00)
> 50 years	6 (6.25)	9 (9.375)	6 (12.00)	5 (16.67)
Holding back urine, n (%)				
No	80 (83.33)	62 (64.58)	43 (86.00)	26 (86.67)
Yes	16 (16.67)	34 (35.42)	7 (14.00)	4 (13.33)
Anxiety or irritability, n (%)				
No	57 (59.375)	30 (31.25)	31 (62.00)	13 (43.33)
Yes	39 (40.625)	66 (68.75)	19 (38.00)	17 (56.67)
Contraception, n (%)				
No	62 (64.58)	50 (52.08)	32 (64.00)	13 (43.33)
Yes	34 (35.42)	46 (47.92)	18 (36.00)	17 (56.67)
Smoking, n (%)				
No	70 (72.92)	6 (6.25)	40 (80.00)	2 (6.67)
≤ 10 cigarettes/d	19 (19.79)	19 (19.79)	7 (14.00)	9 (30.00)
> 10 cigarettes/d	7 (7.29)	71 (73.96)	3 (6.00)	19 (63.33)

BMI Body Mass Index (obtained as weight divided by height squared)

from CP/CPPS, but the morbidity of the disease is more common in men who are younger than 50 years old [1]. Although the clinical presentations are diverse, the main clinical features of prostatitis are pelvic pain and lower urinary tract symptoms [22]. Thus, CP/CPPS is defined as pelvic pain that has presented for at least three months and for which no apparent cause has been found [23].

From recent research, we found that engagement in sedentary work and alcohol consumption had a negative influence while marriage had a positive impact on the prognosis of CP/CPPS [24]. Therefore, the questionnaire we designed included age, BMI, white cells in the urine, NIH-CPSI scores, sedentary, urinary retention, anxiety or irritability, sex life, contraception, past medical history, alcohol consumption, and smoking. Currently, nomograms are prognostic methods that can increase accuracy and make prognoses easier to understand, resulting in better clinical decision making; they are widely used in oncology and medicine [25]. Therefore, in our study, we used multivariate logistic regression analysis to figure out the risk factors for the pain severity in patients with CP/CPPS and used a nomogram device to predict pain severity in CP/CPPS patients. Through using logistic regression analysis to measure the variables, we found that age, urinary retention, anxiety or irritability, contraception,

and smoking were related to the pain severity in patients with CP/CPPS and enrolled those variables in the predictive model. Incorporating these five variables into the nomogram allowed the prediction of pain severity in CP/CPPS patients and resulted in the construction of an accurate prediction model of pain severity in CP/CPPS patients. The validation cohort demonstrated good discrimination and calibration power.

For many diseases, age is a potential risk factor. Previous research showed that CP/CPPS was more prevalent in older people [26, 27]. Other research showed that younger age had been associated with more CP/CPPS symptoms [28] and worse QoL [29]. In our study, we found that age is a risk factor for pain severity in CP/CPPS patients, but the age ranges from 40 to 50 years had a higher risk for pain severity in CP/CPPS patients. In some opinions, sedentary and urinary retention could not cause CP/CPPS, but these variables could intensify pain severity among CP/CPPS due to the distention of the venous plexus of the prostate peripheral zone or chronic congestion of the pelvic cavity when in a sitting position [30]. In our study, we found that urinary retention had a significant correlation with the pain severity in CP/CPPS patients. In previous studies, alcohol consumption was related to unchanged or worse symptoms in CP/

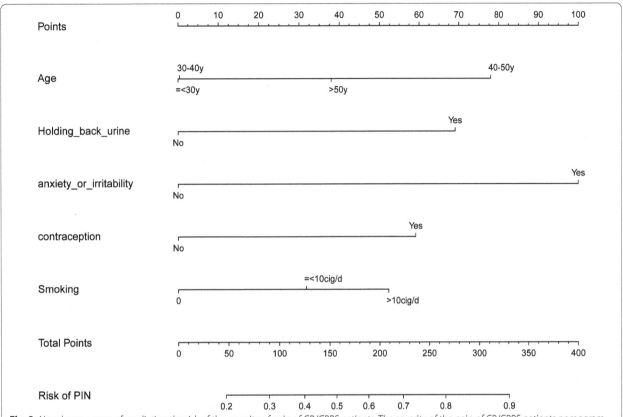

Fig. 2 Novel nomogram of predicting the risk of the severity of pain of CP/CPPS patients. The severity of the pain of CP/CPPS patients nomogram was developed in the cohort, with the use of age, holding back urine, anxiety or irritability, contraception, and smoking

CPPS patients [24]. In our research, through the logistic regression analysis, we found that alcohol consumption was not connected with the pain severity in CP/CPPS patients.

Some researches showed that the frequency of sexual activity, especially the excessive number of sexual intercourse, was related to CP/CPPS [31]. So, we investigate the influence of sexual activity and contraception. In our study, we did not find the relationship between sexual activity with the pain severity in CP/CPPS patients. But we found that contraception was significantly related to the pain severity in CP/CPPS patients. According to previous research, condoms could delay ejaculation resulting in sex lasting longer [32]. In the process of a sexual impulse in humans, the pelvic congestion will regress in about 15–30 min after an orgasm or may last longer without an orgasm [30]. Prolonged sexual activity could increase pelvic congestion. So, one of the possible reasons that condoms could intensify pain severity among CP/CPPS may be due to increased pelvic congestion. Smoking tended to enhance pain sensitivity. However, whether smoking affects CP/CPPS is still controversial. In Chen's study, they found that smoking is a harmful

factor for CP/CPPS [11], but another study found that smoking resulted in a better symptom relief rate [24]. In our research, we found that smoking is a risk factor for pain severity in CP/CPPS patients.

The correlation between stress and pain severity in CP/CPPS patients has been rarely reported. One study showed that people who are under stress at home or work are 1.5-fold more likely to suffer from CP/CPPS than unstressed people [30]. Recently researches showed that biopsychosocial stress had a significant association with chronic pelvic pain in men [33]. In our study, we found that stress is a risk factor for pain severity in CP/CPPS patients. However, whether stress causes or results from the pain in CP/CPPS patients was difficult to decide in the present study.

A 2009 revision of the NIH-CPSI called the GU problem index (GUPI) is now the recommended index as it includes questions on pain with bladder filling and bladder emptying [34]. The questions on pain with bladder filling and bladder emptying did not include in the questionnaire we used according to the previous vision of NIH-CPSI. Then, we will add these two questions in our follow-up research.

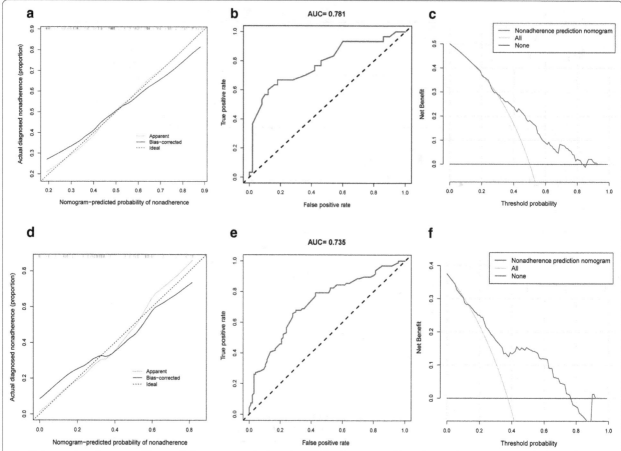

Fig. 3 Apparent performance of the predictive nomogram in the cohort. Calibration curves of the pain severity nomogram prediction in the training cohort (**a**) and the validation cohort (**d**): The x-axis represents the predicted pain severity of CP/CPPS patients. The y-axis represents the actual pain severity of CP/CPPS patients. Receiver operating characteristic (ROC) curves of the nomogram in the training cohort (**b**) and the validation cohort (**e**): The ROC curve is displayed in solid line, and the reference is displayed in dotted line. The ROCs of the predictive nomogram in the training and validation cohorts, with the AUC of 0.781 and 0.735, respectively. Decision curve analysis (DCA) of the nomogram in the training cohort (**c**) and the validation cohort (**f**): The y-axis measures the net benefit. The blue solid line represents the pain severity predictive nomogram. The thin solid line represents the hypothesis that all patients are mild pain. The thin thick solid line represents the assumption that patients are moderate to severe pain. The DCA showed that if the threshold probability of a patient and a doctor are > 25% and < 83% in training cohort (**c**) and > 16% and < 78% in the validation cohort (**f**), respectively. Using this predictive nomogram to predict the pain severity of CP/CPPS patients adds more benefit than the intervention-all-patients scheme or the intervention-none scheme

Conclusion

In summary, age, holding back urine, anxiety or irritability, contraception and smoking were related to the pain severity in patients with CP/CPPS, and the establishment of the nomogram model could accurately assess the pain severity in patients with CP/CPPS to provide novel inspirations for clinicians to design the personalized treatment plan for each CP/CPPS patient who has suffered different encounters.

Supplementary information

Additional file 1: Table S1. Eleven variables were selected for analysis and variables tested.

Abbreviations

CP/CPPS: Chronic Prostatitis/Chronic Pelvic Pain Syndrome; NIH: The National Institutes of Health; BPH: Benign prostatic hyperplasia; SAS: Self-Rating Anxiety Scale; CI: Confidence interval; ROC: Receiver operating characteristic curve; AUC: Area under the curve; DCA: Decision curve analyses; OR: Odds ratio.

Acknowledgments

Not applicable.

Authors' contributions

CL and MZ designed the research and revised the paper. HZ, DN, HL,KW collected and summaried the data. MZ, JC, LZ, LL, XZ analysied and interpreted the data. JC, MZ drafted the paper. All authors contributed substantial intellectual contributions. All authors read and approved the final manuscript.

Author details

[1] Department of Urology, The First Affiliated Hospital of Anhui Medical University, Hefei, People's Republic of China. [2] The Institute of Urology, Anhui Medical University, Hefei, People's Republic of China. [3] The Second Clinical College of Anhui Medical University, Hefei, Anhui, People's Republic of China. [4] Anhui Province Key Laboratory of Genitourinary Diseases, Anhui Medical University, Hefei, People's Republic of China. [5] Department of Urology, b Reproductive Medicine Center, Xiangya Hospital, Central South University, Changsha, People's Republic of China. [6] Institute of Urology of Shenzhen University, The Third Affiliated Hospital of Shenzhen University, Shenzhen Luohu Hospital Group, Shenzhen, People's Republic of China.

References

1. Collins MM, Stafford RS, O'Leary MP, Barry MJ. How common is prostatitis? A national survey of physician visits. J Urol. 1998;159(4):1224–8.
2. Schwartz ES, Xie A, La JH, Gebhart GF. Nociceptive and inflammatory mediator upregulation in a mouse model of chronic prostatitis. Pain. 2015;156(8):1537–44. https://doi.org/10.1097/j.pain.0000000000000201.
3. Rees J, Abrahams M, Doble A, Cooper A, Prostatitis Expert Reference Group (PERG). Diagnosis and treatment of chronic bacterial prostatitis and chronic prostatitis/chronic pelvic pain syndrome: a consensus guideline. BJU Int. 2015;116(4):509–25. https://doi.org/10.1111/bju.13101.
4. Liang CZ, Li HJ, Wang ZP, et al. The prevalence of prostatitis-like symptoms in China. J Urol. 2009;182(2):558–63. https://doi.org/10.1016/j.juro.2009.04.011.
5. Krieger JN, Nyberg L Jr, Nickel JC. NIH consensus definition and classification of prostatitis. JAMA. 1999;282(3):236–7. https://doi.org/10.1001/jama.282.3.236.
6. Murphy SF, Schaeffer AJ, Thumbikat P. Immune mediators of chronic pelvic pain syndrome. Nat Rev Urol. 2014;11(5):259–69. https://doi.org/10.1038/nrurol.2014.63.
7. Magistro G, Wagenlehner FME, Grabe M, Weidner W, Stief CG, Nickel JC. Contemporary management of chronic prostatitis/chronic pelvic pain syndrome. Eur Urol. 2016;69(2):286–97. https://doi.org/10.1016/j.eururo.2015.08.061.
8. Magri V, Wagenlehner FM, Marras E, et al. Influence of infection on the distribution patterns of NIH-Chronic Prostatitis Symptom Index scores in patients with chronic prostatitis/chronic pelvic pain syndrome (CP/CPPS). Exp Ther Med. 2013;6(2):503–8. https://doi.org/10.3892/etm.2013.1174.
9. Tadros NN, Shah AB, Shoskes DA. Utility of trigger point injection as an adjunct to physical therapy in men with chronic prostatitis/chronic pelvic pain syndrome. Transl Androl Urol. 2017;6(3):534–7. https://doi.org/10.21037/tau.2017.05.36.
10. Wagenlehner FM, van Till JW, Magri V, et al. National Institutes of Health Chronic Prostatitis Symptom Index (NIH-CPSI) symptom evaluation in multinational cohorts of patients with chronic prostatitis/chronic pelvic pain syndrome. Eur Urol. 2013;63(5):953–9. https://doi.org/10.1016/j.eururo.2012.10.042.
11. Chen X, Hu C, Peng Y, et al. Association of diet and lifestyle with chronic prostatitis/chronic pelvic pain syndrome and pain severity: a case–control study. Prostate Cancer Prostatic Dis. 2016;19(1):92–9. https://doi.org/10.1038/pcan.2015.57.
12. Zhang R, Sutcliffe S, Giovannucci E, et al. Lifestyle and risk of chronic prostatitis/chronic pelvic pain syndrome in a cohort of United States male health professionals. J Urol. 2015;194(5):1295–300. https://doi.org/10.1016/j.juro.2015.05.100.
13. Magistro G, Wagenlehner FME, Grabe M, et al. Contemporary management of chronic prostatitis/chronic pelvic pain syndrome. Eur Urol. 2016;69(2):286–97. https://doi.org/10.1016/j.eururo.2015.08.061.
14. Lee SH, Lee BC. Electroacupuncture relieves pain in men with chronic prostatitis/chronic pelvic pain syndrome: three-arm randomized trial. Urology. 2009;73(5):1036–41. https://doi.org/10.1016/j.urology.2008.10.047.
15. Litwin MS, McNaughton-Collins M, Fowler FJ Jr, et al. The National Institutes of Health chronic prostatitis symptom index: development and validation of a new outcome measure. Chronic Prostatitis Collaborative Research Network. J Urol. 1999;162(2):369–75. https://doi.org/10.1016/s0022-5347(05)68562-x

16. Barry MJ, Simmons LH. Prevention of prostate cancer morbidity and mortality: primary prevention and early detection. Med Clin North Am. 2017;101(4):787–806. https://doi.org/10.1016/j.mcna.2017.03.009.
17. Manuel RG, Zelber SS, Trenell M. Treatment of NAFLD with diet, physical activity and exercise. J Hepatol. 2017;67(4):829–46. https://doi.org/10.1016/j.jhep.2017.05.016.
18. Anwar T, Cooper CS, Lockwood G, Storm DW, et al. Assessment and validation of a screening questionnaire for the diagnosis of pediatric bladder and bowel dysfunction. J Pediatr Urol. 2019;15(5):528.e1–.e8. https://doi.org/10.1016/j.jpurol.2019.07.016.
19. Dunstan DA, Scott N, Todd AK. Screening for anxiety and depression: reassessing the utility of the Zung scales. BMC Psychiatry. 2017;17(1):329. https://doi.org/10.1186/s12888-017-1489-6.
20. Nelson PR, Chen P, Battista DR, et al. Randomized trial to compare smoking cessation rates of snus, with and without smokeless tobacco health-related information, and a nicotine lozenge. Nicotine Tob Res. 2019;21(1):88–94. https://doi.org/10.1093/ntr/nty011.
21. Bajpayee P, Kumar K, Sharma S, et al. Prostatitis: prevalence, health impact and quality improvement strategies. Acta Pol Pharm. 2012;69(4):571–9.
22. Nickel JC, Nyberg LM, Hennenfent M. Research guidelines for chronic prostatitis: consensus report from the first National Institutes of Health International Prostatitis Collaborative Network. Urology. 1999;54(2):229–33. https://doi.org/10.1016/s0090-4295(99)00205-8.
23. Nickel JC, Alexander R, Anderson R, et al. Prostatitis unplugged? Prostatic massage revisited. Tech Urol. 1999;5(1):1–7.
24. Zhang J, Zhang X, Cai Z, Li N, Li H. The lifetime risk and prognosis of chronic prostatitis/chronic pelvic pain syndrome in the middle-aged Chinese males. Am J Mens Health. 2019;13(4):1557988319865380. https://doi.org/10.1177/1557988319865380.
25. Wei L, Champman S, Li X, et al. Beliefs about medicines and non-adherence in patients with stroke, diabetes mellitus and rheumatoid arthritis: a cross-sectional study in China. BMJ Open. 2017;7(10):e017293. https://doi.org/10.1136/bmjopen-2017-017293.
26. Cheah PY, Liong ML, Yuen KH, et al. Chronic prostatitis: symptom survey with follow-up clinical evaluation. Urology. 2003;61(1):60–4. https://doi.org/10.1016/s0090-4295(02)02081-2.
27. Wang Y, He L, Zhou Z, et al. The association between metabolic syndrome and the National Institutes of Health Chronic Prostatitis Symptom Index: results from 1673 men in China. Urology. 2013;82(5):1103–7. https://doi.org/10.1016/j.urology.2013.06.007.
28. Schaeffer AJ, Landis JR, Knauss JS, et al. Demographic and clinical characteristics of men with chronic prostatitis: the national institutes of health chronic prostatitis cohort study. J Urol. 2002;168(2):593–8.
29. McNaughton Collins M, Pontari MA, O'Leary MP, et al. Quality of life is impaired in men with chronic prostatitis: the Chronic Prostatitis Collaborative Research Network. J Gen Intern Med. 2001;16(10):656–62. https://doi.org/10.1111/j.1525-1497.2001.01223.x.
30. Pavone C, Caldarera E, Liberti P, et al. Correlation between chronic prostatitis syndrome and pelvic venous disease: a survey of 2,554 urologic outpatients. Eur Urol. 2000;37(4):400–3. https://doi.org/10.1159/000020185.
31. Gallo L. Effectiveness of diet, sexual habits and lifestyle modifications on treatment of chronic pelvic pain syndrome. Prostate Cancer Prostatic Dis. 2014;17(3):238–45. https://doi.org/10.1038/pcan.2014.18.
32. Randolph ME, Pinkerton SD, Bogart LM, Cecil H, Abramson PR. Sexual pleasure and condom use. Arch Sex Behav. 2007;36(6):844–8. https://doi.org/10.1007/s10508-007-9213-0.
33. Anderson RU, Orenberg EK, Morey A, Chavez N, Chan CA. Stress induced hypothalamus-pituitary-adrenal axis responses and disturbances in psychological profiles in men with chronic prostatitis/chronic pelvic pain syndrome. J Urol. 2009;182(5):2319–24. https://doi.org/10.1016/j.juro.2009.07.042.
34. Clemens JQ, Calhoun EA, Litwin MS, et al. Validation of a modified National Institutes of Health chronic prostatitis symptom index to assess genitourinary pain in both men and women. Urology. 2009;74(5):983–987.e9873. https://doi.org/10.1016/j.urology.2009.06.078.

Body size throughout the life-course and incident benign prostatic hyperplasia-related outcomes and nocturia

Saira Khan[1*†], K. Y. Wolin[2†], R. Pakpahan[3], R. L. Grubb[4], G. A. Colditz[3], L. Ragard[5], J. Mabie[6], B. N. Breyer[7], G. L. Andriole[8] and S. Sutcliffe[3]

Abstract

Background: Existing evidence suggests that there is an association between body size and *prevalent* Benign Prostatic Hyperplasia (BPH)-related outcomes and nocturia. However, there is limited evidence on the association between body size throughout the life-course and *incident* BPH-related outcomes.

Methods: Our study population consisted of men without histories of prostate cancer, BPH-related outcomes, or nocturia in the intervention arm of the Prostate, Lung, Colorectal, and Ovarian Cancer Screening Trial (PLCO) (n = 4710). Associations for body size in early- (age 20), mid- (age 50) and late-life (age ≥ 55, mean age 60.7 years) and weight change with incident BPH-related outcomes (including self-reported nocturia and physician diagnosis of BPH, digital rectal examination-estimated prostate volume ≥ 30 cc, and prostate-specific antigen [PSA] concentration > 1.4 ng/mL) were examined using Poisson regression with robust variance estimation.

Results: Men who were obese in late-life were 25% more likely to report nocturia (Relative Risk (RR): 1.25, 95% Confidence Interval (CI): 1.11–1.40; p-trend$_{for continuous BMI}$ < 0.0001) and men who were either overweight or obese in late-life were more likely to report a prostate volume ≥ 30 cc (RR$_{overweight}$: 1.13, 95% CI 1.07–1.21; RR$_{obese}$: 1.10, 95% CI 1.02–1.19; p-trend$_{for continuous BMI}$ = 0.017) as compared to normal weight men. Obesity at ages 20 and 50 was similarly associated with both nocturia and prostate volume ≥ 30 cc. Considering trajectories of body size, men who were normal weight at age 20 and became overweight or obese by later-life had increased risks of nocturia (RR$_{normal to overweight}$: 1.09, 95% CI 0.98–1.22; RR$_{normal to obese}$: 1.28, 95% CI 1.10–1.47) and a prostate volume ≥ 30 cc (RR$_{normal to overweight}$: 1.12, 95% CI 1.05–1.20). Too few men were obese early in life to examine the independent effect of early-life body size. Later-life body size modified the association between physical activity and nocturia.

Conclusions: We found that later-life body size, independent of early-life body size, was associated with adverse BPH outcomes, suggesting that interventions to reduce body size even late in life can potentially reduce the burden of BPH-related outcomes and nocturia.

Keywords: Benign Prostatic Hyperplasia (BPH), Body size, Obesity, Nocturia, Prostate volume, PLCO

*Correspondence: khans@udel.edu
†Saira Khan and K. Y. Wolin are co-first authors
[1] Epidemiology Program, College of Health Sciences, University of Delaware, 100 Discovery Blvd., 7th floor, Newark, DE 19713, USA
Full list of author information is available at the end of the article

Introduction

Benign prostatic hyperplasia (BPH)-related outcomes and lower urinary tract symptoms (LUTS) are extremely common among middle- and older-aged American men. By the time men reach their sixties approximately half are believed to have prevalent BPH/LUTS [1–3]. LUTS contribute to considerable bother and decreased quality of life among older men [4], and may lead to severe complications [5] as well as high healthcare costs [6].

Body size and obesity are risk factors for many inextricably linked conditions, including many sex-hormone related diseases, through a complex set of interrelated mechanisms. Specifically, recent interest in the role of body size in BPH/LUTS prevention has grown [7–9]. Greater body size, particularly obesity, may promote BPH/LUTS through several possible mechanisms. First, obesity increases the ratio of estrogens to testosterone and its metabolites, thus possibly exaggerating the natural increase that occurs with aging in men. This increase in the estrogen to testosterone ratio has been shown to contribute to BPH in dogs [10] and proposed to contribute to BPH/LUTS development in men. Second, obese individuals have higher levels of systemic inflammation and oxidative stress. Both systemic inflammation and oxidative stress have been proposed to promote unregulated prostate growth based on the frequent observation of inflammation in BPH tissue, and the observed correlation between the extent and severity of inflammation and the degree of prostate enlargement [11]. Finally, excess body weight may exert increased intra-abdominal pressure on the bladder and increased intravesical pressure, causing or exacerbating LUTS [12].

Consistent with these mechanisms, recent epidemiological reviews have observed positive associations between body mass index (BMI) and the presence of BPH and LUTS [13]. However, most of these studies did not exclude men with LUTS at baseline from their analyses. This approach is concerning because LUTS may cause men to alter their behaviors (e.g., reduce physical activity), which in turn may influence their BMI and contribute to misleading positive associations. Interestingly, fewer studies have investigated *incident* BPH-related outcomes in men free of LUTS at baseline to avoid the concern of reverse causation. Findings from this smaller number of incident (rather than prevalent) studies have been variable [14–23].

As the underlying pathology of BPH/LUTS is believed to begin in men as early as their twenties or thirties [24], early-life body size may also potentially contribute to BPH/LUTS risk. However, only a few studies, to our knowledge, have investigated body size earlier in life or across the life-course in relation to BPH/LUTS [10, 17, 23, 25–27], and most were limited to prevalent disease. Therefore, many of these early-life studies are still subject to the same methodologic concerns as described above for studies of later-life body size. Accurately assessing the relationship between earlier-life BMI and BPH/LUTS development is important to inform the necessary timing of future preventive interventions, i.e., whether body size

reduction must be addressed earlier in life or whether a reduction in body size even later in life may still reduce BPH/LUTS risk.

Finally, results from investigations of other disease outcomes have suggested that obesity and physical inactivity may act synergistically on disease processes [28]. Our previous analyses in this cohort found significant reductions in the incidence of some BPH-related outcomes for men who were physically active [29]. However, few studies have examined whether the benefits of physical activity are the same for obese and lean men.

We investigated the relationship between body size and risk of BPH-related outcomes and nocturia in the large Prostate, Lung, Colorectal, and Ovarian Cancer Screening Trial (PLCO). Importantly, this is one of the first studies to examine early-, mid-, and late-life body size, as well changes in body size throughout the life-course, with *incident* BPH/LUTS.

Methods
Study population
PLCO is a large, ongoing clinical trial designed to investigate the effects of prostate, lung, colorectal, and ovarian cancer screening on cancer-specific mortality [30]. From 1993 to 2001, men were recruited into PLCO at 10 screening centers across the U.S. Each site obtained IRB approval and consented participants. All men 55–74 years of age with no reported histories of prostate cancer or prostatectomy were eligible. Men who had used finasteride in the prior 6 months were not eligible. Half of recruited male participants were randomized to the intervention arm, which included annual prostate-specific antigen (PSA) testing for 5 years and digital rectal examinations (DREs) for 3 years after baseline, and half were randomized to the control arm, which consisted of routine medical care.

At baseline, participants in both arms of PLCO completed a baseline questionnaire, which included questions on weight history, height, and BPH/LUTS. Participants in the intervention arm also completed a food frequency and physical activity questionnaire. In 2004–2008, participants completed a supplemental questionnaire, which included additional questions about BPH/LUTS. Finally, from baseline until active data collection ended in 2015, participants completed brief annual questionnaires to update their cancer information and provide information on finasteride use.

We restricted our analysis to men in the intervention arm (n = 38,340), as only these men provided complete baseline information on physical activity and diet, and underwent annual PSA tests and DREs. We also excluded participants with a history of cancer or evidence of BPH-related outcomes at baseline, missing baseline data, or who did not complete the supplemental questionnaire. Detailed exclusion information is available in the Additional file 1. These exclusion criteria resulted in an incident cohort of 4710 men. Because of the large number of excluded men, we also performed sensitivity analyses excluding only men with the BPH-related outcome of interest from the analysis (e.g., excluding only men with nocturia at baseline from the incident nocturia analysis). These analyses resulted in similar findings as the main analysis.

Weight and physical activity assessment

On the baseline questionnaire, participants reported their weight in pounds at ages 20, 50, and currently (mean age at baseline = 60.7 years), and their height in feet and inches. We used these values to calculate BMI at ages 20, 50, and baseline, and weight change from ages 20 and 50 to baseline. BMI was categorized as underweight (< 18.5), normal (18.5–24.9), overweight (25–29.9), or obese (≥ 30). Because of small numbers, underweight and normal were combined for analysis. Weight change was categorized as weight loss (> 5 lb), weight maintenance (5 lb loss to 4 lb gain), and increments of weight gain depending on the range of weight gain: 5–14, 15–24, 25–34, 35–44, 45–54, 55–64, 65–74, and ≥ 75 lbs. Participants reported their current levels of "vigorous activities, such as swimming, brisk walking, etc." and categories of

hours per week (none, < 1, 1, 2, 3, and 4 + h/wk) on the baseline questionnaire. We dichotomized physical activity as ≥ 1 versus < 1 h per week.

BPH-related outcomes and nocturia

Methods used to define BPH-related outcomes are described in detail elsewhere [29, 31]. Briefly, the presence of BPH-related outcomes at baseline was determined using three items from the baseline questionnaire (waking during the night to urinate during the past year [nocturia]; a history of surgical procedures of the prostate, including transurethral resection of the prostate [TURP] and prostatectomy for benign disease; and a history of a physician diagnosis of "an enlarged prostate or benign prostatic hypertrophy"), DRE examiner-estimated baseline prostate volume ≥ 30 cc, and baseline PSA > 1.4 ng/mL [32–35]. Additional details about baseline outcome definitions are noted in Table 1.

Incident BPH-related outcomes and nocturia were defined using data from the supplemental questionnaire, the annual study update questionnaires, and follow-up examinations (Table 1). Two sets of BPH-related questions were included on the supplemental questionnaire: average frequency of waking during the night to urinate in the past year and a physician diagnosis of an enlarged prostate or BPH. We used this information to define incident nocturia [32] and physician diagnosis of an enlarged

Table 1 Definitions of incident benign prostatic hyperplasia (BPH)-related outcomes and nocturia

	Nocturia	Physician diagnosis	Finasteride use	Prostate volume ≥ 30 cc	PSA elevation
Baseline questionnaire					
Wake 2 + times/night to urinate during a typical night in the past year? (Nocturia)	×	×	×	×	×
Ever been told by a doctor that they have an enlarged prostate or BPH?	×	×	×	×	×
Ever had TURP or prostatectomy for benign disease?	×	×	×	×	×
Baseline examination					
Prostate volume[a] ≥ 30 cc	×	×	×	×	×
PSA > 1.4 ng/mL and no known cancer	×	×	×	×	×
Supplemental questionnaire					
Wake 2 + times/night to urinate during a typical night in the past year? (Nocturia)	*				
Ever been told by a doctor that they have an enlarged prostate or BPH?		*			
Annual study update					
Taken Proscar or Propecia (Finasteride) in the past year?	×		*	×	×
Follow-up examination					
Prostate volume[a] ≥ 30 cc on any of three DREs				*	
PSA > 1.4 ng/mL on any one of five PSA tests					*
Total	1515	1446	881	2499	1322

× = exclusion criteria; * = inclusion criteria; DRE = digital rectal examination; PSA = prostate-specific antigen

[a] Calculated as (π/6) × width^2 × length, where width is the transverse measurement and length is the sagittal measurement. Both measurements were estimated by palpation by the trained DRE examiner

prostate/BPH. Data from the annual study update questionnaires were used to define incident finasteride use, and data from the follow-up examinations were used to define incident prostate volume ≥ 30 cc), and incident PSA > 1.4 ng/mL.

Statistical analysis

We investigated associations for body size with incident BPH-related outcomes and nocturia by calculating relative risks (RRs) using Poisson regression with robust variance estimation. All regression models included age. In addition, models for incident self-reported outcomes included time between the dates of completion of the baseline and supplemental questionnaires; those for incident prostate volume ≥ 30 cc included number of follow-up DREs and time between participants' first and last DRE; and those for incident PSA elevation included number of follow-up PSA tests and time between participants' first and last PSA test. We investigated as potential confounders factors that might be associated with frequency of medical care including demographic factors, chronic medical conditions, physical activity, and suspected risk-factors for BPH-related outcomes including nutritional factors (see Table 2 for a complete list).

To investigate the possible influence of body size throughout the life-course on BPH/LUTS risk, we examined associations for (1) early-life (BMI at age 20), (2) mid-life (BMI at age 50), and (3) later-life (baseline BMI) with incident BPH-related outcomes. These analyses were not mutually adjusted for BMI at different ages, because the small number of men who lost weight over time resulted in small cell sizes and unstable models (Additional file 2: Figure S1).

To further examine associations for body size and weight change throughout the life-course, we investigated associations for weight change from (1) age 20 to baseline and (2) age 50 to baseline with incident BPH-related outcomes. Weight change throughout the life-course was examined in two ways. First, we examined the impact of changing BMI categories throughout the life-course (e.g., a man who went from the normal BMI category at age 20 to the overweight category at baseline compared to a man who remained normal weight throughout the life-course). Second, we examined the impact of smaller increments of weight change throughout the life-course (loss > 5, loss or gain of 5, gain 5–14, gain 15–24, gain 25–34, gain 35–44, gain 45–54, gain 55–64, gain 65–74, gain ≥ 75 lbs) from both (1) age 20 to baseline and (2) age 50 to baseline. These models were adjusted for starting BMI at age 20 or 50 depending on the time interval examined (i.e., models examining weight change from age 20 to baseline were adjusted for BMI at age 20). In secondary analyses, we restricted the

analysis to men who did not change BMI category over the time period of interest to further examine the influence of weight change independent of BMI category (i.e., smaller amounts of weight change insufficient to cause a change in BMI category).

To examine the joint influence of body size and physical activity, we performed analyses of baseline physical activity (< 1 vs. ≥ 1 h of activity per week [29]) and incident BPH-related outcomes stratified by baseline BMI category.

Results

Of the 4710 men in the incident analysis, 1204 (25.6%) participants were under/normal weight, 2399 (50.9%) were overweight, and 1107 (23.5%) were obese at baseline (Table 2). Compared to normal weight men, obese men tended to be younger, and were less likely to be Asian/Pacific Islander, have a college degree or higher, be married, engage in physical activity 4 h/week, and be current smokers, although they were more likely to be former smokers. The most common comorbid chronic conditions were hypertension (26.7%), arthritis (24.1%), and coronary heart disease (9.2%). Obese men were more likely to have hypertension, diabetes, arthritis, and gall bladder stone or inflammation as compared to normal weight men.

Considering BMI earlier in life, 3541 (75.2%) participants were normal weight at age 20 and only 102 (2.2%) were obese. At age 50, 1544 (32.8%) participants were normal weight and 724 (15.4%) were obese. Most participants gained weight over the course of their lives (89.6% gained at least 5 lbs since age 20 with a mean weight gain of 35.9 lbs among those who gained more than 5 lbs), and only a small percentage lost weight (4.0% lost at least 5 lbs since age 20 with a mean weight loss of 17.1 lbs among those who lost more than 5 lbs).

Over the course of follow-up (median = 9 years, range: 5–13), 1515 participants developed nocturia, 1446 reported a new physician diagnosis of BPH, and 881 reported finasteride use (Table 1). With respect to outcomes measured at the follow-up examinations, 2499 men developed a prostate volume ≥ 30 cc over a median of 4 years of follow-up (median number of follow-up DREs = 3) and 1322 developed an elevated PSA over a median of 6 years of follow-up (median number of follow-up PSA tests = 5).

Later-life (baseline) BMI

Baseline BMI was associated with several definitions of incident BPH-related outcomes (Table 3). Men who were obese were 25% more likely to report nocturia (RR: 1.25, 95% CI 1.11–1.40; p-trend$_{for\ continuous\ BMI}$ < 0.0001) than normal weight men. Overweight and obese men were also

Table 2 Age-adjusted baseline characteristics of 4710 male participants eligible for the analysis of body mass index and incident benign prostatic hyperplasia (BPH)-related outcomes and nocturia in the intervention arm of the Prostate, Lung, Colorectal, and Ovarian Cancer Screening Trial by baseline body mass index (BMI), 1993–2001

	Baseline body mass index (kg/m^2)			All participants
	< 25	25–29	≥ 30	
N	1204	2399	1107	4710
Age (mean, years)	61.1	60.8	60.2	60.7
Race/ethnicity (%)				
White	88.3	92.2	92.9	91.3
Black	2.0	1.3	3.0	1.9
Asian/Pacific Islander	8.8	5.2	2.2	5.4
Other	0.9	1.3	1.9	1.4
Education (%)				
Less than high school degree	3.8	5.4	6.4	5.2
High school graduate	12.3	18.4	21.6	17.6
Some college/post high school training	28.3	32.5	36.2	32.3
College degree or higher	55.6	43.8	35.9	44.9
Marital status (%)				
Married or living as married	83.9	86.7	87.6	86.2
Not currently married	16.1	13.3	12.4	13.8
Current physical activity (h/week, %)				
None	11.0	12.4	18.3	13.4
One	24.1	29.5	34.4	29.2
Two to three	30.9	33.0	29.7	31.7
Four or more	34.1	25.1	17.7	25.7
Smoking history (%)				
Never smoker	34.4	29.1	24.1	29.3
Current cigarette smoker	13.8	11.0	6.9	10.7
Former cigarette smoker	45.3	51.5	60.3	52.0
Cigar or pipe smoker only	6.5	8.3	8.8	8.0
Current mean intakes of				
Energy (kcal/day)	2255.0	2320.4	2445.4	2333.0
Carbohydrates (g/day)	292.3	292.8	300.0	294.3
Fat (g/day)	74.4	79.7	87.0	80.0
Poly-unsaturated fatty acid (g/day)	15.2	15.9	17.0	16.0
Protein (g/day)	85.7	90.7	97.9	91.1
Alcohol (g/day)	18.0	17.1	17.1	17.3
Fruit (servings/day)	2.5	2.3	2.3	2.3
Vegetables (servings/day)	3.8	3.7	3.8	3.8
Red meat (g/day)	87.5	102.3	124.3	103.7
Dietary				
Alpha-carotene (mcg/day)	1283.8	1280.5	1316.3	1289.8
Beta-carotene equivalents (mcg/day)	5632.7	5566.4	5611.4	5593.9
Lycopene (mcg/day)	11,205.0	11,839.0	12,667.0	11,716.3
Total (from the diet and supplements)				
Beta-carotene (mcg/day)	5463.9	5282.4	5276.2	5327.3
Selenium (mcg/day)	117.6	122.1	130.3	122.9
Vitamin A (IU/day)	15,230.0	14,949.0	14,987.0	15,030.0
Vitamin C (mg/day)	441.8	418.8	377.6	415.0
Vitamin E (IU/day)	164.7	153.3	152.5	156.0
Zinc (mg/day)	20.3	20.3	21.0	20.5

Table 2 (continued)

	Baseline body mass index (kg/m^2)			All participants
	< 25	25–29	≥ 30	
Multivitamin use (%)	48.8	42.7	39.5	43.5
Medical history (%)				
Hypertension	15.8	26.9	38.1	26.7
Coronary heart disease	6.8	9.4	11.5	9.2
Stroke	1.0	1.0	1.6	1.2
Diabetes	3.7	4.7	8.7	5.4
Arthritis	19.1	23.5	30.8	24.1
Emphysema	2.0	1.8	1.6	1.8
Bronchitis	2.1	2.0	2.0	2.0
Gall bladder stone or inflammation	3.4	5.6	9.0	5.8
Cirrhosis	0.1	0.2	0.2	0.2
Diverticulosis	3.7	4.3	4.1	4.1
Hepatitis	3.5	3.5	3.1	3.4
Colon polyps and polyp syndromes	6.8	6.6	8.1	7.0
Clinical prostatitis	3.7	3.0	3.3	3.2

g/day: grams per day; h/week: hour per week; IU/day: international unit per day; kcal/day: kilocalories per day; kg/m^2: kilograms per meter^2; mcg/day: micrograms per day; mg/day: milligrams per day

more likely to have a prostate volume ≥ 30 cc (RR$_{overweight}$: 1.13, 95% CI 1.07–1.21; RR$_{obese}$: 1.10, 95% CI 1.02–1.19; p-trend$_{for continuous BMI}$ = 0.017). However, men who were overweight or obese were less likely to have an elevated PSA (RR$_{overweight}$: 0.89, 95% CI 0.80–0.99; RR$_{obese}$: 0.75, 95% CI 0.65–0.85; p-trend$_{for continuous BMI}$ < 0.0001), and no more likely to report a physician diagnosis of an enlarged prostate/BPH than normal weight men. Associations for finasteride use were difficult to interpret because of the small number of men who used finasteride, but they tended to be consistent in direction and magnitude to associations for nocturia and a prostate volume ≥ 30 cc. Adjusting for covariates did not change any of the associations. However, it is important to note that these findings are not independent of BMI in early- or mid-life (i.e., BMI at ages 20 and 50).

Early- and mid-life BMI

Similar to the results for baseline BMI, BMI at age 20 was associated with an increased risk of BPH-related outcomes (Table 3). Obese men were 20% more likely to develop nocturia (RR = 1.20, 95% CI 0.93–1.55; p-trend = 0.026) and 21% more likely to develop a prostate volume ≥ 30 cc (RR = 1.21 95% CI 1.05–1.39; p-trend = 0.0006). Results for BMI at age 50 were similar to those for BMI at age 20 with significant findings for nocturia (RR$_{obese}$ = 1.18, 95% CI 1.04–1.34; p-trend = 0.0021) and a prostate volume ≥ 30 cc (RR$_{obese}$ = 1.11, 95% CI 1.02–1.20; p-trend = 0.0048).

BMI across the life-course

As our findings for BMI at specific ages (i.e., age 20, age 50, and baseline) might reflect the fact that men who are overweight or obese as young men tend to remain overweight or obese throughout life, we next sought to determine the independent effects of BMI at different ages on risk of BPH-related outcomes. This is important to determine the necessary timing of future prevention interventions. Compared to men who remained normal weight throughout life, those who were normal weight at age 20 and became overweight by baseline had slightly increased risks of nocturia (RR = 1.09, 95% CI 0.98–1.22) and a prostate volume ≥ 30 cc (RR = 1.12, 95% CI 1.05–1.20) and those who were normal weight at age 20 and became obese had an increased risk of nocturia (RR = 1.28, 95% CI 1.10–1.47, Table 4). Men who were overweight at age 20 who became obese also had an increased risk of nocturia relative to those who remained overweight throughout life (RR = 1.49, 95% CI 1.00–2.21). Generally similar findings were observed for cross-categories of BMI at age 50 and baseline BMI. Together, these findings suggest that later-life overweight and obesity (i.e., at ≥ 55 years of age, the minimum age of entry into PLCO) contributes independently, of early-life body size, to nocturia, and that later-life overweight contributes independently to a prostate volume ≥ 30 cc.

Too few men were overweight or obese in early-life and too few men lost large amounts of weight through the life-course to investigate the independent effects of early-life overweight and obesity with confidence.

Table 3 Age-adjusted risk ratios (RRs) and 95% confidence intervals (CIs) of incident benign prostatic hyperplasia (BPH)-related outcomes and nocturia by body mass index (BMI) across the life-course; Prostate, Lung, Colorectal, and Ovarian Cancer Screening Trial

	< 25		25–29		≥ 30		Per 5 kg/m² increase		p-trend[a]
	RR	95% CI	RR	95% CI	RR	95% CI	RR	95% CI	
Baseline BMI									
Nocturia[b]	1.00	Referent	1.07	0.96, 1.18	1.25	1.11, 1.40	1.11	1.06, 1.16	< 0.0001
No. of cases	363		763		389				
Physician Diagnosis[b]	1.00	Referent	1.00	0.90, 1.11	0.95	0.84, 1.07	0.97	0.92, 1.02	0.26
No. of cases	377		748		321				
Finasteride[b]	1.00	Referent	1.07	0.71, 1.61	1.44	0.91, 2.27	1.17	0.96, 1.42	0.11
No. of cases	32		67		40				
Prostate volume ≥ 30 cc[c]	1.00	Referent	1.13	1.07, 1.21	1.10	1.02, 1.19	1.04	1.01, 1.07	0.017
No. of cases	604		1351		544				
Elevated PSA[d]	1.00	Referent	0.89	0.80, 0.99	0.75	0.65, 0.85	0.86	0.81, 0.92	< 0.0001
No. of cases	381		682		259				
BMI at age 20									
Nocturia[b]	1.00	Referent	1.09	0.99, 1.20	1.20	0.93, 1.55	1.08	1.01, 1.16	0.026
No. of cases	1124		353		38				
Physician diagnosis[b]	1.00	Referent	0.98	0.88, 1.09	0.88	0.64, 1.22	0.98	0.91, 1.05	0.57
No. of cases	1098		320		28				
Finasteride[b]	1.00	Referent	1.18	0.81, 1.71	[e]		1.09	0.86, 1.39	0.49
No. of cases	103		35						
Prostate volume ≥ 30 cc[c]	1.00	Referent	1.05	0.99, 1.11	1.21	1.05, 1.39	1.07	1.03, 1.12	0.0006
No. of cases	1871		566		62				
Elevated PSA[d]	1.00	Referent	0.98	0.88, 1.10	0.70	0.47, 1.04	0.93	0.86, 1.01	0.074
No. of cases	1006		296		20				
BMI at age 50									
Nocturia[b]	1.00	Referent	1.07	0.98, 1.18	1.18	1.04, 1.34	1.09	1.03, 1.15	0.0021
No. of cases	480		794		241				
Physician diagnosis[b]	1.00	Referent	0.92	0.84, 1.01	0.92	0.80, 1.05	0.95	0.93, 1.01	0.13
No. of cases	504		730		212				
Finasteride[b]	1.00	Referent	1.07	0.73, 1.57	1.49	0.93, 2.41	1.18	0.96, 1.46	0.12
No. of cases	42		70		27				
Prostate volume ≥ 30 cc[c]	1.00	Referent	1.08	1.02, 1.15	1.11	1.02, 1.20	1.05	1.02, 1.09	0.0048
No. of cases	796		1341		362				
Elevated PSA[d]	1.00	Referent	0.91	0.82, 1.00	0.75	0.64, 0.89	0.85	0.79, 0.90	< 0.0001
No. of cases	476		682		164				

BPH: benign prostatic hyperplasia; CI: Confidence Interval; BMI: body mass index; RR: risk ratio

[a] For continuous BMI

[b] Also adjusted for time between completion of the baseline and supplemental questionnaires

[c] Also adjusted for number of DREs and time between participants' first and last DRE

[d] Also adjusted for number of PSA tests and time between participants' first and last PSA test

[e] Too few cases (n = 1) to estimate

Incremental and within BMI category weight change across the life-course

Findings for weight change from ages 20 and 50 (Table 5) were consistent with those from the BMI cross-category analyses. For weight change from age 20 to baseline, risk of nocturia increased slightly for a 35–44 lb weight gain and increased to a greater degree for a ≥ 45 lb gain; smaller amounts of weight gain, particularly those insufficient to cause an increase in BMI category, were not associated with increased nocturia risk. Weight gain sufficient to cause a change in BMI category was also necessary to increase risk of a prostate volume ≥ 30 cc. Similar findings were observed for weight change from age 50 to baseline as for weight change from age 20 to baseline.

Table 4 Age-adjusted risk ratios (RRs) and 95% confidence intervals (CIs) of incident benign prostatic hyperplasia (BPH)-related outcomes and nocturia by body mass index (BMI) change across the life-course; Prostate, Lung, Colorectal, and Ovarian Cancer Screening Trial

| | | Baseline BMI (kg/m^2) | | | | | |
| | | < 25 | | 25–29 | | ≥ 30 | |
		RR	95% CI	RR	95% CI	RR	95% CI
BMI at 20 (kg/m^2)							
< 25	Nocturia[a]	1.00	Referent	1.09	0.98, 1.22	1.28	1.10, 1.47
	No. of cases	336		609		179	
	Prostate volume ≥ 30 cc[b]	1.00	Referent	1.12	1.05, 1.20	1.04	0.94, 1.15
	No. of cases	572		1058		241	
25–29	Nocturia[a]	1.40	1.03, 1.90	1.09	0.93, 1.28	1.25	1.08, 1.45
	No. of cases	26		150		177	
	Prostate volume ≥ 30 cc[b]	0.94	0.73, 1.20	1.16	1.06, 1.26	1.10	1.00, 1.21
	No. of cases	31		280		255	
≥ 30	Nocturia[a]	c		c		1.41	1.07, 1.86
	No. of cases					33	
	Prostate volume ≥ 30 cc[b]	c		1.61	1.32, 1.97	1.25	1.05, 1.48
	No. of cases			13		48	
BMI at 50 (kg/m^2)							
< 25	Nocturia[a]	1.00	Referent	1.09	0.93, 1.28	c	
	No. of cases	317		158			
	Prostate volume ≥ 30 cc[b]	1.00	Referent	1.07	0.98, 1.18	c	
	No. of cases	539		253			
25–29	Nocturia[a]	1.04	0.80, 1.34	1.06	0.94, 1.19	1.30	1.13, 1.49
	No. of cases	44		561		189	
	Prostate volume ≥ 30 cc[b]	0.87	0.72, 1.05	1.13	1.06, 1.21	1.06	0.96, 1.17
	No. of cases	60		1029		252	
≥ 30	Nocturia[a]	c		1.23	0.96, 1.58	1.21	1.05, 1.41
	No. of cases			44		195	
	Prostate volume ≥ 30 cc[b]	c		1.16	1.00, 1.36	1.10	1.00, 1.21
	No. of cases			69		288	

BPH: benign prostatic hyperplasia; CI: Confidence Interval; BMI: body mass index; RR: risk ratio

[a] Also adjusted for time between completion of the baseline and supplemental questionnaires

[b] Also adjusted for number of DREs and time between participants' first and last DRE

[c] Too few cases (n ≤ 5) to estimate

Weight loss did not appear to be protective for either nocturia or a prostate volume ≥ 30 cc, but the amount of weight loss in the cohort was small.

Physical activity and BMI

Physical activity was not associated with nocturia risk among obese men (RR = 0.94, 95% CI 0.80–1.10), but was associated with a reduced risk of nocturia among overweight men (RR = 0.85, 95% CI 0.75–0.96). Normal weight men had a non-significant risk reduction similar to that of overweight men (RR = 0.86, 95% CI 0.71–1.04). No associations were observed for physical activity and a prostate volume ≥ 30 cc in normal weight, overweight, or obese men (RRs = 0.99–1.04).

Discussion

This report expands on previous research on body size and BPH by examining body size in relation to *incident*, as opposed to *prevalent*, BPH-related outcomes and nocturia, and by examining body size across the life-course as opposed to later in life only. Our findings suggest that greater later-life body size (overweight or obesity) is associated with adverse BPH-related outcomes, independent of early-life body size. Specifically, becoming overweight or obese, but not gaining smaller amounts of weight

Table 5 Age-adjusted risk ratios (RRs) and 95% confidence intervals (CIs) of incident benign prostatic hyperplasia (BPH)-related outcomes and nocturia by weight change across the life-course; Prostate, Lung, Colorectal, and Ovarian Cancer Screening Trial

	Loss > 5		Loss or gain of 5		Gain 5–14		Gain 15–24		Gain 25–34		Gain 35–44		Gain 45–54		Gain 55–64		Gain 65–74		Gain ≥ 75		p-trend[a]
	RR	95% CI	RR	95% CI	RR	95% CI	RR	95% CI	RR	95% CI	RR	95% CI	RR	95% CI	RR	95% CI	RR	95% CI	RR	95% CI	
Weight change from age 20 to baseline (lbs)																					
All participants																					
Nocturia[a]	1.15	0.89, 1.48	1.00	Referent	0.96	0.78, 1.18	1.00	0.82, 1.21	1.05	0.87, 1.28	1.08	0.89, 1.32	1.13	0.92, 1.39	1.33	1.07, 1.64	1.16	0.90, 1.49	1.21	0.96, 1.52	0.0028
No. of cases	68		93		183		241		254		219		169		128		67		93		
Prostate volume ≥ 30 cc[b]	1.09	0.93, 1.28	1.00	Referent	1.11	0.98, 1.25	1.10	0.97, 1.24	1.08	0.95, 1.21	1.14	1.00, 1.28	1.16	1.02, 1.32	1.10	0.96, 1.27	1.13	0.96, 1.32	1.11	0.95, 1.29	0.18
No. of cases	106		155		349		431		428		363		273		170		102		122		
Restricted to those who did not change body mass index category from age 20 to baseline																					
Nocturia[a]	1.09	0.79, 1.50	1.00	Referent	0.93	0.74, 1.16	1.04	0.83, 1.31	0.94	0.70, 1.25	0.90[a]	0.64, 1.25									0.97
No. of cases	40		88		134		137		69		51										
Prostate volume ≥ 30 cc[b]	1.10	0.90, 1.33	1.00	Referent	1.06	0.92, 1.21	1.07	0.93, 1.23	1.02	0.85, 1.22	0.92[a]	0.75–1.13									0.76
No. of cases	66		147		258		227		121		81										
Weight change from age 50 to baseline (lbs)																					
All participants																					
Nocturia[a]	1.10	0.89, 1.35	1.00	Referent	0.99	0.89, 1.11	1.17	0.96, 1.42	1.23	0.90, 1.68	1.38[a]	1.01, 1.90									0.0039
No. of cases	194		434		456		242		97		92										
Prostate volume ≥ 30 cc[b]	1.03	0.91, 1.16	1.00	Referent	1.02	0.95, 1.08	1.04	0.92, 1.16	0.93	0.77, 1.14	1.14[a]	0.83, 1.01									0.32
No. of cases	310		777		807		373		125		107										
Restricted to those who did not change body mass index category from age 50 to baseline																					
Nocturia[a]	1.06	0.78, 1.44	1.00	Referent	1.07	0.90, 1.27	1.07[a]	0.80, 1.42													0.28
No. of cases	85		242		155		37														
Prostate volume ≥ 30 cc[b]	0.99	0.83, 1.19	1.00	Referent	1.03	0.93, 1.14	1.03[a]	0.87, 1.23													0.25
No. of cases	146		436		263		55														

a Includes values of weight gain greater than the upper bound of the weight category

throughout the life-course, was associated with increased risks of nocturia and a prostate volume ≥ 30 cc. This is important as it suggests that interventions to reduce overweight or obesity even later in life have the potential to prevent adverse BPH-related outcomes. Too few men were obese early in life or lost large amounts of weight to determine the independent effects of greater early-life body size. While rare in PLCO, early-life obesity will become important to understand with the growing obesity epidemic. Finally, although we found that engaging in physical activity reduced the risk of nocturia for normal and overweight men, it did not reduce the risk for obese men or the risk of a prostate volume ≥ 30 cc for men of any weight, suggesting the need for other prevention strategies.

Later-life body size
Our results for later-life body size are generally consistent with the literature to date, including two meta-analyses [8, 9]. Although a strength of our study is that we specifically examined incident BPH, our findings were generally consistent with those that examined prevalent BPH. Our positive findings for nocturia are similar to those from most existing studies of body size and incident BPH or LUTS (or composite endpoints including LUTS, which likely dominated these endpoints) [8, 15, 17, 20, 21, 36]. Our findings for a prostate volume ≥ 30 cc are also similar to those from most previous studies of prevalent large prostate volume/weight, as well as to those that examined prostate growth over time. [8, 9, 11, 13, 36–42]. In addition, although our findings for finasteride use were not statistically significant, they are still consistent in direction and magnitude to those from most previous studies of incident BPH/LUTS and prevalent prostate volume. Finally, our protective findings for overweight/ obesity and an elevated PSA are similar to those from many previous studies [43–46], and likely reflect the influence of overweight/obesity on blood volume rather than on prostate size.

Despite the similarity of our findings to those from many previous studies, they do still differ from a handful of previous studies [14, 16, 19, 23, 47]. These differences could be partly attributed to differences in patient populations (e.g., Asian versus North American populations); variations in ages of BMI ascertainment (e.g., mid- versus late-life), inconsistencies in both exposure and outcome definitions (e.g., continuous versus categories of BMI, varying composite definitions of BPH, outcomes ascertained by ICD-9 codes versus self-report, and changes in clinical practice over the decades captured by these studies). In addition, our null results for a physician diagnosis of BPH differ from our positive or suggestively positive findings for nocturia and finasteride use. This difference

may possibly be explained by the more stringent criteria required for a physician diagnosis rather than self-report of LUTS.

Body size through the life-course
Despite growing interest in a life-course approach to disease causation, few studies have examined how early-life factors or changes in risk factors may alter risk of BPH-related outcomes. This information is critical for chronic conditions as it provides key information on when interventions should be targeted. In our analyses, we found a clear association between gaining large amounts of weight (at least 45 lbs) and risk of nocturia, similar to findings from one [17], but not another [23] study of weight change and incident BPH-related outcomes. Specifically, in the study by Mondul et al., weight gain from age 21 was significantly associated with risk of moderate or worse LUTS only among men who gained at least 40 lbs, and with progression to severe LUTS among those who gained at least 30 lbs [17]. By contrast, Gupta et al., did not observe an association between weight change per decade (mean weight change per decade 4–5 kg) and the development of BPH [23]. Together, these findings suggest that a sizeable weight gain of at least 30–40 lbs throughout the life-course is needed before the risk for LUTS increases.

Despite the large sample size of PLCO, one limitation in this analysis is that too few men were obese early in life and too few lost weight to inform: (1) the independent contribution of early-life body size on the risks of nocturia and a large prostate, and (2) weight loss as a possible prevention strategy for BPH/LUTS. Cohorts with greater prevalences of early-life obesity, such as more contemporary cohorts, and cohorts with greater prevalences of weight loss will be required to answer these questions. All that we can say with a greater degree of certainty from our analyses is that being overweight or obese as an older man was associated with increased risks of developing nocturia and a prostate volume ≥ 30 cc.

Physical activity
Because previous studies have indicated a role for physical activity in BPH/LUTS [29], we examined the joint association of activity and obesity. Our findings suggest that the physical activity benefit may be limited to normal and overweight men, and that among obese men, the effects of obesity trump any potential benefit of physical activity. This finding, which is consistent with that observed in the Southern Community Study [20], is unfortunate because other management strategies and therapies, such as finasteride, have also had limited efficacy in obese men [40, 48].

Our study results must be interpreted in light of some limitations. First, it is difficult to accurately measure prostate volume, particularly in obese men [43]. This could have contributed to our weaker dose–response for increasing BMI with risk of DRE-estimated prostate volume ≥ 30 cc than for nocturia. In addition, weight was based on self-report and men were asked to recall their weight decades earlier. However, despite this, we were still able to observe significant associations between both early- and mid-life BMI and BPH/LUTS, as well as between weight gain and BPH/LUTS. Previous research has shown that middle-aged men can accurately recall both height and weight 27–37 years later, and, on average, weight gain is only underestimated by 3 kg and BMI by 1 kg/m^2 [49]. It is also important to note that BMI may be a less accurate measure of obesity in younger, muscular men, as it does not distinguish between muscle mass and body fat [50]. Moreover, unmeasured components of medical history, including use of certain medications such as diuretics, could have biased our results. Unmeasured medical conditions could have also impacted our findings, however, our assessment of common comorbidities (see Table 2 for full list) including diabetes, indicated that they were not significant confounders. Finally, our measure of BPH-related outcomes only included one LUTS–nocturia. Thus, men with LUTS other than nocturia, particularly milder storage LUTS (e.g., urinary urgency and frequency) that would be unlikely to contribute to a physician diagnosis of BPH or finasteride use, may not have been captured by our BPH-related outcome definitions.

Despite these limitations, our study has several strengths. These include ascertaining incident rather than prevalent BPH/LUTS, and measuring BMI at multiple-time points including early-, mid-, and later-life.

Conclusion

We found that obesity was associated with incident nocturia and a prostate volume ≥ 30 cc. Importantly, we were able to show that late-life BMI was associated with risk of BPH/LUTS independent of early-life BMI, indicating that interventions later in life have the potential to reduce BPH/LUTS. Our results further suggest that nocturia may be prevented or reduced through weight management, but that exercise alone may not be as effective in reducing nocturia risk in obese men.

Abbreviations

BPH: Benign Prostatic Hyperplasia; PLCO: Prostate, Lung, Colorectal, and Ovarian Cancer Screening Trial; RR: Relative Risk; CI: Confidence Interval; LUTS: Lower Urinary Tract Symptoms; DRE: Digital Rectal Exam; TURP: Transurethral Resection of the Prostate; PSA: Prostate Specific Antigen; BMI: Body Mass Index.

Supplementary Information

Additional file 1. Study exclusion criteria.

Additional file 2: Supporting Figure 1. Average weight change in pounds from ages 20 and 50 to baseline, by BMI Category.

Authors' contributions

KYW and SS contributed to the conception and design. RP conducted the data analysis. SK, RLG, GAC, JM, BNB, and GLA made substantial contributions to interpreting data and drafting manuscript. All authors read and approved the final manuscript.

Author details

[1] Epidemiology Program, College of Health Sciences, University of Delaware, 100 Discovery Blvd., 7th floor, Newark, DE 19713, USA. [2] Coeus Health, 222 W Merchandise Mart Plaza, Chicago, IL 60654, USA. [3] Division of Public Health Sciences, Department of Surgery, Washington University in St. Louis School of Medicine, 660 S. Euclid Ave., Campus Box 8100, St. Louis, MO 63110, USA. [4] Department of Urology, Medical University of South Carolina, 135 Rutledge Ave, Charleston, SC 29425, USA. [5] Westat, 1600 Research Blvd, Rockville, MD 20850, USA. [6] Information Management Services, Inc., 1455 Research Blvd, Suite 315 , Rockville, MD 20850, USA. [7] Departments of Urology and Epidemiology and Biostatistics, University of California - San Francisco, 400 Parnassus Ave # 610, San Francisco, CA 94143, USA. [8] Division of Urologic Surgery, Department of Surgery, Washington University in St. Louis School of Medicine, 4921 Parkway Place, St. Louis, MO 63110, USA.

References

1. Chute CG, Panser LA, Girman CJ, Oesterling JE, Guess HA, Jacobsen SJ, et al. The prevalence of prostatism: a population-based survey of urinary symptoms. J Urol. 1993;150(1):85–9.
2. Wei JT, Schottenfeld D, Cooper K, Taylor JM, Faerber GJ, Velarde MA, et al. The natural history of lower urinary tract symptoms in black American men: relationships with aging, prostate size, flow rate and bothersomeness. J Urol. 2001;165(5):1521–5.
3. Coyne KS, Sexton CC, Thompson CL, Milsom I, Irwin D, Kopp ZS, et al. The prevalence of lower urinary tract symptoms (LUTS) in the USA, the UK and Sweden: results from the epidemiology of LUTS (EpiLUTS) study. BJU Int. 2009;104(3):352–60.
4. Girman CJ, Jacobsen SJ, Tsukamoto T, Richard F, Garraway WM, Sagnier PP, et al. Health-related quality of life associated with lower urinary tract symptoms in four countries. Urology. 1998;51(3):428–36.
5. Roehrborn CG, McConnell JD. Benign prostatic hyperplasia: etiology, pathophysiology, epidemiology, and natural history. Campbell Walsh Urol. 2007;10:2649–73.
6. Wei JT, Calhoun E, Jacobsen SJ. Urologic diseases in America project: benign prostatic hyperplasia. J Urol. 2005;173(4):1256–61.
7. Gacci M, Corona G, Vignozzi L, Salvi M, Serni S, De Nunzio C, et al. Metabolic syndrome and benign prostatic enlargement: a systematic review and meta-analysis. BJU Int. 2015;115(1):24–31.
8. Vignozzi L, Gacci M, Maggi M. Lower urinary tract symptoms, benign prostatic hyperplasia and metabolic syndrome. Nat Rev Urol. 2016;13(2):108–19.
9. Wang S, Mao Q, Lin Y, Wu J, Wang X, Zheng X, et al. Body mass index and risk of BPH: a meta-analysis. Prostate Cancer Prostatic Dis. 2012;15(3):265–72.
10. Giovannucci E, Rimm EB, Chute CG, Kawachi I, Colditz GA, Stampfer MJ, et al. Obesity and benign prostatic hyperplasia. Am J Epidemiol. 1994;140(11):989–1002.
11. Parsons JK, Carter HB, Partin AW, Windham BG, Metter EJ, Ferrucci L, et al. Metabolic factors associated with benign prostatic hyperplasia. J Clin Endocrinol Metab. 2006;91(7):2562–8.

12. Cohen PG. Abdominal obesity and intra-abdominal pressure: a new paradigm for the pathogenesis of the hypogonadal-obesity-BPH-LUTS connection. Horm Mol Biol Clin Investig. 2012;11(1):317–20.

13. Parsons JK, Sarma AV, McVary K, Wei JT. Obesity and benign prostatic hyperplasia: clinical connections, emerging etiological paradigms and future directions. J Urol. 2013;189(1 Suppl):S102–6.

14. Glynn RJ, Campion EW, Bouchard GR, Silbert JE. The development of benign prostatic hyperplasia among volunteers in the Normative Aging Study. Am J Epidemiol. 1985;121(1):78–90.

15. Kristal AR, Arnold KB, Schenk JM, Neuhouser ML, Weiss N, Goodman P, et al. Race/ethnicity, obesity, health related behaviors and the risk of symptomatic benign prostatic hyperplasia: results from the prostate cancer prevention trial. J Urol. 2007;177(4):1395–400.

16. Kok ET, Schouten BW, Bohnen AM, Groeneveld FP, Thomas S, Bosch JL. Risk factors for lower urinary tract symptoms suggestive of benign prostatic hyperplasia in a community based population of healthy aging men: the Krimpen Study. J Urol. 2009;181(2):710–6.

17. Mondul AM, Giovannucci E, Platz EA. A prospective study of obesity, and the incidence and progression of lower urinary tract symptoms. J Urol. 2014;191(3):715–21.

18. Parsons JK, Messer K, White M, Barrett-Connor E, Bauer DC, Marshall LM. Obesity increases and physical activity decreases lower urinary tract symptom risk in older men: the Osteoporotic Fractures in Men study. Eur Urol. 2011;60(6):1173–80.

19. Wong SY, Woo J, Leung JC, Leung PC. Depressive symptoms and lifestyle factors as risk factors of lower urinary tract symptoms in Southern Chinese men: a prospective study. Aging Male. 2010;13(2):113–9.

20. Penson DF, Munro HM, Signorello LB, Blot WJ, Fowke JH. Obesity, physical activity and lower urinary tract symptoms: results from the Southern Community Cohort Study. J Urol. 2011;186(6):2316–22.

21. Zhao SC, Xia M, Tang JC, Yan Y. Associations between metabolic syndrome and clinical benign prostatic hyperplasia in a northern urban Han Chinese population: a prospective cohort study. Sci Rep. 2016;6:33933.

22. Jung JH, Ahn SV, Song JM, Chang SJ, Kim KJ, Kwon SW, et al. Obesity as a risk factor for prostatic enlargement: a retrospective cohort study in Korea. Int Neurourol J. 2016;20(4):321–8.

23. Gupta A, Gupta S, Pavuk M, Roehrborn CG. Anthropometric and metabolic factors and risk of benign prostatic hyperplasia: a prospective cohort study of Air Force veterans. Urology. 2006;68(6):1198–205.

24. Berry SJ, Coffey DS, Walsh PC, Ewing LL. The development of human benign prostatic hyperplasia with age. J Urol. 1984;132(3):474–9.

25. Rohrmann S, Smit E, Giovannucci E, Platz EA. Associations of obesity with lower urinary tract symptoms and noncancer prostate surgery in the Third National Health and Nutrition Examination Survey. Am J Epidemiol. 2004;159(4):390–7.

26. Fritschi L, Tabrizi J, Leavy J, Ambrosini G, Timperio A. Risk factors for surgically treated benign prostatic hyperplasia in Western Australia. Public Health. 2007;121(10):781–9.

27. Zucchetto A, Tavani A, Dal Maso L, Gallus S, Negri E, Talamini R, et al. History of weight and obesity through life and risk of benign prostatic hyperplasia. IJO. 2005;29(7):798–803.

28. Lee CD, Jackson AS, Blair SN. US weight guidelines: is it also important to consider cardiorespiratory fitness? Int J Obes Relat Metab Disord. 1998;22(Suppl 2):S2-7.

29. Wolin KY, Grubb RL III, Pakpahan R, Ragard LR, Mabie J, Andriole G, et al. Physical activity and benign prostatic hyperplasia-related outcomes and nocturia. Med Sci Sports Exerc. 2015;47(3):581–92.

30. Prorok PC, Andriole GL, Bresalier RS, Buys SS, Chia D, Crawford ED, et al. Design of the Prostate, Lung, Colorectal and Ovarian (PLCO) cancer screening trial. Control Clin Trials. 2000;21(6 Suppl):273S-309S.

31. Sutcliffe S, Grubb Iii RL, Platz EA, Ragard LR, Riley TL, Kazin SS, et al. Non-steroidal anti-inflammatory drug use and the risk of benign prostatic hyperplasia-related outcomes and nocturia in the Prostate, Lung, Colorectal, and Ovarian Cancer Screening Trial. BJU Int. 2012;110(7):1050–9.

32. Abrams P, Swift S. Solifenacin is effective for the treatment of OAB dry patients: a pooled analysis. Eur Urol. 2005;48(3):483–7.

33. Jacobsen SJ, Jacobson DJ, Girman CJ, Roberts RO, Rhodes T, Guess HA, et al. Treatment for benign prostatic hyperplasia among community dwelling men: the Olmsted County study of urinary symptoms and health status. J Urol. 1999;162(4):1301–6.

34. Pinsky PF, Kramer BS, Crawford ED, Grubb RL, Urban DA, Andriole GL, et al. Prostate volume and prostate-specific antigen levels in men enrolled in a large screening trial. Urology. 2006;68(2):352–6.

35. Siami P, Roehrborn CG, Barkin J, Damiao R, Wyczolkowski M, Duggan A, et al. Combination therapy with dutasteride and tamsulosin in men with moderate-to-severe benign prostatic hyperplasia and prostate enlargement: the CombAT (Combination of Avodart and Tamsulosin) trial rationale and study design. Contemp Clin Trials. 2007;28(6):770–9.

36. Ozden C, Ozdal OL, Urgancioglu G, Koyuncu H, Gokkaya S, Memis A. The correlation between metabolic syndrome and prostatic growth in patients with benign prostatic hyperplasia. Eur Urol. 2007;51(1):199–203.

37. Benjamin RM, Yanovski SZ, Simons-Morton DG. Can primary care physician-driven community programs address the obesity epidemic among high-risk populations? JAMA Intern Med. 2013;173(19):1778–9.

38. Freedland SJ, Platz EA, Presti JCJ, Aronson WJ, Amling CL, Kane CJ, et al. Obesity, serum prostate specific antigen and prostate size: implications for prostate cancer detection. J Urol. 2006;175(2):500–4.

39. Lee S, Min HG, Choi SH, Kim YJ, Oh SW, Kim YJ, et al. Central obesity as a risk factor for prostatic hyperplasia. Obesity. 2006;14(1):172–9.

40. Muller RL, Gerber L, Moreira DM, Andriole G Jr, Hamilton RJ, Fleshner N, et al. Obesity is associated with increased prostate growth and attenuated prostate volume reduction by dutasteride. Eur Urol. 2013;63(6):1115–21.

41. Sarma AV, Jaffe CA, Schottenfeld D, Dunn R, Montie JE, Cooney KA, et al. Insulin-like growth factor-1, insulin-like growth factor binding protein-3, and body mass index: clinical correlates of prostate volume among Black men. Urology. 2002;59(3):362–7.

42. Xie LP, Bai Y, Zhang XZ, Zheng XY, Yao KS, Xu L, et al. Obesity and benign prostatic enlargement: a large observational study in China. Urology. 2007;69(4):680–4.

43. Freedland SJ, Platz EA. Obesity and prostate cancer: making sense out of apparently conflicting data. Epidemiol Rev. 2007;29(1):88–97.

44. Skolarus TA, Wolin KY, Grubb RL. The effect of body mass index on PSA levels and the development, screening and treatment of prostate cancer. Nat Clin Pract Urol. 2007;4(11):605–14.

45. Yang HJ, Doo SW, Yang WJ, Song YS. Which obesity index best correlates with prostate volume, prostate-specific antigen, and lower urinary tract symptoms? Urology. 2012;80(1):187–90.

46. Banez LL, Hamilton RJ, Partin AW, Vollmer RT, Sun L, Rodriguez C, et al. Obesity-related plasma hemodilution and PSA concentration among men with prostate cancer. JAMA. 2007;298(19):2275–80.

47. Burke JP, Rhodes T, Jacobson DJ, McGree ME, Roberts RO, Girman CJ, et al. Association of anthropometric measures with the presence and progression of benign prostatic hyperplasia. Am J Emidemiol. 2006;164(1):41–6.

48. Parsons JK, Schenk JM, Arnold KB, Messer K, Till C, Thompson IM, et al. Finasteride reduces the risk of incident clinical benign prostatic hyperplasia. Eur Urol. 2012;62(2):234–41.

49. Norgan NG, Cameron N. The accuracy of body weight and height recall in middle-aged men. Int J Obes Relat Metab Disord. 2000;24(12):1695–8.

50. Lennon H, Sperrin M, Badrick E, Renehan AG. The obesity paradox in cancer: a review. Curr Oncol Rep. 2016;18(9):56.

25

Prostatic urethral lift (UroLift): A real-world analysis of outcomes using hospital episodes statistics

Toby Page[1]* , Rajan Veeratterapillay[1], Kim Keltie[1,2] , Julie Burn[1] and Andrew Sims[1,2]

Abstract

Background: To determine real-world outcomes of prostatic urethral lift (UroLift) procedures conducted in hospitals across England.

Methods: A retrospective observational cohort was identified from Hospital Episode Statistics data including men undergoing UroLift in hospitals in England between 2017 and 2020. Procedure uptake, patient demographics, inpatient complications, 30-day accident and emergency re-attendance rate, requirement for further treatment and catheterization were captured. Kaplan–Meier and hazard analysis were used to analyse time to re-treatment.

Results: 2942 index UroLift procedures from 80 hospital trusts were analysed; 85.3% conducted as day-case surgery (admitted to hospital for a planned surgical procedure and returning home on the same day). In-hospital complication rate was 3.4%. 93% of men were catheter-free at 30 days. The acute accident and emergency attendance rate within 30 days was 12.0%. Results of Kaplan Meier analysis for subsequent re-treatment (including additional UroLift and endoscopic intervention) at 1 and 2 years were 5.2% [95% CI 4.2 to 6.1] and 11.9% [10.1 to 13.6] respectively.

Conclusions: This real-world analysis of UroLift shows that it can be delivered safely in a day-case setting with minimal morbidity. However, hospital resource usage for catheterization and emergency hospital attendance in the first 30 days was substantial, and 12% required re-treatment at 2 years.

Keywords: Prostatic urethral lift, BPH, LUTS, Urinary retention, UroLift

Background

Prostatic urethral lift (PUL) is a minimally invasive treatment for men with lower urinary tract symptoms (LUTS), which involves placing non-absorbable sutures with a nitinol prostate capsular anchor and a stainless steel urethral end piece to mechanically open the anterior prostatic fossa and disobstruct the urethra [1]. As the treatment does not use thermal energy to excise or ablate tissue it also reduces some adverse effects, such as erectile dysfunction and ejaculatory dysfunction, which can be associated with traditional treatments such as TURP [2]. Other minimally invasive treatments are available; prostate artery embolization (PAE) and iTIND also avoid the use of thermal energy, Rezum therapy uses steam heat energy to remove prostate tissue, whilst Aquablation uses high pressure water jet to remove adenoma. Currently in the UK there is no consensus as to which treatment should be offered to which men and at what point in the treatment pathway. Recent UK National audits suggest the majority of men are still treated with traditional TURP, and that less than 10% of men are being treated with PUL, even less with PAE and Rezum, and that Aquablation is only offered at one centre in the UK [3].

*Correspondence: toby.page@nhs.net
[1] The Newcastle Upon Tyne Hospitals NHS Foundation Trust, Newcastle upon Tyne, UK
Full list of author information is available at the end of the article

PUL marketed as UroLift (manufactured by NeoTract Inc.) was first performed in the United Kingdom (UK) as part of the commercially sponsored BPH-6 trial [4]. The UK National Institute for Health and Care Excellence (NICE) published interventional procedures guidance for urethral lift in January 2014, recommending its use for the treatment of men with lower urinary tract symptoms [5], and Medical Technology Guidance on the UroLift System in September 2015 [6]. This recommended UroLift as an alternative to surgical procedures, in a day-case surgery setting, in men over the age of 50, who have a prostate of less than 100 ml without an obstructing middle lobe. Further studies support the wider use of PUL in men with obstructive median lobes [7], large prostates [8] and in men with retention [9]. Yet despite the positive published outcomes of UroLift, adoption of the procedure in the NHS has been slow. To encourage widespread adoption, UroLift was added to the Innovation Technology Tariff (ITT) in April 2017, and subsequently selected as a Rapid Uptake Product by the National Health Service (NHS) Accelerated Access Collaborative in 2018 [10]. Both schemes aim to support adoption of innovative technologies within the NHS.

Hospital Episode Statistics (HES) is a data warehouse containing episodes of care under a single consultant for patients at NHS hospitals in England. HES datasets include Admitted Patient Care (all admissions including day-case procedures), outpatient appointments and attendance at accident and emergency departments [11]. Clinical coding of procedures uses the Classification of Intervention and Procedures, (OPCS-4) and coding of diagnoses uses the International Classification of Diseases (ICD-10). A specific procedure code was introduced into the UK National Clinical Coding Standards for UroLift in 2017 ("M68.3: Endoscopic insertion of prosthesis to compress lobe of prostate") enabling robust identification of procedures in HES data from that point.

The aim of this study is to use national administrative data from HES to determine uptake as well as real-world in-hospital and longitudinal outcomes of prostatic urethral lift (UroLift) procedures conducted in an NHS hospital setting in England.

Methods

Episodes of UroLift implantation were identified from the presence of procedure code "M68.3: Endoscopic insertion of prosthesis to compress lobe of prostate" in the HES Admitted Patient Care (APC) dataset with a discharge date between 1st April 2017 and 31st January 2020. This dataset also includes day-case surgeries where the patient is admitted to hospital for a planned surgical procedure and returns home on the same day. Individual episodes of care from HES were aggregated into admissions (single

periods of care within a treating hospital) [12]. Analysis was restricted to the earliest UroLift implantation admission for each patient (index admission) conducted within NHS hospitals, which also included a diagnosis code relating to benign prostate hyperplasia (Additional file 1). Those discharged after 1st January 2020 were excluded to ensure 30 day follow up.

Pseudonymised data from HES and the Civil Registration (formerly, the Office of National Statistics) Mortality datasets were supplied under Data Access Request Service (DARS) agreement DARS-NIC-170211-Z1B4J. No patient identifiable information was used and ethical approval was not sought or required. All scripts for applying eligibility criteria, data cleaning, processing and statistical analysis were written in the statistical programming language R [13].

Patient characteristics from the index UroLift procedural admission were summarised using descriptive statistics. Patients catheterized on admission were identified by the presence of ICD10 code Z96.0 "Presence of urogenital implants". In-hospital outcomes included complications [14], catheterization due to retention (procedure code M47 "Urethral catheterization of bladder"), subsequent removal of the catheter (M47.3 "removal of catheter from bladder"), length of hospital stay and death.

All hospital activity (including APC episodes, day-case surgeries, outpatients, and accident and emergency attendances) and all-cause mortality occurring after discharge from the index UroLift implantation were extracted for the cohort. Outcomes at 30-days included catheter status by analyzing catheterization code in both APC and outpatient attendances. Longitudinal outcomes included retreatment (Additional file 2), other bladder/prostate intervention (Additional file 3) and all-cause mortality. Kaplan–Meier analysis was applied to the time from the discharge date of the index UroLift procedure to the date of retreatment (by UroLift of other endoscopic interventions) or date of death. The timing of events was estimated using the hazard function [15]. Patients with no events and known to be alive at the end of the study were considered censored.

Results

Cohort identification

A total of 3433 hospital episodes of care from 3376 patients were identified by the initial search in HES APC. Index UroLift admissions were identified for 3359 patients; exclusions included: 179 treated within private centres, 143 missing discharge date or discharged after 1st January 2020, 95 without eligible diagnoses of BPH (Fig. 1). Following exclusions, 2942 UroLift procedures from 2942 patients, treated across 80 NHS hospital trusts

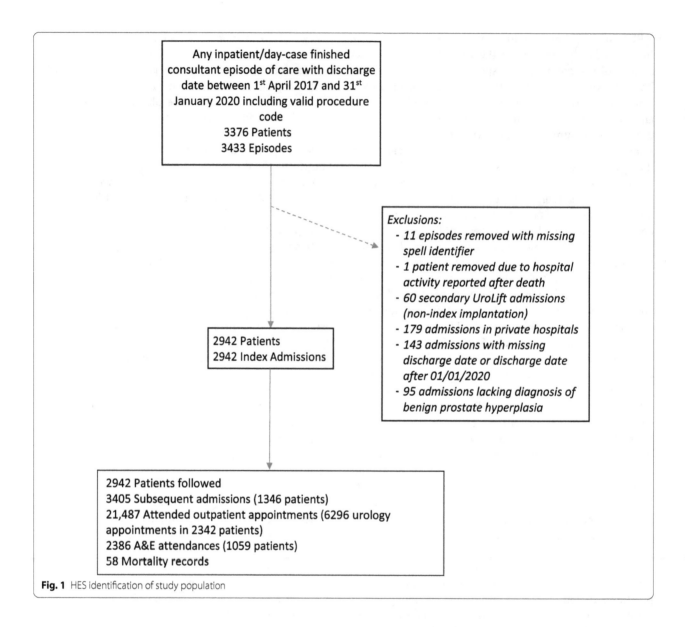

Fig. 1 HES identification of study population

remained for analysis; with an increase in procedure uptake during the study period (Additional file 4).

Patient demographics
The median age at implantation was 69 years [Q1:Q3, 61 to 75] with 108 patients (3.7%) aged less than 50 years at the time of their index UroLift implantation, Table 1. The majority of patients (n = 2509, 85.3%) had the procedure as a day-case surgery.

In-hospital (procedural) outcomes
Inpatient complications were recorded for 99 patients (n = 3.4%) with the most commonly reported complication being urinary retention (n = 40, 1.4%), followed by haematuria/haemorrhage (n = 26, 0.9%) (Additional

file 5). Inpatient infective complications were coded in 3 cases (0.1%) and there was one coded case of bladder injury. No in-hospital deaths occurring during the procedural admission were identified.

Eighty-two patients (2.8%) already had a catheter in place for retention at admission and 135 (4.6%) additional patients were catheterized during their admission. In our cohort of 2942 men, 2747 (93.4%) were catheter-free at discharge.

Longitudinal (post-discharge) outcomes
Within 30 days of discharge from the UroLift implantation, 394 patients (13.4%) had 496 hospital admissions (reasons for readmission described in Additional file 6); 250 of which were an emergency (50%). A total of 881

Table 1 Demographics and in-hospital outcomes

	Patient demographics (n = 2942)
Demographics	
Age, years median, (Q1:Q3); [min–max]	69 (61:75) [35 to 97]
Elective admission (%)	2938 (99.9%)
Day case admission (%)	2317 (78.8%)
Comorbidities (ICD-10)[a]	
Diabetes (E10–E14)	421 (14.3%)
Hypertensive disease (I10–I15)	1066 (36.2%)
Ischaemic heart disease (I20–I25)	373 (12.7%)
Heart failure (I50)	52 (1.8%)
Other chronic obstructive pulmonary disease (J44)	168 (5.7%)
Catheter in place at admission	82 (2.8%)
Outcomes	
In-hospital complication (%)	99 (3.4%)
Catheterisation due to retention (%)	135 (4.6%)
Length of stay	
Day case	2509 (85.3%)
1 night	354 (12.0%)
More than 1 night	79 (2.7%)
In-hospital deaths (%)	0 (0.0%)

[a] ICD10 codes in any DIAG01-20 position, not exclusive

patients (29.9%) attended 1452 outpatient appointments within 30 days. Of these, 336 patients attended 435 urology outpatient appointments within 30 days (106 (24.3%) appointments for removal of catheter, Additional file 7). A total of 352 patients (12.0%) attended A&E 472 times within 30 days (168 A&E attendances in 152 patients resulted in admission). Two patients died within 30 days of UroLift implantation—with main cause of death including "Infection following a procedure" (contributory factors including sepsis) and "Atrial fibrillation and atrial flutter, unspecified" (contributory factors including congestive heart failure, COPD and type 2 diabetes). A total of 2737 men (93.0%) were catheter-free at 30-days.

Analysis of longitudinal outcomes was conducted for all 2942 patients discharged post-UroLift implantation, with a total follow-up of 1,313,627 patient days. The median follow-up per patient was 424 days (Q1:Q3 of 211:653, range 11–1032 days). Throughout follow-up, a total of 3405 subsequent all-cause admissions from 1346 patients were recorded. In addition, 243/2737 men who were catheter-free at 30 days required subsequent catheterization (8.9%) and 42/205 men who had a catheter in place at 30 days had subsequent catheterization (20.5%).

During follow-up, 206 patients required retreatment with 57 patients requiring further UroLift intervention and 158 patients requiring endoscopic intervention (Table 2; Additional file 8). Additional interventions described in Additional file 3. Subsequent UroLift treatment at 1 and 2 years was 1.5 [95% CI 1.0 to 2.0]% and 3.0 [2.1 to 3.8]% respectively, subsequent endoscopic treatment (excluding UroLift) was 3.9 [3.0 to 4.7]% and 9.5 [7.9 to 10.1]% (Table 2). Overall retreatment was 5.2% [95% CI 4.2 to 6.1] and 11.9% [10.1 to 13.6] at 1 and 2 years respectively (Fig. 2, Additional file 9). Two patients died within 30 days of UroLift implantation; the mortality rate in our cohort at year 1 and year 2 post-procedure were 1.4 [0.9 to 1.9]% and 3.1 [2.2 to 4.0]% respectively.

Table 2 Longitudinal outcomes at 1 and 2 years

	Total events	1 year event-free probability [95% CI]	2 year event-free probability [95% CI]
Retreatment	206	0.948 [0.939 to 0.958] (n = 1557)	0.881 [0.864 to 0.899] (n = 497)
UroLift	57	0.985 [0.980 to 0.990] (n = 1620)	0.970 [0.962 to 0.979] (n = 543)
Endoscopic	158	0.961 [0.953 to 0.970] (n = 1579)	0.905 [0.889 to 0.921] (n = 508)
All-cause mortality	58	0.986 [0.981 to 0.991] (n = 1647)	0.969 [0.960 to 0.978] (n = 557)

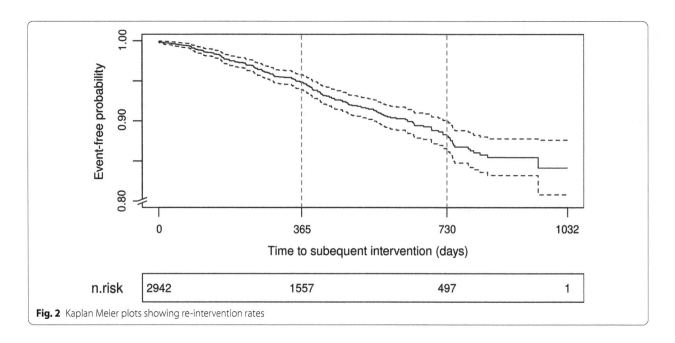

Fig. 2 Kaplan Meier plots showing re-intervention rates

Discussion

This HES analysis represents the largest cohort study of UroLift in a NHS hospital setting, with robust identification of procedures, comprehensive coverage across England, median follow-up of 1.2 years [min 11 days; max 2.8 years]. Our study demonstrates an increase in uptake of the procedure across the NHS during the study period, with 80 NHS trusts providing the procedure in England. In our study 3.7% of patients were aged less than 50 years old, this is higher than the rate reported in a retrospective case review conducted in the US and Australia (17 in 1413, 1.2%) [16]. However, given the major benefit of PUL is to maintain sexual function there continues to be a strong argument for treating younger men who may wish to preserve normal ejaculation for conception. Our results suggest a potential selection bias towards older men as a new procedure is introduced into practice, which may represent a learning curve as clinicians become comfortable with the technique and its results. Additionally in the UK the majority of men opt for pharmaceutical treatment rather than procedure based treatment for mild to moderate symptoms due to national guidelines.

We confirmed that the majority of procedures were conducted as day-case surgeries (85.3%) and that there was a low rate of in-hospital complications (3.4%). This is in keeping with previous reports that UroLift has several advantages including the ability to be undertaken under local anesthesia as a day case, a short learning curve and shorter procedure time (compared with traditional bladder outlet procedures) [17]. The majority (> 95%) of complications reported in the literature have been Clavien grade 1 with the most common being pelvic pain and dysuria [17]. The complication rate we found was low but we are not able to directly compare ICD-10 classification with Clavien–Dindo without introducing reporter bias in the assessment of the severity of the ICD-10 code in the absence of detailed patient notes. The most common adverse event we noted was urinary retention followed by bleeding.

By day 30, 205 men (7.0%) remained catheter dependent, and an additional 243 men required catheterization after 30 days (variable follow-up). In the LIFT study, 32% of patients required catheterization for failed voiding trial with a mean catheter duration of 0.9 days average for the whole cohort of 206 patients across the trial [1]. In the BPH-6 study, 45% of UroLift patients had a postoperative catheter for more than 24 h [4]. The post-operative catheterization rate we report is lower than in the two trials and may represent more cautious patient selection for implementation of a new procedure in an NHS setting compared to a trial setting, however the clinical profile of patients cannot be determined from HES coding. The lower rate may also be due to increasing clinician confidence and experience in the post-operative period after treatment.

Although the overall reported complication rate from UroLift is low, there is a paucity of longitudinal data on emergency re-presentations in the real-life setting. We noted a large proportion of our cohort (12%) attended A&E within 30 days of their PUL procedure. This will be an overestimate of complications, as some attendances maybe unrelated to UroLift, nevertheless it represents an upper limit used to demonstrate hospital service usage following UroLift implantation. However, there is little published data for comparable bladder outlet procedures for A&E admissions in the UK.

Due to large cohort size, our study is able to provide a more robust estimate of retreatment rates (11.9% at 2 years) following UroLift implantation. Retreatment rates were higher than those found in patients randomized to UroLift (n = 140) in the LIFT study (7.5% [95% CI 3.8 to 13.6%] at 2 years [18], but similar to the outcomes at 3 years, 10.7% [95% CI 6.3 to 17.3%] [19]. This may represent a lower threshold to offer retreatment outside of clinical trials.

Whilst this is a retrospective cohort study, it reports real-world outcomes from all UroLift procedures conducted across NHS hospitals in England, with comprehensive follow-up, which reduces both selection and reporting bias [11]. This approach allows normalization of outcome as it reflects both the high volume experienced surgeon and those surgeons who perform fewer cases. Given the large number of cases we have captured and described, the effect of outliers, surgical selection and retreatment bias is minimized, and the overall results offer a valid real-world reflection of the outcomes and hospital resource usage associated with PUL when conducted in an English NHS hospital.

There are however some limitations of using the HES data as it can only be used to produce overall performance indicators (e.g. readmission, complications and length of stay) and it does not allow assessment of all individual patient characteristics as some are not coded (e.g. severity of symptoms, size of prostate, presence of median lobe, International Prostate Symptom Score (IPSS), uroflowmetry, medication etc.) which makes it difficult for our study to comment on efficacy of UroLift. Additionally, due to lack of coding (both procedural and diagnosis) administrative data cannot be used to make meaningful comparisons of outcomes between the different prostate procedures (e.g. TURP, GreenLight, HoLEP etc.). However due to the creation of a procedure code introduced specifically for UroLift, and implemented in 2017, we have been able to use routine administrative data to identify and follow a cohort of men having this intervention across all NHS hospitals in England. This makes HES a powerful tool in investigating patient pathways, hospital resource usage and safety outcomes following an intervention due its comprehensive coverage of hospital activity.

Conclusions

This HES data analysis of UroLift shows that it can be delivered safely in a day-case surgery setting with minimal morbidity. The hospital resource usage in terms of catheterization is lower than in published trial data but emergency hospital attendance in the first 30 days following UroLift implantation is higher than would have been expected for a minimally invasive treatment. The need for further surgical intervention seen in this study appears higher than reported in published trial data at 2 years which may have an impact on the health economic calculations used to assess the place of this treatment in NHS hospital pathways.

Abbreviations

A&E: Accident and emergency; APC: Admitted patient care; HES: Hospital episode statistics; LUTS: Lower urinary tract symptoms; NHS: National Health Service; NICE: National Institute for Health and Care Excellence; PUL: Prostatic urethral lift; UK: United Kingdom.

Supplementary Information

Additional file 1. Online Resource 1: ICD codes for cohort identification.

Additional file 2. Online Resource 2: Subsequent interventions deemed as retreatment, identified by OPCS codes during follow-up.

Additional file 3. Online Resource 3: Additional interventions identified during follow-up (but not included within retreatment rates).

Additional file 4. Online Resource 4: Eligible UroLift procedure uptake in NHS hospitals in England between April 2017 and January 2020.

Additional file 5. Online Resource 5: In-hospital complications recorded during UroLift implantation. Note complications are not mutually exclusive as patients can have multiple complications.

Additional file 6. Online Resource 6: Reason for readmissions occurring within 30 days (using first diagnosis code).

Additional file 7. Online Resource 7: The main procedure conducted during urology outpatient appointment conducted within 30 days (using first procedure code).

Additional file 8. Online Resource 8: Retreatment procedures captured during follow-up.

Additional file 9. Online Resource 9: Hazard rate of retreatment (subsequent UroLift intervention or other endoscopic prostate intervention) following index UroLift implantation procedure. [Note: due to limited number of events kernel-density estimated smoothing was not appropriate, and piecewise exponential hazard function was applied].

Acknowledgements

The study was facilitated by the Academic Health Science Network for the North East and North Cumbria (AHSN NENC). We are grateful to the clinical coding staff at Aintree University Hospital NHS Foundation Trust, Chelsea and Westminster Hospital NHS Foundation Trust, Countess of Chester Hospital NHS Foundation Trust, East Sussex Healthcare NHS Trust, King's College Hospital NHS Foundation Trust, London North West University Healthcare NHS Trust, Oxford University Hospitals NHS Foundation Trust, Royal Liverpool and Broadgreen University Hospitals NHS Trust, Southend University Hospital NHS Foundation Trust, South Warwickshire NHS Foundation Trust, St Helens and Knowsley Teaching Hospitals NHS Trust, Surrey and Sussex Healthcare NHS Trust, Taunton and Somerset NHS Foundation Trust, The Newcastle upon Tyne Hospitals NHS Foundation Trust, University Hospitals of Derby and Burton, West Hertfordshire Hospitals NHS Trust for providing advice. HES data held by NHS Digital (formerly the UK NHS Health and Social Care Information Centre, HSCIC) have been used to help complete the analysis © 2020. Reused with the permission of NHS Digital/HSCIC. All rights reserved.

Authors' contributions

TP: Protocol, Data analysis, Manuscript writing, Read and approved manuscript. KK: Protocol, Data management, Data analysis, Manuscript writing, Read and approved manuscript. RV: Data analysis, Manuscript Writing, Read and approved manuscript. JB: Protocol, Data analysis, Manuscript editing, Read and approved manuscript. AS: Data analysis, Manuscript editing, Supervision, Read and approved manuscript. All authors read and approved the final manuscript.

Author details

[1] The Newcastle Upon Tyne Hospitals NHS Foundation Trust, Newcastle upon Tyne, UK. [2] Faculty of Medical Sciences, Translational and Clinical Research Institute, University of Newcastle Upon Tyne, Newcastle upon Tyne, UK.

References

1. Roehrborn CG, Gange SN, Shore ND, et al. The prostatic urethral lift for the treatment of lower urinary tract symptoms associated with prostate enlargement due to benign prostatic hyperplasia: the L.I.F.T. study. J Urol. 2013;190(6):2161–7.

2. Gratzke C, Barber N, Speakman MJ, et al. Prostatic urethral lift vs transurethral resection of the prostate: 2-year results of the BPH6 prospective, multicentre, randomized study. BJU Int. 2017;119(5):767–75.

3. Joshi H, Sali G, Paramore L, et al. Current process and outcomes of the surgical management of LUTS due to benign prostatic enlargement: how consistent are we?—results from the multi-institutional audit of surgical management of BPE (AuSuM BPE) in the United Kingdom. Scott Med J. 2021;17:36933020977295. https://doi.org/10.1177/0036933020977295.

4. Sonksen J, Barber N, Speakman M, et al. Prospective, randomized, multinational study of prostatic urethral lift versus transurethral resection of the prostate: 12-month results from the BPH6 study. Eur Urol. 2015;68:643–52.

5. National Institute for Health and Care Excellence. Insertion of prostatic urethral lift implants to treat lower urinary tract symptoms secondary to benign prostatic hyperplasia. 2014. https://www.nice.org.uk/guidance/ ipg475 Accessed 16 Sep 2020.

6. National Institute for Health and Care Excellence. UroLift for treating lower urinary tract symptoms of benign prostatic hyperplasia. Medical Technologies Guidance (MTG26). 2015. https://www.nice.org.uk/guida nce/mtg26. Accessed 16 Sep 2020.

7. Rukstalis D, Grier D, Stroup SP, et al. Prostatic Urethral Lift (PUL) for obstructive median lobes: 12 month results of the MedLift Study. Prostate Cancer Prostatic Dis. 2019;22(3):411–9.

8. Shah BB, Tayon K, Madiraju S, et al. Prostatic Urethral Lift: does size matter? J Endourol. 2018;32(7):635–8.

9. Kayes O, Page T, Barber N et al. Prostatic Urethral Lift Treatment in Subject with Acute Urinary Retention (PULSAR). https://www.ics.org/2019/abstr act/679/. Accessed 16 Sep 2020.

10. NHS England. https://www.england.nhs.uk/aac/what-we-do/what-innov ations-do-we-support/rapid-uptake-products/. Accessed 16 Sep 2020.

11. Herbert A, Wijlaars L, Zylbersztejn A, Cromwell D, Hardelid P. Data resource profile: hospital episode statistics admitted patient care (HES APC). Int J Epidemiol. 2017;46(4):1093–1093i.

12. Keltie K, Donne A, Daniel M, et al. Paediatric tonsillectomy in England: a cohort study of clinical practice and outcomes using Hospital Episode Statistics data (2008–2019). Clin Otolaryngol. 2021;00:1–10.

13. R Core Team. R: A language and environment for statistical computing. R Foundation for Statistical Computing, Vienna, Austria. http://www.R-proje ct.org/. Accessed 16 Sep 2020.

14. Aylin P, Tanna S, Bottle A, Jarman B. Dr Foster's case notes: how often are adverse events reported in English hospital statistics? BMJ. 2004;329(7462):369.

15. S original by Kenneth Hess, R port by R. Gentleman. muhaz: Hazard Function Estimation in Survival Analysis. https://CRAN.R-project.org/packa ge=muhaz. Accessed 16 Sep 2020.

16. Eure G, Gange S, Walter P, et al. Real-world evidence of prostatic urethral lift confirms pivotal clinical study results: 2-year outcomes of a retrospective multicenter study. J Endourol. 2019;33(7):576–84.

17. Jones P, Rai BP, Aboumarzouk O, Somani BK. UroLift: a new minimally-invasive treatment for benign prostatic hyperplasia. Ther Adv Urol. 2016;8(6):372–6.

18. Roehrborn CG, Gange SN, Shore ND, et al. Durability of the Prostatic Urethral Lift: 2-year results of the L.I.F.T. study. Urol Pract. 2015;2:1–7.

19. Roehrborn CG, Rukstalis DB, Barkin J, et al. Three year results of the prostatic urethral L.I.F.T. study. Can J Urol. 2015;22(3):7772–82.

26

Pumpkin seed oil (*Cucurbita pepo*) versus tamsulosin for benign prostatic hyperplasia symptom relief: A single-blind randomized clinical trial

Nikan Zerafatjou[1]*[iD], Mohammadali Amirzargar[2], Mahdi Biglarkhani[3], Farzaneh Shobeirian[4] and Ghazal Zoghi[5]

Abstract

Background: Benign prostatic hyperplasia (BPH) is very common in aging men. We aimed to compare the effects of tamsulosin and pumpkin (*Cucurbita pepo*) seed oil on BPH symptoms.

Methods: This single-blind randomized clinical trial included patients with BPH aged $\geq$ 50 years referred to the Urology Clinic of Shahid Beheshti Hospital, Hamadan, Iran, from August 23, 2019 to February 19, 2020. Patients were randomized into two groups. One group received 0.4 mg tamsulosin every night at bedtime and the other received 360 mg pumpkin seed oil twice a day. Patients' age, weight, height, and body mass index (BMI) were recorded. The International Prostate Symptom Score (IPSS) was filled out by the patients at baseline and then 1 month and 3 months after the initiation of treatment. The BPH-associated quality of life (QoL), serum prostate-specific antigen, prostate and postvoid residual volume, and maximum urine flow were also assessed at baseline and 3 months later. Drug side effects were also noted.

Results: Of the 73 patients included in this study with a mean age of 63.59 $\pm$ 7.04 years, 34 were in the tamsulosin group and 39 in the pupkin seed oil group. Patients were comparable with respect to age, weight, height, BMI, and baseline principal variables in both groups. Also, there was no significant difference between groups in terms of principal variables at any time point. However, there was a significant decrease in IPSS and a significant improvement in QoL in both groups. Although the decrease in IPSS from baseline to 1 month and 3 months was significantly higher in the tamsulosin group compared to the pumpkin group ($P = 0.048$ and $P = 0.020$, respectively), the decrease in IPSS from 1 to 3 months was similar ($P = 0.728$). None of the patients in the pumpkin group experienced drug side effects, while dizziness (5.9%), headache (2.9%), retrograde ejaculation (2.9%), and erythema with pruritus occurred in the tamsulosin group.

Conclusions: Pumpkin (*Cucurbita pepo*) seed oil relieved BPH symptoms with no side effects, but was not as effective as tamsulosin. Further studies are required to confirm the role of pumpkin seed oil as an option for the treatment of BPH symptoms.

Trial registration Iranian Registry of Clinical Trials, IRCT20120215009014N340. Registered 19.02.2020. Retrospectively registered, https://en.irct.ir/trial/45335.

---

*Correspondence: nikan.zerafatjou@gmail.com
[1] Department of Urology, School of Medicine, Hamadan University of Medical Sciences, Hamadan, Iran
Full list of author information is available at the end of the article

Keywords: Benign prostatic hyperplasia, Tamsulosin, Pumpkin seed oil

Introduction

Benign prostatic hyperplasia (BPH) is a common age-dependent chronic disease that results from the progressive enlargement of the prostate gland due to the non-malignant proliferation of epithelial prostate cells and smooth muscle cells [1]. A recent systematic review and meta-analysis including data from 25 countries reported a lifetime prevalence of 26.2% for BPH [2]. Patients with BPH become symptomatic when the tissue overgrowth around the urethra constricts its opening leading to lower urinary tract symptoms (LUTS), including incomplete urination, frequency, urgency, nocturia, and decreased urine flow [3]. The prevalence of BPH-associated LUTS increases with age and it has been reported that approximately 80% of men experience BPH-associated LUTS by 70 years of age [4]. However, not every man with BPH symptoms seeks medical attention; most often, BPH patients only seek medical care when BPH-associated LUTS become bothersome or intolerable [1].

There is a variety of treatment strategies for BPH symptoms depending on symptom severity, together with patient discomfort and preference. These treatment strategies include lifestyle alterations, medical therapy, and surgical treatment [5]. Alpha-blockers such as tamsulosin are excellent first-line options of medical therapy [6]. Recently, there has been an increasing tendency towards the use of herbal medicines for different medical conditions. Pumpkin (*Cucurbita*) seeds are traditionally known around the world for their remedial effects on urinary tract complications, such as nocturia, urinary frequency, and stress urinary incontinence [7]. Pumpkins belong to the Cucurbitaceae family which includes various species such as *Cucurbita pepo*, *Cucurbita moschata*, and *Cucurbita maxima* [8]. *Cucurbita pepo* seed oil consists of high amounts of free fatty acids serving as a natural source of vitamins, proteins, trace elements, and polyunsaturated fatty acids, such as omega 3, 6, and 9 [9]. It is the phytosterol content of *Cucurbita pepo* seed oil that appears to interfere with the function of dihydrotestosterone produced by 5α-reductase which plays a major role in the process of BPH [10]. The phytosterol content varies among different *Cucurbita* species, including *Cucurbita pepo* and the previously mentioned *Cucurbita moschata* and *Cucurbita maxima* [11, 12]. However, only *Cucurbita pepo* is available in the Iranian market. Thus, in the current study we aimed to compare the effects of *Cucurbita pepo* with tamsulosin for the treatment of BPH symptoms.

Methods

Participants

This single-blind randomized clinical trial included patients aged ≥ 50 years with the clinical diagnosis of BPH by an expert urologist based on history, digital rectal examination (DRE), and paraclinical tests including serum prostate-specific antigen (PSA), who had been referred to the Urology Clinic of Shahid Beheshti Hospital, Hamadan, Iran, from August 23, 2019 to February 19, 2020. Exclusion criteria were PSA > 10 ng/ml, indications of surgical treatment (patients who were planned to receive surgical treatment for BPH due to absolute or relative indications, including renal insufficiency caused by benign prostatic obstruction, intractable urinary retention, recurrent cystitis, failure of medical therapy, bladder calculi, and persistent hematuria due to prostatic bleeding), previous surgical treatment of BPH, symptom exacerbation during the study period mandating surgical intervention, change in the diagnosis during the study period, any morbidities interfering with the course of treatment, having taken BPH-related medications within the past 6 months, and the development of drug side effects leading to its discontinuation. In patients with PSA > 4 ng/ml and < 10 ng/ml, in order to rule out prostatic cancer, DRE was done and free/total PSA ratio was measured. Also, in suspicious cases, prostatic biopsy was performed. The sample size was calculated as at least 35 patients in each group using a level of significance of 5%, power of 90%, and non-inferiority margin of 50%. The study was approved by the Institutional Review Board of Hamadan University of Medical Sciences (IR.UMSHA.REC.1398.429) and it complies with the statements of the Declaration of Helsinki. Written informed consent was obtained from all the participants. The study has also been retrospectively registered at the Iranian Registry of Clinical Trials (IRCT) under the registration number: IRCT20120215009014N340.

Study design

Initially, 80 patients were eligible to enter the study. Patients were randomized into two equal groups using random generated numbers by the Random Allocation software. Seven patients were lost to follow-up. Details of patient enrollment are demonstrated in Fig. 1. Patients' age, weight, and height were recorded. Body mass index (BMI) was calculated for each patient by dividing their weight (kg) by the square of their height (m). Patients in the tamsulosin group received 0.4 mg tamsulosin capsules (Farabi Pharmaceutical Co., Iran)

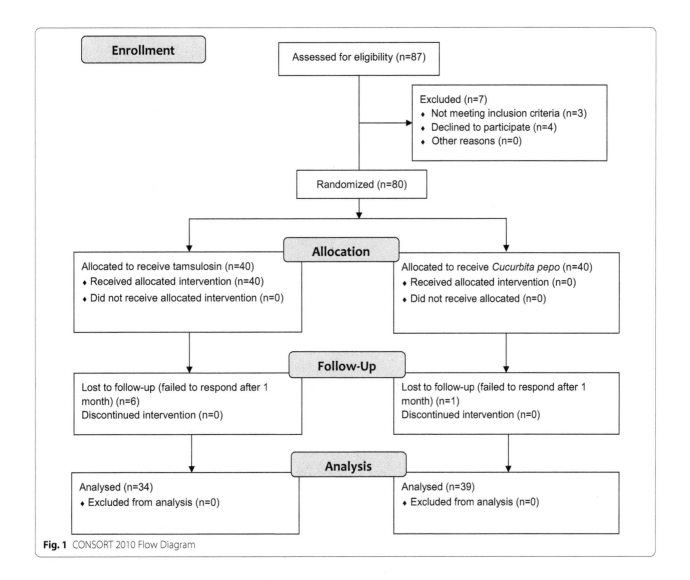

Fig. 1 CONSORT 2010 Flow Diagram

every night at bedtime, while patients in the pumpkin group received 360 mg pumpkin (*Cucurbita pepo*) seed oil capsules (Tehran Darou Pharmaceutical Co., Iran) containing 1% phytosterol, twice a day. The reason for choosing this dose and type of pumpkin (*Cucurbita pepo*) was that it was the only form and dose available in the Iranian market. In previous studies, Vahlensieck et al. and Friedrich et al. used 1000 mg of pumpkin [13, 14]; however, with the available dose per capsule in our study, taking 3 capsules (1080 mg) could have reduced patient compliance. Thus, patients in the pumpkin group received 2 capsules a day (720 mg). Patients in both groups continued taking their medications till the last round of evaluations at 3 months. Patients were asked to fill out the International Prostate Symptom Score (IPSS) for the assessment of BPH symptom

severity, before treatment and then 1 and 3 months later. The BPH-associated quality of life (QoL) scale was also used once before treatment and then at 3 months. The QoL scale evaluates how the patient would feel if he were to spend the rest of his life with his current urinary condition. It is scored from 0 to 6 with 0 indicating the highest and 6 the lowest QoL. Before treatment and at 3 months, all patients underwent ultrasonography for the measurement of postvoid residual (PVR) and prostate volume. Uroflowmetry was also performed for all the participants at the same time points and serum PSA was measured as well. Drug side effects, including dizziness, headache, retrograde ejaculation, and erythema with pruritus during the study period were noted. The laboratory personnel and the individuals in charge of ultrasonography and uroflowmetry were blinded to the grouping of the patients.

Data analysis

We used the Statistical Package for the Social Sciences (SPSS) software (version 25.0, Armonk, NY: IBM Corp.) for data analysis. Mean, standard deviation, frequency, and percentages were used to describe the variables. Based on the results of Kolmogorov–Smirnov normality test, independent t test and Mann–Whitney test were used to compare quantitative variables between groups. Friedman test was used to assess the significance of changes in qualitative variables across different time points. Pairwise comparisons were made using paired t-test and Wilcoxon test. P values ≤ 0.05 were regarded as statistically significant.

Results

Of the 73 patients included in this study with a mean age of 63.59 ± 7.04 years, 39 (53.4%) were in the pumpkin group and 34 (46.6%) in the tamsulosin group. Patients' general characteristics are shown in Table 1. Participants in both groups were comparable regarding age, weight, height, and BMI.

There was no significant difference between groups in terms of baseline IPSS, IPSS at one month, and IPSS at three months (Table 2). However, there was a significant change in IPSS from baseline to the end of three months in both groups ($P < 0.001$). The reduction in IPSS from baseline to 1 month and 3 months was significantly higher in the tamsulosin group compared to the pumpkin group (-3.30 ± 3.15 vs. -1.74 ± 3.02, $P = 0.048$ and -5.33 ± 3.64 vs. -3.19 ± 3.63, $P = 0.020$, respectively). Pairwise comparisons (Additional file 1: Table S1) also showed significant decrease in IPSS between any two time points in both groups. Moreover, although the QoL scores were comparable between groups at baseline and at 3 months, these scores significantly decreased between these time points in both groups (Table 2). Serum PSA was also similar in both groups at baseline and at 3 months. There was a slight increase in serum PSA between these time points in both groups; nevertheless, this was not statistically significant. Prostate volume was comparable between groups at baseline and at 3 months

with no significant increase in any of the groups. The same was true for PVR and maximum urine flow.

Furthermore, none of the patients in the pumpkin group experienced drug side effects, while in the tamsulosin group, dizziness occurred in 2 patients (5.9%), headache in 1 (2.9%), retrograde ejaculation in 1 (2.9%), and erythema with pruritus in 1 (2.9%).

Discussion

In the current study, we found that both tamsulosin and pumpkin (*Cucurbita pepo*) seed oil significantly reduced BPH symptoms assessed by IPSS. However, the decrease in IPSS from baseline to 1 month and 3 months was significantly higher in the tamsulosin group compared to the pumpkin group, while the decrease from 1 to 3 months was similar. Moreover, no patients in the pumpkin group experienced drug side effects, while dizziness (5.9%), headache (2.9%), retrograde ejaculation (2.9%), and erythema with pruritus occurred in the tamsulosin group.

With a global prevalence of 20–62% in men over 50 years, BPH is considered a very common condition [15]. BPH causes LUTS which markedly affect the quality of life in many patients [16, 17]. Multiple strategies have been proposed and used for the relief of BPH-related symptoms. Alpha-blockers such as tamsulosin are regarded as the first-line options. By selectively blocking α_1A-adrenergic receptors leading to the relaxation of the prostate smooth muscles, tamsulosin is reported to improve dysuria and other BPH symptoms [18]. Although tamsulosin is generally preferred due to its lower side effects compared to other alpha-blockers, it can still cause some complications and unwanted reactions, including dizziness, headache, and retrograde ejaculation [19]. We also observed some of these side effects in patients taking tamsulosin.

The effects of tamsulosin and pumpkin seed oil on BPH symptoms have separately been investigated in multiple studies, yet none have compared them with regard to BPH symptom relief. In vitro and in vivo experiments have shown promising results for pumpkin seeds. In their study on Sprague–Dawley rats, Gossell-Williams et al. observed a reduction of prostate size with pumpkin

Table 1 General characteristics of the study population

Variables	Total (n = 73)	Tamsulosin (n = 34)	Pumpkin (n = 39)	P value*
Age (years) mean ± SD	63.59 ± 7.04	62.71 ± 6.63	64.36 ± 7.38	0.320
Height (cm) mean ± SD	169.49 ± 6.74	169.12 ± 6.49	169.82 ± 7.01	0.916†
Weight (kg) mean ± SD	73.04 ± 12.21	71.27 ± 12.11	74.54 ± 12.25	0.261
BMI (kg/m^2) mean ± SD	25.38 ± 3.64	24.89 ± 3.68	25.78 ± 3.61	0.309

n, number; SD, standard deviation; BMI, body mass index

* Analyzed by independent t-test

† Analyzed by Mann–Whitney test

Table 2 Comparison of IPSS, QoL, serum PSA, maximum urine flow, PVR, and prostate volume between groups at different time points

Variables	Tamsulosin (n = 34) Mean ± SD (95% CI)	Pumpkin (n = 39) Mean ± SD (95% CI)	P-value*
Baseline IPSS	10.58 ± 5.70 (8.55–12.60)	11.08 ± 5.71 (9.23–12.93)	0.773
IPSS at 1 month	7.35 ± 4.53 (5.77–8.93)	9.33 ± 5.57 (7.53–11.14)	0.174
IPSS at 3 months	5.65 ± 4.25 (4.09–7.20)	7.46 ± 5.84 (5.51–9.41)	0.231
P-value	<0.001†	<0.001†	
IPSS change from baseline to 1 month	− 3.30 ± 3.15 (− 4.42–− 2.19)	− 1.74 ± 3.02 (− 2.72–− 0.77)	0.048
IPSS change from baseline to 3 months	− 5.33 ± 3.64 (− 6.69–− 3.97)	− 3.19 ± 3.63 (− 4.40–− 1.98)	0.020
IPSS change from 1 to 3 months	− 1.84 ± 2.59 (− 2.79–− 0.89)	− 1.46 ± 3.81 (− 2.73–− 0.19)	0.728
Baseline QoL score	2.35 ± 1.41 (1.86–2.85)	2.41 ± 1.33 (1.98–2.84)	0.767
QoL score at 3 months	1.38 ± 0.99 (1.04–1.73)	1.67 ± 1.06 (1.32–2.01)	0.148
P-value	<0.001‡	0.001‡	
QoL change	− 0.97 ± 1.03 (− 1.33–− 0.61)	− 0.74 ± 1.16 (− 1.12–− 0.37)	0.465
Baseline serum PSA (ng/ml)	2.39 ± 1.57 (1.80–2.99)	2.91 ± 2.54 (2.05–3.77)	0.678
Serum PSA at 3 months (ng/ml)	2.67 ± 2.16 (1.81–3.52)	3.05 ± 2.88 (1.83–4.26)	0.706
P-value	0.194‡	0.903‡	
Serum PSA change (ng/ml)	0.48 ± 1.41 (− 0.11–1.07)	0.13 ± 1.36 (− 0.47–0.73)	0.396¶
Baseline prostate volume (ml)	50.93 ± 22.74 (42.87–58.99)	53.53 ± 23.53 (45.79–61.26)	0.511
Prostate volume at 3 months (ml)	55.00 ± 21.22 (46.21–63.75)	58.32 ± 23.78 (46.85–69.77)	0.629¶
P-value	0.569‡	0.180§	
Prostate volume change (ml)	0.38 ± 11.43 (− 4.44–5.20)	3.22 ± 9.77 (− 1.63–8.08)	0.402¶
Baseline PVR (ml) mean ± SD	67.56 ± 71.32 (38.12–97.00)	67.03 ± 53.67 (46.62–87.45)	0.385
PVR at 3 months (ml)	56.43 ± 81.63 (19.27–93.59)	51.61 ± 33.54 (34.93–68.29)	0.080
P-value	0.723‡	0.087‡	
PVR change (ml)	− 9.56 ± 94.93 (− 56.76–37.65)	− 7.67 ± 21.98 (− 19.84–4.50)	0.563
Baseline maximum urine flow (ml/sec)	12.97 ± 11.41 (8.45–17.48)	9.44 ± 4.92 (7.69–11.18)	0.172
Maximum urine flow at 3 months (ml/sec)	12.27 ± 5.62 (9.83–14.69)	11.18 ± 6.09 (8.61–13.75)	0.344
P-value	0.698‡	0.091‡	
Maximum urine flow change (ml/sec)	0.11 ± 3.09 (− 1.42–1.64)	1.82 ± 4.39 (− 0.12–3.77)	0.328

SD, standard deviation; CI, confidence interval; IPSS: International Prostate Symptom Score; QoL, quality of life; PSA, prostate-specific antigen; PVR, postvoid residual

*Analyzed by Mann–Whitney test

† Analyzed by Friedman test

‡ Analyzed by Wilcoxon test

§ Analyzed by paired t-test

¶ Analyzed by independent t test

seed oil [20]. This effect has been confirmed by other in vitro and animal studies [21–23]. In line with our findings, Vahlensieck et al. demonstrated a clinically relevant reduction of IPSS compared to placebo after 12 months of taking pumpkin seed extract [13]. They used 500 mg *Cucurbita pepo* seed oil extract capsules twice a day. Nevertheless, the period of treatment was much longer in their study reflecting the long-term effects of pumpkin seeds compared to the 3-month period of treatment in our study. In a study on 100 patients by Shirvan et al., pumpkin seed oil (360 mg *Cucurbita pepo* twice a day) was compared with prazosin for the treatment of BPH symptoms [24]. They found pumpkin seed oil to be safe and effective but not as effective as prazosin.

Their findings were consistent with ours. We also found a significant reduction in IPSS with both tamsulosin and pumpkin seed oil from baseline 3 months; nonetheless, the reduction in IPSS from baseline to the end of 1 month and 3 months was significantly higher with tamsulosin. Moreover, they further evaluated patients after 6 months of ttreatment, while we only assessed the results after 3 months. The results of a large study by Friederich et al. on 2245 BPH patients taking pumpkin seed extract (1–2 500 mg *Cucurbita pepo* capsules) for 3 months have also confirmed the effectiveness of this herbal medications showing a 41.4% decrease in IPSS and 46.1% improvement in their QoL [14]. Dihydrotestosterone, converted from testosterone by 5α-reductase, is responsible for the overgrowth of the prostate gland which is characteristic of BPH. [25]. Targeting this pathway has been the mainstay of medical treatment in BPH. Pumpkin seeds appear to affect BPH through the same pathway [10]. Anti-inflammatory properties of pumpkin seeds have been proposed as another mechanism for the effectiveness of pumpkin seed oil in BPH [26]. BPH is associated with the inflammation of the prostate gland and overexpression of cytokines, leukotriene, inducible nitric oxide synthase, NF-κB, and cyclooxygenase-2 is linked with prostatitis [27]. Another proposed mechanism is the diuretic effects of pumpkin seed due to its fatty acids content [28].

Of note, IPSS is a subjective tool to assess the improvement of BPH symptoms. An objective method to evaluate BPH improvement is maximum urine flow and we found no significant change in this variable in any of the groups. One reason for this can be that we had included patients with > 15 ml/s maximum urine flow at baseline only because they complained of BPH symptoms and this could have interfered with the results.

Also, we did not observe significant reductions in PSA and prostate volume with pumpkin seed oil. The results of the study by Hong et al. were similar, as they found no significant reduction in PSA and prostate volume after 3 months in patients receiving 320 mg/day pumpkin seed oil. They did not specify the *Cucurbita* species used in their study (29). As the effect of pumpkin seed oil has been attributed to its phytosterol content, higher doses of pumpkin seed oil potentially include higher amounts of phytosterol leading to increased effects. Nevertheless, patients' adherence to medications would be of concern with higher doses.

The strength of the current study was the homogeneity of patients taking tamsulosin or pumpkin seed oil regarding the potential effectors, as well as baseline characteristics, including symptom severity, QoL, serum PSA, maximum urine flow, and prostate and PVR volumes. This study was not without limitations. First, it has been conducted on a limited number of patients. The study did not reach the minimal sample size of 35; 6 patients were lost to follow-up in the tamsulosin group and 34 patients remained in this group. Further studies with a larger sample size are required to confirm our findings. Second, we only evaluated the efficacy of pumpkin seeds for a 3-month period of treatment and its long-term effects need to be determined in future studies. Also, patients' adherence to treatment, which we failed to assess, is another factor that could have influenced the results. Moreover, we included patients with IPSS < 8 who were mildly symptomatic. Although the initial design of the study was to only include patients with moderate to severe BPH symptoms, we also included mildly symptomatic patients due to the persistent complaint of these

patients of BPH symptoms causing them discomfort, as well as the limited recruitment time.

Conclusions

Both pumpkin seed oil and tamsulosin significantly reduced BPH symptoms; however, due the higher reduction in IPSS scores from baseline to 1 month and 3 months, tamsulosin was more effective. The advantage of pumpkin seed was its lower side effects of pumpkin seeds. Further studies are required to confirm the role of pumpkin seed oil as an option for the treatment of BPH symptoms.

Abbreviations

BMI: Body mass index; BPH: Benign prostatic hyperplasia; DRE: Digital rectal examination; IPSS: International Prostate Symptom Score; IRCT: Iranian Registry of Clinical Trials; LUTS: Lower urinary tract symptoms; PSA: Prostate-specific antigen; PVR: Postvoid residual; QoL: Quality of life.

Supplementary Information

> **Additional file 1.** Pairwise comparisons of IPSS scores at different time points in each group.

Acknowledgements

We sincerely appreciate the dedicated efforts of the investigators, the coordinators, the volunteer patients, and the personnel of the Urology Clinic of Shahid Beheshti Hospital, Hamadan, Iran.

Authors' contributions

Conceptualization and study validation: MA. Study supervision: MB and FS. Implementation: NZ. Data analysis and interpretation: MB and FS. Writing and reviewing: NZ. Editing and revision: GZ. All the authors have read and approved the manuscript.

Author details

[1]Department of Urology, School of Medicine, Hamadan University of Medical Sciences, Hamadan, Iran. [2]Urology and Nephrology Research Center, Hamadan University of Medical Sciences, Hamadan, Iran. [3]Department of Persian Medicine, School of Medicine, Hamadan University of Medical Sciences, Hamadan, Iran. [4]Department of Radiology, School of Medicine, Guilan University of Medical Sciences, Rasht, Iran. [5]Endocrinology and Metabolism Research Center, Hormozgan University of Medical Sciences, Bandar Abbas, Iran.

References

1. Egan KB. The epidemiology of benign prostatic hyperplasia associated with lower urinary tract symptoms: prevalence and incident rates. Urol Clin. 2016;43(3):289–97.
2. Lee SWH, Chan EMC, Lai YK. The global burden of lower urinary tract symptoms suggestive of benign prostatic hyperplasia: a systematic review and meta-analysis. Sci Rep. 2017;7(1):1–10.
3. McVary KT, Roehrborn CG, Avins AL, Barry MJ, Bruskewitz RC, Donnell RF, et al. Update on AUA guideline on the management of benign prostatic hyperplasia. J Urol. 2011;185(5):1793–803.
4. Litman HJ, McKinlay JB. The future magnitude of urological symptoms in the USA: projections using the Boston Area Community Health survey. BJU Int. 2007;100(4):820–5.

5. Nickel JC, Aaron L, Barkin J, Elterman D, Nachabé M, Zorn KC. Canadian Urological Association guideline on male lower urinary tract symptoms/benign prostatic hyperplasia (MLUTS/BPH): 2018 update. Can Urol Assoc J. 2018;12(10):303.

6. Rendon RA, Mason RJ, Marzouk K, Finelli A, Saad F, So A, et al. Canadian Urological Association recommendations on prostate cancer screening and early diagnosis. Can Urol Assoc J. 2017;11(10):298.

7. Medjakovic S, Hobiger S, Ardjomand-Woelkart K, Bucar F, Jungbauer A. Pumpkin seed extract: Cell growth inhibition of hyperplastic and cancer cells, independent of steroid hormone receptors. Fitoterapia. 2016;110:150–6.

8. Lee YK, Chung WI, Ezura H. Efficient plant regeneration via organogenesis in winter squash (Cucurbita maxima Duch.). Plant Sci. 2003;164(3):413–8.

9. Ratnam N, Najibullah M, Ibrahim MD. A review on Cucurbita pepo. Int J Pharm Phytochem Res. 2017;9:1190–4.

10. Perez Gutierrez RM. Review of Cucurbita pepo (pumpkin) its phytochemistry and pharmacology. Med chem. 2016;6(1):012–21.

11. Martínez Aguilar Y, Martínez Yero O, Córdova López J, Valdivié Navarro M, Estarrón EM. Fitoesteroles y escualeno como hipocolesterolémicos en cinco variedades de semillas de Cucurbita maxima y Cucurbita moschata (calabaza). Revista Cubana de Plantas Medicinales. 2011;16(1):72–81.

12. Elias MS, Hassan KD, Odeh S, Mohiaddin SR. Study of growth, yield and phytosterol of squash (Cucurbita pepo L. and medical pumpkin (Cucurbita pepo) an their hybrid. Iraqi J Agric Sci. 2020;51(2):675–84.

13. Vahlensieck W, Theurer C, Pfitzer E, Patz B, Banik N, Engelmann U. Effects of pumpkin seed in men with lower urinary tract symptoms due to benign prostatic hyperplasia in the one-year, randomized, placebo-controlled GRANU study. Urol Int. 2015;94(3):286–95.

14. Friederich M, Theurer C, Schiebel-Schlosser G. Prosta Fink Forte capsules in the treatment of benign prostatic hyperplasia. Multicentric surveillance study in 2245 patients. Res Complement Natural Class Med. 2000;7(4):200–4.

15. Yeboah ED. Prevalence of benign prostatic hyperplasia and prostate cancer in Africans and Africans in the diaspora. J West Afr College Surg. 2016;6(4):1.

16. Bushman W. Etiology, epidemiology, and natural history. Urol Clin. 2009;36(4):403–15.

17. Woodard TJ, Manigault KR, McBurrows NN, Wray TL, Woodard LM. Management of benign prostatic hyperplasia in older adults. The Consultant Pharmacist®. 2016;31(8):412–24.

18. Zhou Z, Cui Y, Wu J, Ding R, Cai T, Gao Z. Meta-analysis of the efficacy and safety of combination of tamsulosin plus dutasteride compared with tamsulosin monotherapy in treating benign prostatic hyperplasia. BMC Urol. 2019;19(1):1–12.

19. Sun Y-h, Liu Z-y, Zhang Z-s, Xu C-l, Ji J-T, Wu Y-Y, et al. Long-term efficacy and safety of tamsulosin hydrochloride for the treatment of lower urinary tract symptoms associated with benign prostatic hyperplasia: data from China. Chin Med Journal. 2011;124(1):56–60.

20. Gossell-Williams M, Davis A, O'Connor N. Inhibition of testosterone-induced hyperplasia of the prostate of sprague-dawley rats by pumpkin seed oil. J Med Food. 2006;9(2):284–6.

21. Abdel-Rahman MK. Effect of pumpkin seed (Cucurbita pepo L.) diets on benign prostatic hyperplasia (BPH): chemical and morphometric evaluation in rats. World J Chem. 2006;1(1):33–40.

22. Tsai Y-S, Tong Y-C, Cheng J-T, Lee C-H, Yang F-S, Lee H-Y. Pumpkin seed oil and phytosterol-F can block testosterone/prazosin-induced prostate growth in rats. Urol Int. 2006;77(3):269–74.

23. Schleich S, Papaioannou M, Baniahmad A, Matusch R. Extracts from Pygeum africanum and other ethnobotanical species with antiandrogenic activity. Planta Med. 2006;72(09):807–13.

24. Shirvan MK, Mahboob MRD, Masuminia M, Mohammadi S. Pumpkin seed oil (prostafit) or prazosin? Which one is better in the treatment of symptomatic benign prostatic hyperplasia. JPMA J Pak Med Assoc. 2014;64(6):683–5.

25. Banerjee PP, Banerjee S, Brown TR, Zirkin BR. Androgen action in prostate function and disease. Am J Clin Experim Urol. 2018;6(2):62.

26. Fahim AT, Abd-El Fattah AA, Agha AM, Gad MZ. Effect of pumpkin-seed oil on the level of free radical scavengers induced during adjuvant-arthritis in rats. Pharmacol Res. 1995;31(1):73–9.

27. Sciarra A, Di Silverio F, Salciccia S, Gomez AMA, Gentilucci A, Gentile V. Inflammation and chronic prostatic diseases: evidence for a link? Eur Urol. 2007;52(4):964–72.

28. Ramak P, Mahboubi M. The beneficial effects of pumpkin (Cucurbita pepo L.) seed oil for health condition of men. Food Rev Int. 2019;35(2):166–76.

29. Hong H, Kim C-S, Maeng S. Effects of pumpkin seed oil and saw palmetto oil in Korean men with symptomatic benign prostatic hyperplasia. Nurs Res Pract. 2009;3(4):323–7.

27

Modified bladder outlet obstruction index for powerful efficacy prediction of transurethral resection of prostate with benign prostatic hyperplasia

Hongming Liu[1], Ye Tian[2*], Guangheng Luo[2], Zhiyong Su[1], Yong Ban[2], Zhen Wang[2] and Zhaolin Sun[2]

Abstract

Background: The correlation between modified bladder outlet obstruction index (MBOOI) and surgical efficacy still remains unknown. The purpose of the study was to investigate the clinical value of the MBOOI and its use in predicting surgical efficacy in men receiving transurethral resection of the prostate (TURP).

Methods: A total of 403 patients with benign prostate hyperplasia (BPH) were included in this study. The International Prostate Symptom Score (IPSS), quality of life (QoL) index, transrectal ultrasonography, and pressure flow study were conducted for all patients. The bladder outlet obstruction index (BOOI) ($P_{det}Q_{max}-2Q_{max}$) and MBOOI ($P_{ves}-2Q_{max}$) were calculated. All patients underwent TURP, and surgical efficacy was accessed by the improvements in IPSS, QoL, and Q_{max} 6 months after surgery. The association between surgical efficacy and baseline factors was statistically analyzed.

Results: A comparison of effective and ineffective groups based on the overall efficacy showed that significant differences were observed in PSA, P_{ves}, $P_{det}Q_{max}$, P_{abd}, BOOI, MBOOI, TZV, TZI, IPSS-t, IPSS-v, IPSS-s, Q_{max}, and PVR at baseline ($p < 0.05$). Binary logistic regression analysis suggested that MBOOI was the only baseline parameter correlated with the improvements in IPSS, QoL, Q_{max}, and the overall efficacy. Additionally, the ROC analysis further verified that MBOOI was more optimal than BOOI, TZV and TZI in predicting the surgical efficacy.

Conclusion: Although both MBOOI and BOOI can predict the clinical symptoms and surgical efficacy of BPH patients to a certain extent, however, compared to BOOI, MBOOI may be a more useful factor that can be used to predict the surgical efficacy of TURP.

Trial registration retrospectively registered.

Keywords: Benign prostatic hyperplasia, Transurethral resection of prostate, Modified bladder outlet obstruction index, Surgical efficacy

*Correspondence: tianye06@foxmail.com
[2] Department of Urology, Guizhou Provincial People's Hospital, Guiyang, China
Full list of author information is available at the end of the article

Background

Benign prostatic hyperplasia (BPH), whose prevalence progressively increases with age, is one of the most common diseases in middle-aged and elderly men [1]. Currently, static and dynamic obstruction due to benign prostatic enlargement (BPE) or/and benign prostatic obstruction (BPO) is considered as the main cause of low urinary tract symptom (LUTS), which has a severe impact on the physical and mental health and quality of life (QoL) of elderly men.

Pressure-flow studies (PFSs) have been recommended as the gold standard for diagnosing bladder outlet obstruction (BOO) by the International Continence Society, among which the BOO index (BOOI) has become best-known and most widely-adopted urodynamic parameter [2, 3]. It is routinely used to evaluate the condition of BPH patients and gauge the efficacy of corrective surgery. Nevertheless, in our previous study, it was observed there was no significant correlation between BOOI and symptoms and the maximum urine flow rate (Q_{max}) in BPH patients [4]. In fact, as the resistance to urination increases with the progression of BOO, many patients undergo abdominal straining to urinate during a PFS. The process of urination involves both detrusor pressure and abdominal pressure, and it is obviously insufficient to only consider the detrusor pressure. Therefore, research has been carried out to assess the correlation between abdominal pressure and BOO, and it has been previously determined that a modified BOOI (MBOOI) that takes into account abdominal pressure can better predict the BOO than the BOOI [5].

The treatments of LUTS secondary to BPH include drug treatment and surgical treatment, among which transurethral resection of prostate (TURP) is still regarded by the current guidelines as the gold standard for surgical treatment [6]. Although TURP is recognized as a safe and effective treatment, significant efficacy is not achieved for all patients. Surgical failure is more likely to occur in patients with detrusor dysfunction and lower baseline BOOI [7]. It has also been found that the degree of preoperative BOO is positively associated with improvement in LUTS and QoL after TURP [8]. Therefore, a preoperative PFS is recommended for optimal selection of patients who are more suitable for surgery by measuring BOOI and assessing detrusor function.

As mentioned above, BOOI ($P_{det}Q_{max}-2Q_{max}$) does not consider the role of abdominal straining in urination, or a predicted BOO may be worse than a MBOOI. Additionally, the correlation between MBOOI and surgical efficacy still remains unknown. Hence, we hypothesized that MBOOI predicts the surgical outcome more optimally than BOOI, and thus, the purpose of this study was to assess the value of MBOOI in predicting the surgical efficacy of TURP by comparing it with BOOI and other parameters.

Methods

Patient cohort

This was a retrospective study that received approval by the Hospital Ethics Committee of GuiZhou Provincial People's Hospital, and written informed consent was obtained (No. 2018054). From November 2015 to March 2020, a total of 403 patients with LUTS/BPH were enrolled in the study. In addition to routine examination, such as digital rectal examination, serum prostate-specific antigen (PSA), and kidney-bladder ultrasound, the International Prostate Symptom Score (IPSS), transrectal ultrasonography (TRUS), and PFS were routinely performed before surgery, otherwise, the patients were not included in the study. The non-inclusion criteria included: (1) bladder calculi, bladder tumor, neurogenic bladder dysfunction, urethral stricture, and other diseases that may affect the function of urination; (2) previous surgery of the prostate and/or bladder and/or urethra; (3) prostate cancer that was confirmed by post-operative pathology. The patients with suspected prostate cancer underwent an ultrasound-guided transrectal prostate biopsy for confirmation or exclusion of cancer. The indications for the operation are as follows: recurrent or refractory urinary retention, overflow incontinence, recurrent urinary tract infections, bladder stones or diverticula, treatment-resistant macroscopic haematuria due to BPH/BPE, or dilatation of the upper urinary tract due to BPO(with or without renal insufficiency), insufficient relief of LUTS after conservative or medical treatments [6]. All patients were followed up and reassessed with IPSS, QoL, and free flowmetry 6 months later.

Assessment of prostatic anatomical parameters

TRUS (Philips EPIQ 5) was used to estimate the total prostate volume (TPV) and transitional zone volume (TZV) by the prostate ellipsoid formula (height × width × length × π/6). The transitional zone index (TZI) was calculated by TPV and TZV (TZI = TZV/TPV) [9].

Assessment of urinary symptoms and urodynamic measurements

Subjective symptoms were assessed by the IPSS and QoL questionnaires, including IPSS total score (IPSS-t), IPSS voiding score (IPSS-v), IPSS storage score (IPSS-s), post-micturitional IPSS score (IPSS-p), and QoL score. A PFS was performed by multichannel urodynamic evaluation (UDS-94-BT, Delphis, Laborie, Canada) to assess objective symptoms. An 8-F double-lumen catheter was transurethrally inserted, and a 10-F single-lumen catheter was transrectally inserted with the patient in a sitting position. The bladder was perfused with physiological saline solution (20–50 ml/

min) until the patient felt a strong desire to urinate (maximum bladder volume), bladder perfusion was then stopped, and the patient was ordered to urinate into the collector. Maximum bladder volume, intravesical pressure (P_{ves}), abdominal pressure (P_{abd}), Q_{max}, and post void residual (PVR) urine volume were simultaneously measured. Detrusor pressure at maximum urine flow rate ($P_{det}Q_{max}$) is equal to P_{ves} minus P_{abd}, and the BOOI ($P_{det}Q_{max}-2Qmax$) and MBOOI ($P_{ves}-2Q_{max}$) were calculated by P_{ves}, $P_{det}Q_{max}$, and Q_{max} [10].

Assessment of surgical efficacy of TURP

Surgical efficacy was determined according to the improvement of IPSS, QoL score, and Q_{max} after surgery. The degree of improvement was judged as poor (level 1), fair (level 2), good (level 3), and excellent (level 4). IPSS improvement > 75% was considered excellent, 50–75% good, 25–50% fair, and $\leq 25\%$ none. A QoL improvement of 4–6 score was classified excellent, 3 score good, 1–2 score fair, and 0 score poor. A Q_{max} improvement ≥ 10.0 ml/s was considered excellent, 5.0–10.0 ml/s good, 2.5–5.0 ml/s fair, and < 2.5 ml/s poor. The median of the three aspects (IPSS, QoL score, and Q_{max}) was defined as the overall efficacy level, in which levels 3 and 4 were defined as effective, and levels 1 and 2 as ineffective (Table 1) [11].

Statistical analysis

All statistical values were reported as the mean ± standard deviation. Kolmogorov–Smirnov test was used to determine whether the continuous variables were in line with normal distribution. If the variables were normally distributed, Student's t-test was applied to compare difference in preoperative factors between two groups according to the overall efficacy. The non-normal distribution variables were conducted with Mann–Whitney U test. Simple linear regression analysis was applied to determine the significant predicting factors for therapeutic effects, and then, stepwise forward binary logistic regression analysis was carried out to determine the factors associated with surgical outcomes of TURP. The receiver operating characteristic (ROC) curves were produced, and the area under the curve (AUC) was subsequently calculated to describe the predictive value of MBOOI in surgical outcomes. All Statistical analysis were processed using IBM SPSS 25.0 for Windows statistical software (Statistical Package for Social Sciences, IBM Corporation, Armonk, NY, USA). All statistical tests were two-sided, $p < 0.05$ was considered to be statistically significant.

Table 1 Surgical efficacy based on the improvements in symptoms, QoL and function

Efficacy grade	Criteria	No. patients (%)
Symptom: Post/pre ratio of IPSS-t		
Excellent	≤ 0.25	161 (39.95)
Good	≤ 0.50	146 (36.23)
Fair	≤ 0.75	69 (17.12)
Poor	> 0.75	27 (6.70)
QoL: Pre-post of QoL index		
Excellent	6,5,4	139 (34.49)
Good	3	125 (31.02)
Fair	2,1	105 (26.05)
Poor	0	34 (8.44)
Function: Post–pre of Q_{max}		
Excellent	≥ 10 mL/s	116 (28.78)
Good	≥ 5 mL/s	172 (42.68)
Fair	≥ 2.5 mL/s	77 (19.11)
Poor	< 2.5 mL/s	38 (9.43)
The overall efficacy: median of efficacy grades of symptom, function and QoL		
Excellent		136 (33.75)
Good		161 (39.95)
Fair		84 (20.84)
Poor		22 (5.46)

IPSS-t = international prostate symptom total score, QoL = quality of life, Q_{max} = maximum urine flow rate

Results

Comparison of baseline characteristics between the effective and ineffective groups based on the overall efficacy

A total of 403 patients between 53–90 years of age diagnosed with BPH were included in the present study. The general characteristics of the study population are shown in Table 2. The surgical efficacy rates according to the improvements in IPSS, QoL, and Q_{max} after surgery were 76.18%, 65.51%, and 71.46% respectively, and the overall efficacy rate of TURP was 73.70%. Kolmogorov–Smirnov test results showed that Q_{max} followed normal distribution, therefore, Student's t-test was applied to compare difference in Q_{max} between two groups according to the overall efficacy. Mann–Whitney U test was applied to compare difference in other preoperative factors between two groups due to these variables in accordance with normal distribution. A comparison of the overall efficacy in the effective and ineffective groups revealed significant differences in PSA ($p=0.021$), P_{ves} ($p<0.001$), $P_{det}Q_{max}$ ($p<0.001$), P_{abd} ($p<0.001$), BOOI ($p<0.001$), MBOOI ($p<0.001$), TZV ($p=0.022$), TZI ($p=0.025$), IPSS-t ($p<0.001$), IPSS-v ($p=0.014$), IPSS-s ($p<0.001$), Q_{max} ($p=0.010$), and PVR ($p=0.006$) at baseline, but significant differences were not observed in age ($p=0.105$),

Table 2 Baseline clinical characteristics and comparison of preoperative characteristics between the two groups classified by the overall surgical efficacy

Variables	Baseline (n = 403)	Effective (n = 297)	Ineffective (n = 106)	p Value
Age (year)	70.94 ± 7.50	71.30 ± 7.44	69.94 ± 7.62	0.105
PSA (umol/L)	4.86 ± 4.98	5.21 ± 5.30	3.88 ± 3.83	0.021
Ultrasonography				
TPV (mL)	52.84 ± 27.63	54.19 ± 28.06	49.05 ± 26.12	0.074
TZV (mL)	24.90 ± 19.45	26.09 ± 19.92	21.59 ± 17.73	0.022
TZI	0.43 ± 0.14	0.44 ± 0.15	0.40 ± 0.12	0.025
Urodynamics				
P_{ves} (cmH$_2$O)	102.72 ± 40.04	110.38 ± 40.58	81.23 ± 29.38	< 0.001
$P_{det}Q_{max}$(cmH$_2$O)	84.92 ± 35.23	90.57 ± 36.07	69.10 ± 27.22	< 0.001
P_{abd} (cmH$_2$O)	17.79 ± 16.40	19.81 ± 17.98	12.13 ± 8.65	< 0.001
Q_{max}(mL/s)	8.10 ± 3.37	7.84 ± 3.31	8.82 ± 3.43	0.010
BOOI	68.73 ± 35.66	74.89 ± 36.41	51.47 ± 26.90	< 0.001
MBOOI	86.52 ± 40.59	94.71 ± 41.04	63.59 ± 28.96	< 0.001
PVR (mL)	74.36 ± 78.10	79.54 ± 78.75	59.85 ± 74.73	0.006
International prostate symptom score (IPSS)				
IPSS-t	22.51 ± 5.22	23.10 ± 5.17	20.84 ± 5.03	< 0.001
IPSS-v	8.72 ± 3.45	8.99 ± 3.46	7.98 ± 3.34	0.014
IPSS-s	10.25 ± 2.71	10.61 ± 2.65	9.24 ± 2.61	< 0.001
IPSS-p	3.51 ± 1.54	3.48 ± 1.54	3.59 ± 1.54	0.520
IPSS QoL	4.73 ± 1.03	4.77 ± 0.99	4.62 ± 1.14	0.357

PSA = prostate-specific antigen, TPV = total prostate volume, TZV = transitional zone volume, TZI = transitional zone index, P_{ves} = intra-vesical pressure, $P_{det}Q_{max}$ = detrusor pressure at maximum urine flow rate, P_{abd} = abdominal pressure, Q_{max} = maximum urine flow rate, BOOI = bladder outlet obstruction index, MBOOI = modified BOOI, PVR = post void residual urine volume, IPSS-t = IPSS total score, IPSS-v = IPSS voiding score, IPSS-s = IPSS storage score, IPSS-p = post-micturitional IPSS score, QoL = quality of life

TPV ($p = 0.074$), IPPS-p ($p = 0.520$), or QoL ($p = 0.357$) (Table 2).

Association of surgical efficacy with preoperative variables

As presented in Table 3, simple linear regression analysis was used to analyze the correlations between preoperative factors and the surgical efficacy in IPSS, QoL, and Q_{max}. All preoperative variables that were significantly correlated with surgical efficacy in IPSS, QoL, and Q_{max} using simple linear regression analysis were analyzed by stepwise forward binary logistic regression. From the results, MBOOI ($p < 0.001$) and IPSS-t ($p < 0.001$) were correlated with improvement of IPSS-t ($p < 0.05$). MBOOI ($p < 0.001$), P_{abd} ($p = 0.035$) and QoL ($p < 0.001$) with improvement of QoL. Meanwhile, MBOOI ($p < 0.001$) and Q_{max} ($p < 0.001$) with improvement of Q_{max}. In addition, improved MBOOI ($p < 0.001$) and IPSS-t ($p = 0.009$) were correlated with the overall efficacy of TURP. Particularly, MBOOI was the only preoperative factor correlated with the surgical efficacy in IPSS, QoL, Q_{max}, and the overall both (Table 3).

Furthermore, as shown in Fig. 1, the ROC curve was plotted, and the AUC was calculated. ROC analysis further demonstrated that MBOOI (AUC = 0.744,

95% CI 0.691–0.798) was more optimal than BOOI (AUC = 0.701, 95% CI 0.645–0.757), TZV (AUC = 0.575, 95% CI 0.513–0.636), and TZI (AUC = 0.573, 95% CI 0.513–0.634) in predicting the overall surgical efficacy

Table 3 Relationship between the baseline factors and surgical efficacy in IPSS-t, Q_{max}, QoL and the overall surgical efficacy in binary logistic regression

Variables	OR	(95% CI)	p Value
Surgical efficacy in IPSS-t			
MBOOI	1.021	(1.012–1.029)	< 0.001
IPSS-t	1.101	(1.049–1.156)	< 0.001
Surgical efficacy in QoL index			
P_{abd} (cmH$_2$O)	1.022	(1.001–1.043)	0.035
MBOOI	1.021	(1.013–1.030)	< 0.001
QoL	1.962	(1.541–2.498)	< 0.001
Surgical efficacy in Q_{max}			
MBOOI	1.026	(1.018–1.035)	< 0.001
Qmax (mL/s)	0.793	(0.733–0.857)	< 0.001
The overall surgical efficacy			
MBOOI	1.027	(1.018–1.036)	< 0.001
IPSS-t	1.064	(1.016–1.115)	0.009

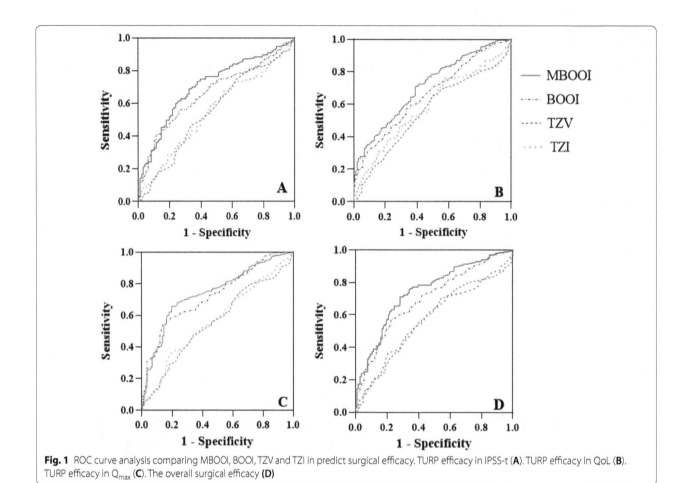

Fig. 1 ROC curve analysis comparing MBOOI, BOOI, TZV and TZI in predict surgical efficacy. TURP efficacy in IPSS-t (**A**). TURP efficacy in QoL (**B**). TURP efficacy in Q_{max} (**C**). The overall surgical efficacy (**D**)

of TURP. With a larger AUC, there was a higher correlation of MBOOI (AUC = 0.708, 95% CI 0.652–0.765) with the improvement in IPSS-t than BOOI (AUC = 0.664, 95% CI 0.606–0.721), TZV (AUC = 0.556, 95% CI 0.491–0622), and TZI (AUC = 0.543, 95% CI 0.484–0.618). Similarly, compared with BOOI (AUC = 0.661, 95% CI 0.608–0.715), TZV (AUC = 0.558, 95% CI 0.501–0.616), and TZI (AUC = 0.582, 95% CI 0.252–0.639), MBOOI (AUC = 0.710, 95% CI 0.659–0.761) had a larger AUC in improvement in QoL. With regard to the surgical efficacy in Q_{max}, the AUC was 0.742 (95% CI 0.691–0.794) for MBOOI, 0.728 (95% CI 0.676–0.779) for BOOI, 0.559 (95% CI 0.499–0.619) for TZV, and 0.570 (95% CI 0.510–0.630) for TZI (Fig. 1).

Discussion

BOO is one of the main causes of LUTS. IPSS is currently recognized as the most effective method to evaluate the severity of subjective symptoms in BPH patients, and PFS is an objective examination to quantify the condition as well as pre-surgical and post-surgical efficacy. The degree of BOO is classified into three grades by BOOI:

unobstructed (BOOI ≤ 20), equivocal (20 < BOOI ≤ 40), and obstructed (BOOI > 40) [12]. However, Han et al. noted that BOOI is often inconsistent with endoscopically proven obstruction due to exclusion of the role of abdominal pressure in urination, and thus, they proposed the concept of modified BOOI and proved that modified BOOI can better predict BOO in patients with LUTS/BPH [5]. This finding is consistent with the results of our study, where MBOOI, when compared with BOOI, exhibited a higher correlation not only with IPSS, QoL, and Q_{max}, but also with PSA, TPV, and TZI.

TURP is the standard surgical method for the treatment of BPH in prostate volume ≤ 80 ml. With the improvement of surgical proficiency and technology, TURP is also commonly used in patients with larger prostate, and it is equally safe and effective in large size prostate (> 80 ml) as compare in small size (≤ 80 ml) [6, 13, 14]. TURP is not only the mainstream surgical method at present, but also often the preferred surgical method for BPH. Therefore, in this study, we did not limit the volume of prostate in the included patients. The mean prostate volume (52.84 ± 27.63) in this study was small, but this is consistent with the results of related studies, the mean PV in each 10- year age group was lower that reported in studies in Asian populations than that in studies on Caucasians and African Americans [15–17]. However, further studies are needed to clarify whether the same results can be obtained from a separate study of large prostate patients, especially prostate volume larger than 80 ml. This study mainly focuses on the prediction of TURP efficacy by MBOOI. Nonetheless, 5–35% of patients postoperatively report persistent symptoms after TURP [18]. Therefore, in clinical practice, it is highly necessary to predict whether invasive surgery will be beneficial for patients. Traditionally, to select appropriate patients for surgery, BOOI with a PFS is recommended. In a study by Seki et al., multiple logistic regression analysis indicated that a higher baseline level of BOOI was associated with greater improvements in IPSS and QoL. Huang et al. conducted a study to establish an efficacy prediction model for transurethral prostatectomy, and found that there was a positive correlation between surgical efficacy with a higher degree of BOO and secondary detrusor cell hypertrophy [19]. Similarly, previous studies have shown that patients with definite BOO derive greater benefit from TURP surgery than those with equivocal and unobstruction [20, 21]. Previous studies indicated that BOOI is an extremely important method for predicting the surgical outcome of TURP.

The limitations of BOOI are emerging. Han et al. followed up 71 patients from 12 to 55 months, and found that 64% of patients were satisfied with the surgical results in the unobstructed and weak bladder contractility group [22]. Although the surgical effect in the BOO-positive group was significantly better than that of those in the BOO-negative group, Kim indicated that being BOO-positive might not be the absolute surgical indication for TURP [23]. Han et al. found that abdominal pressure was correlated with the degree of BOO as defined by cystourethroscopy [5]. In our study, abdominal pressure was a predictive factor for improvement of QoL. Sekido stated that abdominal pressure serves as a compensatory mechanism to promote urination with impaired detrusor and bladder contractions, and an increase in abdominal pressure would reduce the detrusor pressure required to achieve the same flow rate [24]. Consequently, $P_{det}Q_{max}$, which is obtained by subtracting the P_{abd} from P_{ves} for analysis of pressure flow, may lead to a vague interpretation of the P-Q diagrams and an incorrect assessment of outflow impedance [25]. However, the specific mechanism governing abdominal straining in urination remains unknown.

Therefore, in order to better evaluate patients' conditions and predict surgical efficacy, it is vital to determine more valuable parameters that take into account abdominal pressure. Here, we compared the results of a simple modified method with the traditional BOOI, and the present findings confirm that MBOOI appears to be better at predicting surgical outcomes than BOOI. In one respect, MBOOI, providing clearly better results than BOOI, was significantly related to the changes in IPSS (including IPSS-v, IPSS-s, IPSS-p, IPSS-t), QoL, Q_{max}, and PVR after TURP. However, superior results were observed for the association between MBOOI and surgical outcomes, which were accessed by the improvement in IPSS, QoL, and Q_{max} using binary logistic regression analysis. The result was further verified by ROC analysis with a larger AUC in MBOOI. Additionally, to a certain extent, although some preoperative factors are related to surgical outcomes, such as P_{ves}, $P_{det}Q_{max}$, P_{abd}, BOOI, IPSS-t, QoL, and Q_{max}, they are significantly less effective than MBOOI. Particularly, contrary to the findings of the previous study, an additional finding is that a significant correlation between TZI and surgical efficacy was not observed [26]. In addition, related studies have shown that the surgical effect of TURP is similar to that of green-light laser photo-selective vaporization of the prostate (PVP) and holmium laser enucleation of the prostate (HoLEP), and the PVP and HoLEP were not significantly better than the former [27–29]. Of course, A larger resected prostate tissue weight that is present after enucleation techniques, however, similar efficacy has been reported for enucleation techniques and TURP in the treatment of BPH. One RCT comparing holmium laser enucleation of the prostate (HoLEP) with TURP in BPH patients who completed the 7-yr follow-up found that the functional long-term results of HoLEP were comparable with TURP [28]. Therefore, we boldly assume that MBOOI can be applied to predict the surgical efficacy of enucleation techniques, but there is no relevant research at present, and more studies are needed to further clarify.

To the best of our knowledge, this is the first study to investigate the correlation between MBOOI and efficacy of TURP, and the results confirmed that MBOOI may be a potential candidate that can be used to predict surgical outcomes. The pathophysiology of male LUTS/BPH is highly complex and multifactorial, and the disease and efficacy are unlikely to be determined by a single factor [30]. For more optimal diagnosis and treatment of BPH, our task is to continuously explore the pathophysiological mechanism and determine more valuable indicators. This study provides new directions and ideas for this purpose.

There are several limitations to this study. First of all, one limitation of our implementation is that this is a retrospective study, and compared with non-invasive examination such as ultrasound, PFS as invasive examination may bring the risk of trauma to the patient. However, as the gold standard for diagnosing BOO, its status in urology is irreplaceable. We routinely completed this examination before TURP surgery, and the surgical efficacy was confirmed by reexamination 3 months after surgery. This study was retrospective and did not cause additional trauma to patients. In addition, some parameters that may influence the surgical outcome reported in the previous studies were not evaluated, such as intravesical prostatic protrusion, prostatic urethral angulation and ultrasonic estimation of bladder weight, detrusor wall thickness, and resistive index, et al. [31–34]. Further studies should carry out to compare the value of those parameters and MBOOI in predicting surgical efficacy. Thirdly, although Park et al. did not find a correlation between the resected prostate tissue ratio and surgical efficacy, there was no insufficient evidence to support this [35]. For example, Milonas et al. found that the volume of resected tissue was an important factor influencing the degree of symptom improvement [36]. Although the relationship between resected prostate tissue weight and surgical efficacy was not considered in our study, we tried to achieve completeness of resection intraoperatively. Additionally, resected prostate tissue weight is closely related to TZV, and our study shows that TZV has little effect in predicting surgical efficacy. Therefore, it is unlikely to radically change our study results. Finally, additional studies with larger samples are needed to further elucidate the relationship and mechanism between MBOOI and abdominal pressure with BPH and the surgical effect.

Conclusions

Although both MBOOI and BOOI can predict the urinary symptoms in men with LUTS/BPH to a certain extent, however, there was a stronger correlation between MBOOI and LUTS. In addition, both AUC of MBOOI and BOOI for surgical efficacy was between 0.70 and 0.8, but MBOOI was slightly higher than that of BOOI. Meanwhile, our study indicates that MBOOI is significantly associated with improvements in IPSS, QoL, and Qmax after TURP. In general, these findings suggest that MBOOI may have greater potential than BOOI for evaluating disease and predicting surgical efficacy in patients with LUTS/BPH. Further research could quite beneficial to explain the role of MBOOI in the progression of disease and surgical prognosis in men with LUTS/BPH.

Abbreviations

BPH: Benign prostatic hyperplasia; BPO: Benign prostatic obstruction; BPE: Benign prostatic enlargement; LUTS: Low urinary tract symptom; QoL: Quality of Life; PFSs: Pressure-flow studies; BOO: Bladder outlet obstruction; BOOI: Bladder outlet obstruction index; Qmax: Maximum urine flow rate; MBOOI: Modified bladder outlet obstruction index; TURP: Transurethral resection of the prostate; PSA: Prostate-specific antigen; TRUS: Transrectal ultrasonograpy;

TPV: Total prostate volume; TZV: Transitional zone volume; TZI: Transitional zone index; IPSS-s: Storage IPSS; IPPS-t: Total IPSS; IPSS-v: Voiding IPSS; IPSS-p: Post-micturitional IPSS; PVR: Post void residual urine volume; P_{ves}: Intra-vesical pressure; P_{abd}: Abdominal pressure; $P_{det}Q_{max}$: Detrusor pressure at maximum urine flow rate; ROC: Receiver operating characteristic; AUC: Area under the curve; PVP: Green-light laser photo-selective vaporization of the prostate; HoLEP: Holmium laser enucleation of the prostate.

Acknowledgements

We thank Denise R, Jason Qee, from editorbar language editing, Beijing, China (www.leditorbar.com), for editing the English text of a draft of this manuscript.

Authors' contributions

Conceived and designed the study: HML and YT. Collected the data: HML, ZYS, YB, ZW. Analyzed and interpreted data: HML, YT and GHL. Drafted the manuscript: HML and ZYS. Critical revision of the manuscript: GHL, ZLS. All authors read and approved the final manuscript.

Author details

[1]Department of Urology, The Affiliated Hospital of Guizhou Medical University, Guiyang, China. [2]Department of Urology, Guizhou Provincial People's Hospital, Guiyang, China.

References

1. Cao N, Lu Q, Si J, Wang X, Ni J, Chen L, Gu B, Hu B. The characteristics of transitional zone in prostate growth with age. Urology. 2017;105:136–40. https://doi.org/10.1016/j.urology.2017.03.010.
2. Zhao J, Zhao Z, Song J, Ji Z, Tian Y. The diagnostic accuracy and lower cutoff value of three methods for quantifying urethral resistance in men. Urol Int. 2011;86:90–4. https://doi.org/10.1159/000319968.
3. Nitti VW. Pressure flow urodynamic studies: the gold standard for diagnosing bladder outlet obstruction. Rev Urol. 2015;7:S14-21.
4. Tian Y, Su ZY, Liu DY, Yang B, Liu HM, Lei J, Luo GH, Sun ZL, Sun F, Xia SJ. The clinical application value study of bladder outlet obstruction index on benign prostate hyperplasia. Nat J Androl. 2020;26:513–7. https://doi.org/10.13263/j.cnki.nja.2020.06.005.
5. Han JH, Yu HS, Lee JY, Kim J, Kang DH, Kwon JK, Choi YD, Cho KS. Simple modification of the bladder outlet obstruction index for better prediction of endoscopically-proven prostatic obstruction: a preliminary study. PLoS ONE. 2015;10(10):e0141745. https://doi.org/10.1371/journal.pone.0141745.
6. Oelke M, Bachmann A, Descazeaud A, Emberton M, Gravas S, Michel MC, N'dow J, Nordling J, de la Rosette JJ. EAU guidelines on the treatment and follow-up of non-neurogenic male lower urinary tract symptoms including benign prostatic obstruction. Eur Urol. 2013;6:118–40. https://doi.org/10.1016/j.eururo.2013.03.004.
7. van Venrooij GE, van Melick HH, Eckhardt MD, Boon TA. Diagnostic and predictive value of voiding diary data versus prostate volume, maximal free urinary flow rate, and Abrams-Griffiths number in men with lower urinary tract symptoms suggestive of benign prostatic hyperplasia. Urology. 2008;71:469–74. https://doi.org/10.1016/j.urology.2007.11.033.
8. Seki N, Takei M, Yamaguchi A, Naito S. Analysis of prognostic factors regarding the outcome after a transurethral resection for symptomatic benign prostatic enlargement. Neurourol Urodyn. 2006;25:428–32. https://doi.org/10.1002/nau.20262.
9. Aarnink RG, de la Rosette JJ, Debruyne FM, Wijkstra H. Formula-derived prostate volume determination. Eur Urol. 1996;29:399–402. https://doi.org/10.1159/000473786.
10. Abrams PH, Griffiths DJ. The assessment of prostatic obstruction from urodynamic measurements and from residual urine. Br J Urol. 1979;51:129–34. https://doi.org/10.1111/j.1464-410x.1979.tb02846.x.
11. Homma Y, Kawabe K, Tsukamoto T, Yamaguchi O, Okada K, Aso Y, Watanabe H, Okajima E, Kumazawa J, Yamaguchi T, Ohashi Y. Estimate criteria for efficacy of treatment in benign prostatic hyperplasia. Int J Urol. 1996;3:267–73. https://doi.org/10.1111/j.1442-2042.1996.tb00532.x.

12. Griffiths D, Höfner K, van Mastrigt R, Rollema HJ, Spångberg A, Gleason D. Standardization of terminology of lower urinary tract function: pressure-flow studies of voiding, urethral resistance, and urethral obstruction. Neurourol Urodyn. 1997;16:1–18. https://doi.org/10.1002/(sici)1520-6777(1997)16:1%3c1:aid-nau1%3e3.0.co;2-i.

13. Joshi HN, De Jong IJ, Karmacharya RM, Shrestha B, Shrestha R. Outcomes of transurethral resection of the prostate in benign prostatic hyperplasia comparing prostate size of more than 80 grams to prostate size less than 80 grams. Kathmandu Univ Med J (KUMJ). 2014;12(47):163–7. https://doi.org/10.3126/kumj.v12i3.13708.

14. Kumar A, Vasudeva P, Kumar N, Nanda B, Jha SK, Mohanty N. A prospective randomized comparative study of monopolar and bipolar transurethral resection of the prostate and photoselective vaporization of the prostate in patients who present with benign prostatic obstruction: a single center experience. J Endourol. 2013;27(10):1245–53. https://doi.org/10.1089/end.2013.0216.

15. Rhodes T, Girman CJ, Jacobsen SJ, Roberts RO, Guess HA, Lieber MM. Longitudinal prostate growth rates during 5 years in randomly selected community men 40 to 79 years old. J Urol. 1999;161(4):1174–9.

16. Sarma AV, Jaffe CA, Schottenfeld D, Dunn R, Montie JE, Cooney KA, Wei JT. Insulin-like growth factor-1, insulin-like growth factor binding protein-3, and body mass index: clinical correlates of prostate volume among Black men. Urology. 2002;59(3):362–7. https://doi.org/10.1016/s0090-4295(01)01546-1.

17. Park JS, Koo KC, Kim HK, Chung BH, Lee KS. Impact of metabolic syndrome-related factors on the development of benign prostatic hyperplasia and lower urinary tract symptoms in Asian population. Medicine. 2019. https://doi.org/10.1097/MD.0000000000017635.

18. Kanik EA, Erdem E, Abidinoglu D, Acar D, Akbay E, Ulusoy E. Can the outcome of transurethral resection of the prostate be predicted preoperatively? Urology. 2004;64:302–5. https://doi.org/10.1016/j.urology.2004.03.035.

19. Huang T, Yu YJ, Qi J, Xu D, Duan LJ, Ding J, Zhu YP. Establishment and value assessment of efficacy prediction model about transurethral prostatectomy. Int J Urol. 2015;22:854–60. https://doi.org/10.1111/iju.12836.

20. Oh MM, Kim JW, Kim JJ, du Moon G. Is there a correlation between the outcome of transurethral resection of prostate and preoperative degree of bladder outlet obstruction? Asian J Androl. 2012;14:556–9. https://doi.org/10.1038/aja.2011.157.

21. Min DS, Cho HJ, Kang JY, Yoo TK, Cho JM. Effect of transurethral resection of the prostate based on the degree of obstruction seen in urodynamic study. Korean J Urol. 2013;54:840–5. https://doi.org/10.4111/kju.2013.54.12.840.

22. Han DH, Jeong YS, Choo MS, Lee KS. The efficacy of transurethral resection of the prostate in the patients with weak bladder contractility index. Urology. 2008;71:657–61. https://doi.org/10.1016/j.urology.2007.11.109.

23. Kim M, Jeong CW, Oh SJ. Diagnostic value of urodynamic bladder outlet obstruction to select patients for transurethral surgery of the prostate: systematic review and meta-analysis. PLoS ONE. 2017;12(2):e0172590. https://doi.org/10.1371/journal.pone.0172590.

24. Sekido N. Bladder contractility and urethral resistance relation: what does a pressure flow study tell us? Int J Urol. 2012;19:216–28. https://doi.org/10.1111/j.1442-2042.2011.02947.x.

25. Mijailovich SM, Sullivan MP, Yalla SV, Venegas JG. Theoretical analysis of the effects of viscous losses and abdominal straining on urinary outlet function. Neurourol Urodyn. 2004;23:76–85. https://doi.org/10.1002/nau.10146.

26. Milonas D, Saferis V, Jievaltas M. Transition zone index and bothersomeness of voiding symptoms as predictors of early unfavorable outcomes after transurethral resection of prostate. Urol Int. 2008;81:421–6. https://doi.org/10.1159/000167840.

27. Thomas JA, Tubaro A, Barber N, d'Ancona F, Muir G, Witzsch U, Grimm MO, Benejam J, Stolzenburg JU, Riddick A, Pahernik S, Roelink H, Ameye F, Saussine C, Bruyère F, Loidl W, Larner T, Gogoi NK, Hindley R, Muschter R, Thorpe A, Shrotri N, Graham S, Hamann M, Miller K, Schostak M, Capitán C, Knispel H, Bachmann A. A multicenter randomized noninferiority trial comparing GreenLight-XPS laser vaporization of the prostate and transurethral resection of the prostate for the treatment of benign prostatic obstruction: two-yr outcomes of the GOLIATH study. Eur Urol. 2016;69(1):94–102. https://doi.org/10.1016/j.eururo.2015.07.054.

28. Gilling PJ, Wilson LC, King CJ, Westenberg AM, Frampton CM, Fraundorfer MR. Long-term results of a randomized trial comparing holmium laser enucleation of the prostate and transurethral resection of the prostate: results at 7 years. BJU Int. 2012;109(3):408–11. https://doi.org/10.1111/j.1464-410X.2011.10359.x.

29. Zhou Y, Xue B, Mohammad NA, Chen D, Sun X, Yang J, Dai G. Greenlight high-performance system (HPS) 120-W laser vaporization versus transurethral resection of the prostate for the treatment of benign prostatic hyperplasia: a meta-analysis of the published results of randomized controlled trials. Lasers Med Sci. 2016;31(3):485–95. https://doi.org/10.1007/s10103-016-1895-x.

30. Wasson JH, Reda DJ, Bruskewitz RC, Elinson J, Keller AM, Henderson WG. A comparison of transurethral surgery with watchful waiting for moderate symptoms of benign prostatic hyperplasia. The veterans affairs cooperative study group on transurethral resection of the prostate. N Engl J Med. 1995;332(2):75–9. https://doi.org/10.1056/NEJM199501123320202.

31. Lee JW, Ryu JH, Yoo TK, Byun SS, Jeong YJ, Jung TY. Relationship between intravesical prostatic protrusion and postoperative outcomes in patients with benign prostatic hyperplasia. Korean J Urol. 2012;53:478–82. https://doi.org/10.4111/kju.2012.53.7.478.

32. Shim M, Bang WJ, Oh CY, Lee YS, Cho JS. Correlation between prostatic urethral angulation and symptomatic improvement after surgery in patients with lower urinary tract symptoms according to prostate size. World J Urol. 2020;38:1997–2003. https://doi.org/10.1007/s00345-019-02990-6.

33. Huang T, Qi J, Yu YJ, Xu D, Jiao Y, Kang J, Chen YQ, Zhu YK. Predictive value of resistive index, detrusor wall thickness and ultrasound estimated bladder weight regarding the outcome after transurethral prostatectomy for patients with lower urinary tract symptoms suggestive of benign prostatic obstruction. Int J Urol. 2012;19(4):343–50. https://doi.org/10.1111/j.1442-2042.2011.02942.x.

34. Shinbo H, Kurita Y, Nakanishi T, Imanishi T, Otsuka A, Furuse H, Mugiya S, Ozono S. Resistive index: a newly identified predictor of outcome of transurethral prostatectomy in patients with benign prostatic hyperplasia. Urology. 2010;75(1):143–7. https://doi.org/10.1016/j.urology.2009.08.017.

35. Park HK, Paick SH, Lho YS, Jun KK, Kim HG. Effect of the ratio of resected tissue in comparison with the prostate transitional zone volume on voiding function improvement after transurethral resection of prostate. Urology. 2012;79(1):202–6. https://doi.org/10.1016/j.urology.2011.07.1397.

36. Milonas D, Verikaite J, Jievaltas M. The effect of complete transurethral resection of the prostate on symptoms, quality of life, and voiding function improvement. Cent Eur J Urol. 2015;68(2):169–74. https://doi.org/10.5173/ceju.2015.507.

28

Free combination of dutasteride plus tamsulosin for the treatment of benign prostatic hyperplasia in South Korea: Analysis of drug utilization and adverse events using the National Health Insurance Review and Assessment Service database

Zrinka Lulic[1], Hwancheol Son[2], Sang-Bae Yoo[3], Marianne Cunnington[1], Pratiksha Kapse[4*], Diane Miller[5], Vanessa Cortes[6], Suna Park[7], Rachel H. Bhak[7] and Mei Sheng Duh[7]

Abstract

Objective: To assess the use and safety of free combination therapy (dutasteride and tamsulosin), dutasteride monotherapy, or tamsulosin monotherapy in patients with benign prostatic hyperplasia (BPH).

Methods: This non-interventional retrospective cohort study used claims data from the Korea Health Insurance Review and Assessment-National Patient Sample database. Patients with BPH $\geq$ 40 years of age receiving combination therapy (dutasteride 0.5 mg and tamsulosin 0.4 mg daily) or dutasteride 0.5 mg, or tamsulosin 0.4 mg daily dose between 2012 and 2017 were included. The frequency, duration of treatment and risk of any adverse event (AE) or serious AE (SAE) was compared for combination therapy versus each monotherapy using non-inferiority testing.

Results: Of 14,755 eligible patients, 1529 (10.4%) received combination therapy, 6660 (45.1%) dutasteride monotherapy, and 6566 (44.5%) tamsulosin monotherapy. The proportion of patients treated with combination therapy exceeded the pre-specified 3% threshold for 'frequent' use. Safety results indicated a similar risk of any AE and SAE irrespective of treatment group. The adjusted relative risk for any AE over the treatment observation period comparing combination therapy with dutasteride monotherapy was 1.07 (95% confidence interval [CI] 1.03, 1.12), and with tamsulosin monotherapy was 0.98 (95% CI 0.95, 1.02) demonstrating non-inferiority. The adjusted relative risk for any SAE was 1.07 (95% CI 0.66, 1.74) and 0.90 (95% CI 0.56, 1.45), compared with dutasteride and tamsulosin monotherapy, respectively. Although the SAE results did not statistically demonstrate non-inferiority of combination therapy based on pre-specified margins, the 95% CI for the risk ratio estimates included the null with a lower limit below the non-inferiority margins, indicating no meaningful differences in SAE risk between groups. Absolute SAE risks were low.

Conclusion: Combination therapy with dutasteride and tamsulosin is frequently used in real-world practice in South Korea for treatment of BPH and demonstrates a safety profile similar to either monotherapy.

*Correspondence: pratiksha.j.kapse@gsk.com
[4] GlaxoSmithKline, Mumbai, India
Full list of author information is available at the end of the article
Diane Miller was affiliated with GSK at the time of the study.

Introduction

Benign prostatic hyperplasia (BPH) is one of the most common non-malignant conditions in older men [1, 2]. A nationwide survey from the United States (US) reported BPH prevalence of 25% in men > 50 years of age [3]. In a population-based, cross-sectional survey conducted in the US, the United Kingdom (UK) and Sweden, symptoms suggestive of possible BPH were highly prevalent in men, reported in up to 46% of the population studied [4]. Notably, BPH prevalence increases with age, from 14.8% in men aged 40–49 years to 36.8% in those ≥ 80 years [1]. Although current data are limited for Southeast Asia, the overall incidence of BPH in South Korea was reported to be 2105 per 100,000 men based on data from patients diagnosed with BPH in 2008, using a nationwide South Korean database, Health Insurance Review and Assessment (HIRA) [5]. As expected, the prevalence of BPH increased with age; the highest incidence was in patients ≥ 70 years of age.

A common manifestation of BPH is lower urinary tract symptoms (LUTS), including difficulty in voiding, and nocturia [6, 7]. These have considerable negative impacts on health-related quality of life and sexual functioning [6, 8, 9]. The short-term aim of LUTS/BPH therapy is to provide relief of symptoms by improving flow of urine [10]; long-term treatment goals are to alleviate bothersome LUTS, prevent acute urinary retention, and reduce the risk of complications [7, 11, 12].

A fixed-dose combination of dutasteride 0.5 mg plus tamsulosin 0.4 mg therapy (5α-reductase inhibitor (5-ARI) and α1-blocker) is currently approved in over 90 countries, including the US, UK, and Australia, for symptomatic BPH [13–15]. Fixed-dose combination therapy has only recently been approved in South Korea (May 2021) [16], although for several years now the Korean Urological Association guidelines for BPH have endorsed α1-blocker plus 5-ARI combination therapy as being more effective than α1-blocker monotherapy for improving LUTS [17]. The availability of real-world data representative of national populations offers the opportunity to generate country-specific evidence on the benefit:risk of new medicine indications and combinations more rapidly than was previously possible through more traditional clinical study approaches.

The current study assessed real-world use and safety of dutasteride 0.5 mg and tamsulosin 0.4 mg in free combination (ie, administered concomitantly) therapy among patients with BPH using the South Korean HIRA claims database.

Methods

Study design

This was a non-interventional retrospective cohort study using claims data from the HIRA-National Patient Sample (HIRA-NPS) database. The NPS database comprises random 3% annual samples from the overall HIRA database with patients followed for a maximum of 1 year. Eligible patients from each year (2012 − 2017) were pooled into one population. More details are provided in Additional file 1. From the overall population, three treatment cohorts were defined: patients treated with free combination therapy (dutasteride 0.5 mg and tamsulosin 0.4 mg daily), dutasteride 0.5 mg monotherapy (0.5 mg once daily), and tamsulosin 0.4 mg monotherapy (0.4 mg once daily or 0.2 mg twice daily). The study period comprised the baseline period, index date (administration of therapy), and observation period (Fig. 1).

This non-interventional retrospective study was exempted from Institutional Review Board or ethics review committee approval. Patients were not contacted, and patient data were anonymized in compliance with current privacy laws and data de-identification guidelines in South Korea. The study sponsor did not have access to patient identifiers. Additional study information is available in the GlaxoSmithKline Clinical Study Register, Study ID Number: 212907.

Study population

Patients were included from the HIRA-NPS database from 2012 to 2017 if they had: at least one medical claim with a primary or secondary diagnosis for BPH at any time during the year; ≥ 1 prescription dispensed for free combination therapy, dutasteride 0.5 mg monotherapy or tamsulosin 0.4 mg monotherapy; were ≥ 40 years of age on the index date; and were observed for ≥ 6 months while receiving treatment. Patients were excluded from the analysis if they had a record of a primary diagnosis of BPH-related surgery (no specific surgical procedure codes were available), or if they had a medical claim with a primary or secondary diagnosis for prostate cancer, during the baseline period.

Study objectives

The primary objectives were to describe the frequency and duration of treatment, overall risk of any adverse event/serious adverse event (AE/SAE) during the treatment observation period, and the demographic and clinical characteristics of prevalent patients with BPH at treatment initiation.

Evaluated AEs were restricted to those that were identifiable with Korean Classification of Disease codes and were included in the global datasheet for

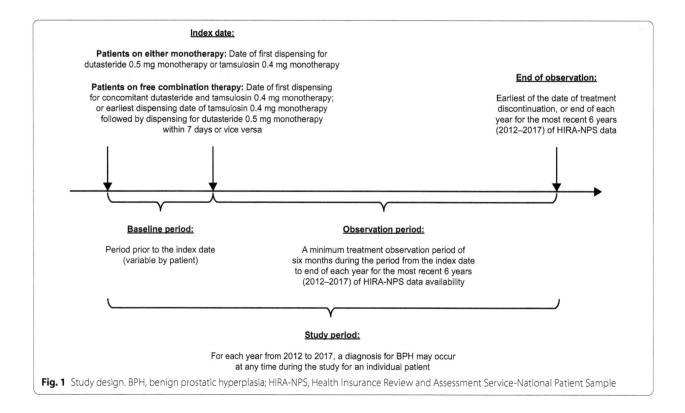

Fig. 1 Study design. BPH, benign prostatic hyperplasia; HIRA-NPS, Health Insurance Review and Assessment Service-National Patient Sample

dutasteride-tamsulosin hydrochloride (Additional file 2). SAEs were any condition from the list of AEs that was the primary diagnosis associated with hospitalization or death during the observation period.

Prostate cancer was included in the global datasheet under 'warnings' as an area of potential risk associated with 5α-reductase inhibitors that needs to be monitored (ie, not a confirmed drug-related AE).

Statistical analysis

Inverse-probability-of-treatment weighting (IPTW) was used to adjust for imbalances in the distribution of baseline characteristics across all cohorts before conducting comparisons. Standardized differences in baseline characteristics of < 10% were deemed as denoting meaningful balance across treatment cohorts [18].

Frequency and duration of treatment with free combination therapy and each monotherapy were summarized using descriptive statistics. In a previous study, the prevalence of moderate or severe LUTS among patients with BPH was reported to be 17.4%, and 33.7% of those patients received treatment for BPH [19]. Based on this it was estimated that 5.9% of patients would be eligible for receiving a BPH medical treatment in the population of interest. In the absence of a pre-defined threshold, this estimate was halved (ie, 3%) and used as a threshold to

define frequent use for the free combination therapy of dutasteride and tamsulosin in our study population.

To assess safety, non-inferiority testing with a one-sided α-error level of 0.025 was conducted to test the hypothesis that the overall risk of any AE or SAE with free combination therapy was no greater than with either monotherapy. Risk ratios (RRs) for any AE and any SAE were estimated using IPTW-adjusted log-binomial regression models, with a single variable for the treatment cohort. Robust variance estimators were used to obtain the corresponding 95% confidence intervals (CIs). Non-inferiority was confirmed if the upper limit of the 95% CIs of the RRs fell below the pre-specified non-inferiority margin of 1.64 and 1.30 for AEs and 0.84 and 0.77 for SAEs for comparisons with dutasteride and tamsulosin monotherapy, respectively. Non-inferiority margins were based on results from the subgroup of South Korean patients in the pivotal CombAT trial. The RR values for any AE for patients receiving free combination therapy compared with dutasteride 0.5 mg monotherapy and with tamsulosin 0.4 mg monotherapy were 2.7 and 1.7, respectively. In addition, the RR values for any SAE for patients receiving free combination therapy compared with dutasteride 0.5 mg monotherapy and tamsulosin 0.4 mg monotherapy were 0.7 and 0.6, respectively. The non-inferiority margins were estimated using the point-estimate method and taking a preserved effect of 50% of the log RRs, which is in line with regulatory guidance [20, 21].

A subgroup analysis by age (40–59, 60–69, and ≥ 70 years of age), sensitivity analysis among patients without AEs or SAEs during the baseline period, and evaluation of specific AEs using superiority testing with a two-sided α-level of 0.05 were also conducted. No adjustments were made for multiple comparisons. Analyses were conducted using SAS Enterprise Guide Software Version 7.1 (SAS Institute Inc., Cary, NC).

Results

Patient population

A total of 246720 patients with ≥ 1 medical claim for a primary diagnosis for BPH were identified from the HIRA-NPS database from January 1, 2012 to December 31, 2017. Of these, 14,755 (6.0%) patients were eligible and included in the analysis (Additional file 3): 1529 (10.4%) patients received daily treatment with free combination therapy, 6660 (45.1%) received dutasteride monotherapy 0.5 mg daily, and 6566 (44.5%) received tamsulosin monotherapy 0.4 mg daily.

Prior to IPTW adjustment, several baseline demographic and clinical characteristic imbalances were observed between treatment groups with standardized differences of 10% or above. Patients treated with free combination therapy were more likely to have polyuria (13.9% vs 9.9%, standardized difference = 12.6%), a higher number of symptoms or findings associated with BPH (0.3% vs 0.2%, standardized difference = 11.0%), and BPH with LUTS (17.9% vs 12.3%, standardized difference = 15.7%), than those treated with dutasteride 0.5 mg. The free combination and tamsulosin groups were more balanced; however, patients treated with free combination therapy were less likely to be 50–59 years of age (7.7% vs 12.9%, standardized difference = 17.3%) and more likely to be ≥ 70 years of age (60.6% vs 51.6%, standardized difference = 18.3%) at baseline, than those treated with tamsulosin 0.4 mg.

Following IPTW adjustment, baseline demographics and clinical characteristics were balanced across all treatment cohorts with standardized differences of < 10% (Table 1). Most patients (> 87%) were aged ≥ 60 years; BPH with LUTS affected 13.3% to 18.6% of patients, and polyuria was the most common symptom associated with BPH, affecting 10.6% to 14.6% of the IPTW-adjusted samples. The most common medications used during the baseline period were non-steroidal anti-inflammatory drugs (NSAIDS; 34.6−37.9%), calcium channel blockers (21.0−24.2%), and antihypertensives (21.8−23.4%).

Treatment frequency and duration

The proportion of patients treated with free combination therapy was 10.4%, compared with 45.1% (dutasteride monotherapy) and 44.5% (tamsulosin monotherapy); this exceeded the threshold of 3% selected to define frequent combined use. The mean ± standard deviation (SD) duration of treatment was similar for patients treated with free combination therapy (292.5 ± 54.1 days) and either monotherapy (297.1 ± 54.0 days for dutasteride; 295.8 ± 54.0 days for tamsulosin) (Table 2).

Overall risk of any AE or SAE

The risk of any AE occurring was 71.5% (free combination therapy), 64.6% (dutasteride 0.5 mg) and 71.6% (tamsulosin 0.4 mg). The adjusted RR for any AE over the treatment observation period comparing free combination therapy with dutasteride 0.5 mg monotherapy was 1.07 (95% CI 1.03, 1.12) (Fig. 2A) and comparing free combination therapy with tamsulosin 0.4 mg monotherapy was 0.98 (95% CI 0.95, 1.02) (Fig. 2B). The risk of any AE with free combination therapy was non-inferior to that of both monotherapy groups based on non-inferiority margins (non-inferiority $P < 0.001$ each comparison).

The incidence of any SAE in the overall patient population was rare and similar across treatment groups: 1.6% (free combination therapy), 1.3% (dutasteride 0.5 mg monotherapy), and 1.7% (tamsulosin 0.4 mg monotherapy). The adjusted RR for any SAE over the treatment observation period comparing free combination therapy with dutasteride 0.5 mg monotherapy was 1.07 (95% CI 0.66, 1.74) (Fig. 2C), and comparing free combination therapy with tamsulosin 0.4 mg monotherapy was 0.90 (95% CI 0.56, 1.45) (Fig. 2D). Non-inferiority was not shown for either comparison (non-inferiority $P = 0.852$ and 0.762 for comparison with dutasteride and tamsulosin monotherapies, respectively). However, the 95% CI for the RR estimate included the null value of one and had a lower limit below the non-inferiority margins, indicating no meaningful differences in the risk of SAE between treatment groups.

Sensitivity analysis among patients without baseline AEs or SAEs

Results relating to the frequency and duration of treatment and risk of any AE or SAE were consistent with the primary results when patients with AEs or SAEs during the baseline period were excluded from the analysis. For comparison of AEs with free combination therapy versus dutasteride 0.5 mg monotherapy, the adjusted RR was 1.10 (95% CI 1.04, 1.16), indicating a small meaningful difference in favor of dutasteride monotherapy. For comparison of free combination therapy with tamsulosin

Table 1 Baseline characteristics of patients treated with free combination therapy compared with those treated with dutasteride 0.5 mg or tamsulosin 0.4 mg monotherapy, after adjustment using inverse probability of treatment weight

	Free combination therapy versus dutasteride monotherapy			Free combination therapy versus tamsulosin monotherapy		
	Free combination of dutasteride plus tamsulosin therapy (n = 1527)	Dutasteride monotherapy (n = 6661)	Std. diff* (%)	Free combination of dutasteride plus tamsulosin therapy (n = 1544)	Tamsulosin monotherapy (n = 6574)	Std. diff* (%)
Age, n (%)						
40–49 years	29 (1.9)	150 (2.2)	2.3	20 (1.3)	90 (1.4)	0.7
50–59 years	165 (10.8)	704 (10.6)	0.8	182 (11.8)	777 (11.8)	0.2
60–69 years	488 (32.0)	2133 (32.0)	0.1	517 (33.5)	2201 (33.5)	0.0
≥ 70 years	844 (55.3)	3675 (55.2)	0.3	826 (53.5)	3506 (53.3)	0.3
Clinical characteristics, n (%)						
Any AE[†]	422 (27.7)	1857 (27.9)	0.5	476 (30.8)	2030 (30.9)	0.1
Cardiovascular disease[‡]	565 (37.0)	2475 (37.2)	0.3	622 (40.3)	2612 (39.7)	1.2
Hyperlipidemia	304 (19.9)	1361 (20.4)	1.3	338 (21.9)	1433 (21.8)	0.3
Chronic pulmonary disease	221 (14.5)	988 (14.8)	0.9	258 (16.7)	1088 (16.5)	0.4
BPH with LUTS	210 (13.7)	889 (13.3)	1.1	288 (18.6)	1193 (18.2)	1.2
Polyuria[§]	167 (10.9)	709 (10.6)	1.0	225 (14.6)	936 (14.2)	1.0
Concomitant medications, n (%)						
NSAIDs	530 (34.7)	2302 (34.6)	0.4	585 (37.9)	2417 (36.8)	2.3
Calcium channel blockers	330 (21.6)	1400 (21.0)	1.4	374 (24.2)	1500 (22.8)	3.3
Antihypertensives	334 (21.9)	1454 (21.8)	0.1	361 (23.4)	1459 (22.2)	2.8

AE, adverse event; BPH, benign prostatic hyperplasia; LUTS, lower urinary tract symptoms; NSAIDs, nonsteroidal anti-inflammatory drugs; Std. diff, standardized difference

* For continuous variables, the standardized difference was calculated by dividing the absolute difference in means of the free combination therapy cohort and reference monotherapy cohorts by the pooled standard deviation (SD) of both groups, for each comparison. The pooled SD was the square root of the average of the squared SD. For dichotomous variables, the standardized difference was calculated using the following equation where P is the respective proportion of participants in each treatment cohort: $[(P_{freecombination\ therapy} - P_{reference})/ \sqrt{(P_{freecombinationtherapy} \times (1 - P_{freecombinationtherapy}) + P_{reference} \times (1 - P_{reference}))/ 2}]$

[†] For the purpose of this analysis, the data on prostate cancer were included in any AE. See Additional file 2 for list of AEs

[‡] Three categories of Quan–Charlson comorbidities (ie, congestive heart failure, peripheral vascular disease, and myocardial infarction) are listed under cardiovascular disease

[§] Polyuria includes nocturia and urinary frequency

0.4 mg monotherapy, the adjusted RR for any AE was 0.98 (95% CI 0.93, 1.04), indicating no meaningful difference. The RR for any SAE of free combination therapy versus dutasteride 0.5 mg monotherapy was 1.13 (95% CI 0.58, 2.24), and versus tamsulosin 0.4 mg monotherapy was 0.80 (95% CI 0.42, 1.51), indicating no meaningful differences.

Subgroup analysis by age

Treatment frequency with free combination therapy was lowest in patients 40–59 years of age (6.3%) and highest in patients > 70 years of age (11.7%). Among patients aged 60–69 years, 9.8% used free combination therapy. The average duration of treatment was similar for patients treated with free combination therapy and each

monotherapy across all age groups (Additional file 4). The risk of any AE and SAE within each age category was similar to that for the overall population, with no meaningful differences between treatment groups (Additional file 5).

Overall risk of specific AEs and SAEs

The most common AEs throughout the treatment observation period among free combination therapy, dutasteride 0.5 mg monotherapy, and tamsulosin 0.4 mg monotherapy were constipation (26.2%, 19.1%, 24.3%, respectively), depressed mood (14.3%, 11.9%, 15.6%, respectively), urticaria (14.1%, 12.4%, 15.6%, respectively) and dizziness (13.2%, 12.5%, 13.5%, respectively) (Table 3). The 95% CI of the RR for most specific AEs

Table 2 Frequency and duration of treatment with free combination therapy, dutasteride 0.5 mg monotherapy, or tamsulosin 0.4 mg monotherapy in patients with prevalent BPH in South Korea

	Free combination of dutasteride plus tamsulosin therapy (n = 1529)	Free combination therapy versus dutasteride monotherapy		Free combination therapy versus tamsulosin monotherapy	
		Dutasteride monotherapy (n = 6660)	Std. diff*	Tamsulosin monotherapy (n = 6566)	Std. diff*
Treatment duration (days)					
Mean ± SD	292.5 ± 54.1	297.1 ± 54.0	8.6	295.8 ± 54.0	6.1
Median, IQR	305.0 (249.0, 341.0)	310.0 (260.0, 342.0)		310.0 (255.0, 343.0)	
Treatment duration, n (%)					
6–9 months	519 (33.9)	2020 (30.3)	7.7	2085 (31.8)	4.7
9–12 months	1010 (66.1)	4640 (69.7)	7.7	4481 (68.2)	4.7

BPH, benign prostatic hyperplasia; IQR, interquartile range; SD, standard deviation; Std. Diff, standardized difference

* For continuous variables, the standardized difference was calculated by dividing the absolute difference in means of the free combination therapy cohort and reference monotherapy cohorts by the pooled standard deviation (SD) of both groups, for each comparison. The pooled SD was the square root of the average of the squared SD. For dichotomous variables, the standardized difference was calculated using the following equation where P is the respective proportion of participants in each treatment cohort: $[(P_{freecombination\ therapy} - P_{reference}) / \sqrt{(P_{freecombinationtherapy} \times (1 - P_{freecombinationtherapy}) + P_{reference} \times (1 - P_{reference})) / 2}]$

overlapped with 1, indicating no meaningful differences between treatment groups.

The risk of specific SAEs was low (< 1% each) in all treatment groups. The most commonly reported SAEs in the free combination therapy, dutasteride monotherapy and tamsulosin monotherapy groups, respectively, were dizziness (0.5%, 0.3%, 0.4%), cardiac failure (0.3%, 0.1%, 0.2%), arrhythmia (0.2%, 0.2%, 0.2%), and vertigo (0.1%, 0.2%, 0.2%).

Prostate cancer

Prostate cancer was observed in 12.6%, 9.4%, and 12.0% of patients in the free combination therapy, dutasteride 0.5 mg monotherapy, and tamsulosin 0.4 mg monotherapy groups, respectively, throughout the treatment observation period.

Discussion

This retrospective, real-world study was based on a large sample of patients from the South Korean HIRA-NPS database, which includes information on 50 million patients and covers 98% of the total population through the universal coverage system [22]. Although previous studies have assessed BPH treatments using Korean national databases [23–25], to our knowledge this is the first study to analyze the use and safety of free combination therapy (dutasteride and tamsulosin), dutasteride monotherapy, and tamsulosin monotherapy within the Korean population. It also shows the potential for real-world data to inform benefit:risk assessments outside of traditional clinical trial approaches that may capture relatively small country-specific population numbers. Dutasteride and tamsulosin are widely administrated

as a free combination therapy outside of Korea [13–15]. Similarly, the results from our analyses demonstrated frequent use of this free combination therapy for treatment of BPH in the Korean population, without increased risk of any AE or SAE in comparison to either monotherapy. These findings enhance our understanding of BPH treatment in a country with an aging population and elevating prescription for BPH medication [24, 26]. Additionally, these findings support the current evidence from clinical trials on the safety of free combination therapy for treatment of BPH as well as underscoring the benefits of this treatment.

Our analysis demonstrates use of free combination dutasteride 0.5 mg and tamsulosin 0.4 mg was in 10.4% of patients with BPH, which is classified as frequent use (> 3%), based on pre-specified criteria. This is consistent with a previous analysis in South Korea using the HIRA database from 2007–2011, which found that 12–17% of newly diagnosed patients with BPH were prescribed combination therapy [25]. Importantly, combination therapy with an α1-blocker and a 5-ARI is recommended by international BPH treatment guidelines [27, 28] as well as the 2016 Korean clinical practice guideline for BPH [17]. In Korea, tamsulosin 0.4 mg has only recently been approved for use in patients with BPH and there has since been an increase in the use of combination therapy that includes this dose [29, 30]. Continued increase in the use of the combination of dutasteride 0.5 mg and tamsulosin 0.4 mg is expected, particularly given the low satisfactory relief of symptoms observed in patients using tamsulosin 0.2 mg [31]. However, studies have shown inferior medication compliance with free- versus fixed-dose combination therapy [32, 33]. Therefore, clinical

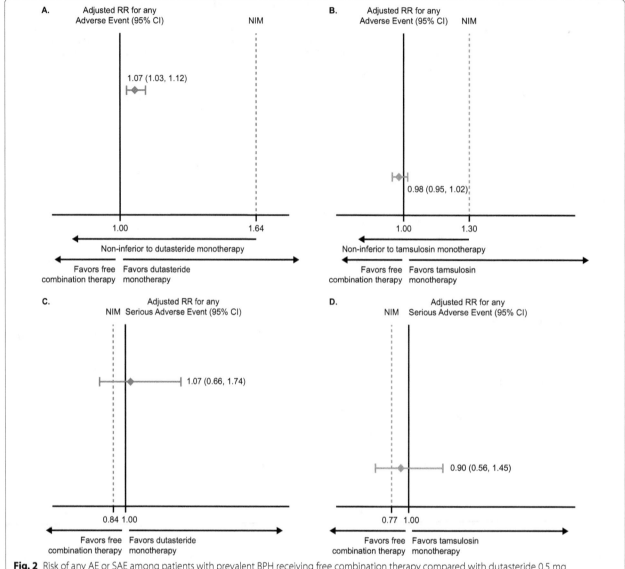

Fig. 2 Risk of any AE or SAE among patients with prevalent BPH receiving free combination therapy compared with dutasteride 0.5 mg monotherapy (**A**: AE, **C**: SAE) or tamsulosin 0.4 mg monotherapy (**B**: AE, **D**: SAE). For the purpose of this analysis, the data on prostate cancer were included in the risk calculations for any AE and any SAE. AE, adverse event; BPH, benign prostatic hyperplasia; CI, confidence interval; NIM, non-inferiority margin; RR, risk ratio; SAE, serious adverse event

outcomes may improve for patients with BPH by increasing compliance and lessening the pill burden on an aging population through fixed-dose combination, which has recently been approved in Korea.

In this analysis, the risk of any AE was similar for those treated with free combination therapy and dutasteride or tamsulosin monotherapies as demonstrated through non-inferiority testing and various subgroup and sensitivity analyses. The risk of any SAE was uniformly low. These results are consistent with the CombAT study, which observed a similar safety profile between combination and monotherapy of dutasteride and tamsulosin

[34]. The most common AEs in the CombAT study were related to sexual function; however, these waned over time. Although our study did not assess AEs longitudinally, there was a numerically higher adjusted relative risk of impotence and breast disorders in the combination groups; however, no statistical analysis was applied to these data. Nonetheless, the risk of any AE and SAE was similar between combination and monotherapy, which extends the evidence of the acceptability of the safety profiles for the dutasteride 0.5 mg and tamsulosin 0.4 mg combination in the BPH population from a real-world setting in South Korea.

Table 3 Risk of specific AEs with free combination therapy compared with dutasteride or tamsulosin monotherapy

	Free combination of dutasteride plus tamsulosin therapy (n = 1529)	Free combination therapy versus dutasteride monotherapy		Free combination therapy versus tamsulosin monotherapy	
		Dutasteride monotherapy (n = 6600)	Adjusted RR (95% CI)*	Tamsulosin monotherapy (n = 6566)	Adjusted RR (95% CI)*
Specific AE, n (%)					
Constipation	401 (26.2)	1271 (19.1)	1.31 (1.17, 1.45)	1595 (24.3)	1.05 (0.94, 1.16)
Depressed mood	219 (14.3)	794 (11.9)	1.05 (0.90, 1.22)	1025 (15.6)	0.91 (0.78, 1.05)
Urticaria	216 (14.1)	828 (12.4)	1.02 (0.87, 1.18)	1024 (15.6)	0.89 (0.76,1.03)
Dizziness	202 (13.2)	833 (12.5)	1.01 (0.87, 1.19)	889 (13.5)	0.98 (0.84, 1.14)
Arrhythmia	188 (12.3)	608 (9.1)	1.33 (1.13, 1.57)	638 (9.7)	1.24 (1.05, 1.46)
Vertigo	176 (11.5)	643 (9.7)	1.20 (1.01, 1.42)	735 (11.2)	1.05 (0.89, 1.24)
Diarrhea	166 (10.9)	702 (10.5)	0.99 (0.83, 1.17)	765 (11.7)	0.94 (0.80, 1.12)
Pruritus	146 (9.5)	624 (9.4)	0.98 (0.81, 1.18)	757 (11.5)	0.83 (0.69, 1.00)
Cardiac failure	137 (9.0)	400 (6.0)	1.37 (1.12, 1.68)	442 (6.7)	1.23 (1.01, 1.49)
Vomiting	117 (7.7)	374 (5.6)	1.29 (1.03, 1.62)	513 (7.8)	0.99 (0.80, 1.22)
Rhinitis	103 (6.7)	422 (6.3)	1.11 (0.89, 1.39)	454 (6.9)	0.97 (0.78, 1.22)
Dyspnea	74 (4.8)	266 (4.0)	1.10 (0.84, 1.44)	288 (4.4)	1.00 (0.77, 1.30)
Asthenia	51 (3.3)	196 (2.9)	1.06 (0.77, 1.47)	204 (3.1)	1.06 (0.75, 1.50)
Localized edema	30 (2.0)	130 (2.0)	0.84 (0.55, 1.29)	149 (2.3)	0.80 (0.52, 1.21)
Impotence	21 (1.4)	88 (1.3)	1.15 (0.69, 1.93)	108 (1.6)	1.09 (0.66, 1.79)
Epistaxis	19 (1.2)	84 (1.3)	1.10 (0.65, 1.87)	87 (1.3)	1.08 (0.60, 1.95)
Syncope orthostatic	13 (0.9)	62 (0.9)	0.83 (0.45, 1.53)	70 (1.1)	0.74 (0.41, 1.34)
Hypotension	11 (0.7)	35 (0.5)	1.34 (0.67, 2.70)	34 (0.5)	1.24 (0.62, 2.46)
Rash	9 (0.6)	22 (0.3)	1.45 (0.65, 3.26)	23 (0.4)	1.33 (0.57, 3.09)
Alopecia	5 (0.3)	34 (0.5)	0.87 (0.33, 2.28)	28 (0.4)	1.09 (0.41, 2.91)
Breast disorder	5 (0.3)	25 (0.4)	1.12 (0.39, 3.19)	18 (0.3)	1.53 (0.47, 4.99)
Dry mouth	5 (0.3)	17 (0.3)	0.98 (0.34, 2.83)	23 (0.4)	0.83 (0.30, 2.31)
Visual impairment	2 (0.1)	16 (0.2)	0.44 (0.10, 1.97)	17 (0.3)	0.41 (0.10, 1.79)
Other specified disorders of male genital organ	1 (0.1)	8 (0.1)	0.92 (0.12, 7.37)	10 (0.2)	0.54 (0.07, 4.25)
Vision blurred	0 (0.0)	5 (0.1)	–	7 (0.1)	–
Angioedema	0 (0.0)	4 (0.1)	–	2 (0.0)	–
Erythema multiforme	0 (0.0)	2 (0.0)	–	4 (0.1)	–
Premature ejaculation	0 (0.0)	2 (0.0)	–	1 (0.0)	–
Breast cancer	0 (0.0)	1 (0.0)	–	1 (0.0)	–
Hypertrichosis	0 (0.0)	1 (0.0)	–	0 (0.0)	–
Loss of libido	0 (0.0)	1 (0.0)	–	0 (0.0)	–
Dermatitis exfoliative	0 (0.0)	0 (0.0)	–	3 (0.0)	–
Priapism	0 (0.0)	0 (0.0)	–	1 (0.0)	–

AE, adverse event; CI, confidence interval; RR, risk ratio.*RRs of any or specific AEs among patients receiving free combination therapy compared to each monotherapy were estimated using log-binomial regression models adjusted for inverse probability of treatment weights. A robust variance estimator was used to derive the 95% CIs

Our study has some limitations. Although IPTW-adjustment was used for comparisons of safety endpoints, the potential for bias may remain. For example, the HIRA-NPS database does not include information on variables that influence the choice of BPH treatment strategy, such as prostate volume, total serum prostate-specific antigen, and LUTS. This may lead to unmeasured or residual confounding of data interpretation. Furthermore, key information may have been missed as the baseline period for capturing covariates differed across patients and was short. Additionally, this study relied on diagnosis codes associated with medical claims to determine a BPH diagnosis, clinical characteristics, AEs and SAEs. As such, any miscoding within the database may have resulted in misclassification of BPH clinical characteristics, AEs (particularly of milder, self-limiting events), and SAEs. Furthermore, the HIRA database does not include information on whether AEs and SAEs were treatment related, which may have resulted in miscoding or AEs and SAEs not being reported in this study. This was mitigated by evaluating specific AEs and SAEs related to the therapies under investigation in this study, based on prior clinical trials, post-marketing surveillance studies, and real-world studies [14]. Despite these potential limitations that are associated with real-world data, the results were comparable to those from randomized controlled trials (for example, CombAT and CONDUCT) that would not be subject to the same biases.

The strengths of this study are the generalizability of the findings to the wider BPH population in South Korea resulting from the large sample size and use of the most commonly used database in South Korea, the robustness of the comparative analyses through IPTW, inclusion of subgroup analyses, and consistency with available BPH literature [22].

The results of this study based on real-world evidence suggest that dutasteride 0.5 mg and tamsulosin 0.4 mg free combination is frequently used in South Korea for the treatment of BPH and the safety profile for free combination therapy is similar to either monotherapy.

Abbreviations

5-ARI: 5α-reductase inhibitor; AE: adverse event; BPH: benign prostatic hyperplasia; CI: confidence interval; HIRA: Health Insurance Review and Assessment; IPTW: inverse-probability-of-treatment weighting; IQR: interquartile range; LUTS: lower urinary tract symptoms; NPS: National Patient Sample; RR: risk ratio; SAE: serious adverse event; SD: standard deviation; UK: United Kingdom; US: United States.

Supplementary Information

Additional file 1. Health Insurance Review and Assessment-National Patient Sample (HIRA-NPS) claims database.

Additional file 2. Adverse events from the Global Datasheet for dutasteride-tamsulosin hydrochloride.

Additional file 3. Identification of treatment cohorts for eligible patients with BPH from the South Korean HIRA-NPS database.

Additional file 4. Frequency and duration of treatment with free combination therapy, dutasteride monotherapy, or tamsulosin monotherapy among patients with prevalent BPH in South Korea by age group.

Additional file 5. Risk of AEs and SAEs with free combination therapy compared with dutasteride or tamsulosin monotherapy*, by patient age group.

Acknowledgements

The authors would like to thank Kale Kponee-Shovein, Louise Yu, Yuqian Gu, and Jensen Vu from Analysis Group for their support on the statistical analyses. Editorial support in the form of development of the initial draft, collating author comment, assembling tables and figures, copyediting and referencing was provided by Lisa Auker, PhD, and Alistair Jones, PhD, of Fishawack Indicia Ltd. part of Fishawack Health and funded by GSK.

Authors' contributions

All authors contributed towards the development of the manuscript or revising it for intellectual content, have approved the final version to be submitted and agreed to be listed as authors. HS, S-BY, ZL, MC, VC, SP, RHB and MSD were responsible for conception and design of the study and data acquisition, analysis and interpretation. PK was responsible for data acquisition, analysis and interpretation. DM was responsible for data analysis and interpretation. All authors read and approved the final manuscript.

Author details

[1]GlaxoSmithKline, Brentford, Middlesex, UK. [2]Department of Urology, Seoul National University College of Medicine, Boramae Hospital, Seoul, Korea. [3]GlaxoSmithKline, Seoul, Korea. [4]GlaxoSmithKline, Mumbai, India. [5]GlaxoSmithKline, Collegeville, PA, USA. [6]GlaxoSmithKline, Bogotá, Colombia. [7]Analysis Group, Inc., Boston, MA, USA.

References

1. Lee SWH, Chan EMC, Lai YK. The global burden of lower urinary tract symptoms suggestive of benign prostatic hyperplasia: a systematic review and meta-analysis. Sci Rep. 2017;7(1):7984.
2. Madersbacher S, Sampson N, Culig Z. Pathophysiology of benign prostatic hyperplasia and benign prostatic enlargement: a mini-review. Gerontology. 2019;65(5):458–64.
3. Roehrborn CG, Marks L, Harkaway R. Enlarged prostate: a landmark national survey of its prevalence and impact on US men and their partners. Prostate Cancer Prostatic Dis. 2006;9(1):30–4.
4. Coyne KS, Sexton CC, Thompson CL, Milsom I, Irwin D, Kopp ZS, Chapple CR, Kaplan S, Tubaro A, Aiyer LP, et al. The prevalence of lower urinary tract symptoms (LUTS) in the USA, the UK and Sweden: results from the Epidemiology of LUTS (EpiLUTS) study. BJU Int. 2009;104(3):352–60.
5. Lee YJ, Lee JW, Park J, Seo SI, Chung JI, Yoo TK, Son H. Nationwide incidence and treatment pattern of benign prostatic hyperplasia in Korea. Investig Clin Urol. 2016;57(6):424–30.
6. Roehrborn CG. Benign prostatic hyperplasia: an overview. Reviews in urology. 2005;7(Suppl 9):S3–14.
7. Speakman M, Kirby R, Doyle S, Ioannou C. Burden of male lower urinary tract symptoms (LUTS) suggestive of benign prostatic hyperplasia (BPH) - focus on the UK. BJU Int. 2015;115(4):508–19.
8. Carbone DJ Jr, Hodges S. Medical therapy for benign prostatic hyperplasia: sexual dysfunction and impact on quality of life. Int J Impot Res. 2003;15(4):299–306.
9. Kim TH, Han DH, Ryu DS, Lee KS. The impact of lower urinary tract symptoms on quality of life, work productivity, depressive symptoms, and sexuality in Korean men aged 40 years and older: a population-based survey. Int Neurourol J. 2015;19(2):120–9.
10. Marberger M. The MTOPS study: new findings, new insights, and clinical implications for the management of BPH. Eur Urol Suppl. 2006;5:628–33.
11. Foster HE, Barry MJ, Dahm P, Gandhi MC, Kaplan SA, Kohler TS, Lerner LB, Lightner DJ, Parsons JK, Roehrborn CG, et al. Surgical management of lower urinary tract symptoms attributed to benign prostatic hyperplasia: AUA guideline. J Urol. 2018;200(3):612–9.
12. Emberton M, Cornel EB, Bassi PF, Fourcade RO, Gómez JMF, Castro R. Benign prostatic hyperplasia as a progressive disease: a guide to the risk factors and options for medical management. Int J Clin Pract. 2008;62(7):1076–86.
13. Jalyn (dutasteride and tamsulosin hydrochloride). https://www.accessdata.fda.gov/drugsatfda_docs/label/2010/022460s000lbl.pdf

14. Combodart 0.5 mg / 0.4 mg hard capsules. https://www.medicines.org.uk/emc/medicine/22943.

15. Australian Department of Health: Australian PI - Duodart (Dutasteride/Tamsulosin Hydrochloride) capsule. In., February 2018 edn; 2018.

16. MFDS duo dart capsule drug details. https://nedrug.mfds.go.kr/pbp/CCBBB01/getItemDetail?itemSeq=202103982.

17. Yeo JK, Choi H, Bae JH, Kim JH, Yang SO, Oh CY, Cho YS, Kim KW, Kim HJ. Korean clinical practice guideline for benign prostatic hyperplasia. Investig Clin Urol. 2016;57(1):30–44.

18. Austin PC. Balance diagnostics for comparing the distribution of baseline covariates between treatment groups in propensity-score matched samples. Stat Med. 2009;28(25):3083–107.

19. Jo JK, Kim KS, Nam JW, Choi BY, Moon HS. Sociodemographic factors related to lower urinary tract symptoms in men: a Korean community health survey. Int Neurourol J. 2017;21(2):143–51.

20. Choice of a non-inferiority margin. https://www.ema.europa.eu/en/documents/annual-report/annual-report-european-medicines-agency-2009_en.pdf.

21. Non-Inferiority Clinical Trials to Establish Effectiveness Guidance for Industry. https://www.fda.gov/regulatory-information/search-fda-guidance-documents/non-inferiority-clinical-trials.

22. Kim JA, Yoon S, Kim LY, Kim DS. Towards actualizing the value potential of korea health insurance review and assessment (HIRA) data as a resource for health research: strengths, limitations, applications, and strategies for optimal use of HIRA data. J Korean Med Sci. 2017;32(5):718–28.

23. Jo JK, Shinn SH, Kim KS, Moon HS. Changes in prevalence and treatment pattern of benign prostatic hyperplasia in Korea. J Korean Continence Soc. 2021.

24. Kang JY, Min GE, Son H, Kim HT, Lee HL. National-wide data on the treatment of BPH in Korea. Prostate Cancer Prostatic Dis. 2011;14(3):243–7.

25. Park J, Lee YJ, Lee JW, Yoo TK, Chung JI, Yun SJ, Hong JH, Seo SI, Cho SY, Son H. Comparative analysis of benign prostatic hyperplasia management by urologists and nonurologists: a Korean nationwide health insurance database study. Korean J Urol. 2015;56(3):233–9.

26. Phang H. Issues and challenges facing population ageing in Korea: productivity, economic growth, and old-age income security. J Comp Soc Welfare. 2011;27(1):51–62.

27. McVary KT, Roehrborn CG, Avins AL, Barry MJ, Bruskewitz RC, Donnell RF, Foster HE, Gonzalez CM, Kaplan SA, Penson DF, et al. Update on AUA guideline on the management of benign prostatic hyperplasia. J Urol. 2011;185(5):1793–803.

28. Management of Non-neurogenic Male LUTS. https://uroweb.org/guideline/treatment-of-non-neurogenic-male-luts.

29. Chung JH, Oh CY, Kim JH, Ha US, Kim TH, Lee SH, Han JH, Bae JH, Chang IH, Han DH, et al. Efficacy and safety of tamsulosin 0.4 mg single pills for treatment of Asian patients with symptomatic benign prostatic hyperplasia with lower urinary tract symptoms: a randomized, double-blind, phase 3 trial. Curr Med Res Opin. 2018;34(10):1793–801.

30. GlaxoSmithKline: Real-world Evidence on Free Combination Therapy DUT-TAM in Korea to Support Duodart NDA for Treatment of Benign Prostatic Hyperplasia (data on file). In.; 2020.

31. Choi H, Sim JS, Park JY, Bae JH. Assessment of tamsulosin 0.2 mg for symptomatic bladder outlet obstruction secondary to benign prostatic enlargement: data from a korean multicenter cross-sectional study. Urol Int. 2015;95(1):50–5.

32. Du LP, Cheng ZW, Zhang YX, Li Y, Mei D. The impact of fixed-dose combination versus free-equivalent combination therapies on adherence for hypertension: a meta-analysis. J Clin Hypertens (Greenwich). 2018;20(5):902–7.

33. Gupta AK, Arshad S, Poulter NR. Compliance, safety, and effectiveness of fixed-dose combinations of antihypertensive agents. Hypertension. 2010;55(2):399–407.

34. Roehrborn CG, Barkin J, Siami P, Tubaro A, Wilson TH, Morrill BB, Gagnier RP. Clinical outcomes after combined therapy with dutasteride plus tamsulosin or either monotherapy in men with benign prostatic hyperplasia (BPH) by baseline characteristics: 4-year results from the randomized, double-blind Combination of Avodart and Tamsulosin (CombAT) trial. BJU Int. 2011;107(6):946–54.

29

Significant relationship between parameters measured by transrectal color Doppler ultrasound and sexual dysfunction in patients with BPH 12 months after TURP

Li K. Chen[1,2], Yu W. Lai[3,4], Li P. Chiu[5,6] and Saint Shiou-Sheng Chen[4,6,7,8]*

Abstract

Background: A link between sexual dysfunction and lower urinary tract symptoms due to benign prostatic hyperplasia (BPH) has been noticed. Transurethral resection of the prostate (TURP) remains the standard treatment for symptomatic BPH, whether TURP causes sexual dysfunction is still uncertain. In this retrospective study, we investigated the relationship between parameters measured by color Doppler ultrasound (CDU) and sexual dysfunction in patients with BPH 12 months after TURP.

Methods: The parameters include presumed circle area ratio (PCAR), maximal horizontal area of seminal vesicles (MHA), resistive index of the prostate (RIP), and peak systolic velocity in the flaccid penis (PSV). The international prostate symptom score was used to evaluate the lower urinary tract symptoms and the five-item version of the International Index of Erectile Function was used to evaluate sexual function before and after TURP.

Results: Of the 103 patients without sexual dysfunction before TURP, 11 (10.7%) had erectile dysfunction (ED) after TURP. These 11 patients had significantly lower PCAR, RIP, PSV and MHA than those without ED. The patients with retrograde ejaculation after TURP had significantly lower PCAR than those without retrograde ejaculation, and the patients with premature ejaculation after TURP had significantly lower MHA than those without premature ejaculation. Comparing the parameters between baseline and after TURP, PCAR, RIP, and MHA decreased significantly in the patients with sexual dysfunction, but no significant differences were noted in the patients without sexual dysfunction after TURP.

Conclusions: More extended TURP can lead to a higher incidence of ED and retrograde ejaculation in BPH patients without sexual dysfunction before TURP. Patients with a lower volume of seminal vesicles after TURP may have a higher incidence of premature ejaculation.

Keywords: Benign prostatic hyperplasia, Erectile dysfunction, Sexual dysfunction, Transrectal color doppler ultrasound, transurethral resection of the prostate

Background

A link between sexual dysfunction and lower urinary tract symptoms (LUTS) due to benign prostatic hyperplasia (BPH) has been reported [1]. Sexual dysfunction includes erectile dysfunction (ED) and ejaculatory dysfunction, and ejaculatory dysfunction includes premature

*Correspondence: eric.yoyo@msa.hinet.net
[4] Department of Urology, National Yang-Ming University School of Medicine, Taipei, Taiwan
Full list of author information is available at the end of the article

ejaculation, retrograde ejaculation, delayed ejaculation, painful ejaculation, and decreased force of ejaculation [1]. Transurethral resection of the prostate (TURP) remains the standard treatment for symptomatic BPH, which occurs in about 10% to 20% of men over 40 years of age [2–4]. Some patients may experience complications of TURP including TURP syndrome, bladder neck contracture (BNC), bleeding, incontinence, ED and ejaculatory dysfunction, some of which have been reported to be associated with prostate size and surgical time [2, 5]. However, Pavone et al. suggested that TURP did not have a negative impact on ED in contrast to ejaculatory dysfunction [6]. In addition, Muntener et al. reported that TURP did not have a negative influence on sexual activity [7]. Therefore, whether TURP causes sexual dysfunction is still uncertain.

Many methods have been used to measure prostate size, including a digital rectal examination (DRE), cystourethroscopy and retrograde urethrography, however the results of these modalities are poor compared to transrectal ultrasound [8, 9]. Watanabe et al. reported good results using transrectal ultrasound to measure prostate volume [10]. Presumed circle area ratio (PCAR) has been shown to be correlated with LUTS, and especially obstructive symptoms [11, 12]. Changes in prostate size on transrectal ultrasound after TURP for patients with BPH have been reported [13], and our previous study showed a reduction in prostate volume 12 weeks after TURP [14]. Nevertheless, the clinical significance of such changes on transrectal ultrasound is still unclear.

Few studies have assessed the correlation between changes in prostate and seminal vesicle size and blood flow in the prostate and penis after TURP and sexual dysfunction. We hypothesize that TURP will cause morphological change in the prostatic fossa which may compromise the blood flow in the prostate, seminal vesicle and penis and result in sexual dysfunction. Therefore, we conducted this retrospective study by using parameters such as PCAR, resistive index in the prostate (RIP), and maximal horizontal area of seminal vesicles (MHA) measured by transrectal color Doppler ultrasound (TRUS); and peak systolic velocity in the flaccid penis (PSV) measured by color Doppler ultrasound (CDU) to evaluate the possible mechanism of sexual dysfunction after TURP in BPH patients without sexual dysfunction before TURP.

Methods
Patients
The Institutional Review Board of Taipei City Hospital approved this study (TCHIRB-10506107-E). Between August 2004 and November 2010, 154 men with symptomatic BPH who received TURP were evaluated. All the

patients received α-blocker treatment and no patients took 5-α-reductase inhibitor or phosphodiesterase-5 inhibitors before TURP. They agreed to provide regular follow-up including TRUS and CDU of flaccid penis for at least one year following written informed consent. In this period, we used a monopolar cutting loop and 5% glucose water as irrigating fluid to perform TURP, including in diabetic patients who had blood sugar monitored after surgery. Two experienced urologists preformed TURP and removed all the prostate tissue completely until they visualized the surgical capsule of the prostate. Fifty one patients were excluded including 8 did not have complete data, 38 had ED and 5 had poorly controlled diabetes mellitus (DM, fasting blood sugar > 300 or HbA1c > 8.0) before TURP. The remaining 103 patients were included for evaluation, and they were sexually active and did not have sexual dysfunction including ED or ejaculatory dysfunction before medical treatment or TURP, and they all wanted to maintain sexual function after TURP.

Measurement of transrectal color Doppler ultrasound (TRUS) and color Doppler ultrasound (CDU)
TRUS and CDU were performed in all patients using a real-time scanner with a rotating 7.5 MHz transducer (Bruel & Kjaer, Copenhagen, Denmark) 1 month before and 12 months after TURP. Two surgeons performed all of the procedures and ultrasound examinations. PCAR was defined as the ratio of the area of the maximum horizontal section of the prostate measured by TRUS to the area of a presumed circle of which the circumference was equal to the circumference of the maximum horizontal section (to calculate how closely the section approaches a circle), and a PCAR of 1.0 reveals that the section is equal to a circle [11, 12]. MHA was defined as the maximal horizontal area of seminal vesicles by TRUS, and was calculated as maximal length x maximal width of the seminal vesicle. We routinely evaluate seminal vesicles during TRUS at our hospital. RIP (peak systolic velocity—end diastolic velocity/peak systolic velocity) was used to detect blood flow in the prostate by TRUS. Peak systolic velocity in the flaccid penis (PSV) was measured by CDU one month before and 12 months after TURP. The international prostate symptom score (IPSS) was used to evaluate the lower urinary tract symptoms (LUTS), and the five-item version of the International Index of Erectile Function (IIEF-5) was used to evaluate sexual function one month before and 12 months after TURP in all of the patients. Retrograde ejaculation was defied as no semen was found when ejaculated and premature ejaculation was defined as you almost ejaculated before you wished and were very difficult to delay ejaculation 12 months after TURP according to the record of chart.

Statistical analysis

The Mann–Whitney U test was used for statistical analysis, and a P value < 0.05 was regarded to indicate statistical significance. The Mann–Whitney U test is a nonparametric test of the null hypothesis. It does not require the assumption of normal distributions and is nearly as efficient as the t-test on normal distributions. IBM SPSS Statistics for Windows, Version 20.0 (Armonk, NY: IBM Corp.) was used for the statistical analysis.

Results

The total number of TURP procedures performed during this period was 1205. The mean prostate volume was 68.5 cm^3 and the median was 67.5 cm^3, and the mean resected weight was 52.5 g and the median was 51.1 g. The mean operative time was 90.5 min. Of the 103 patients (mean age 70.3 years, range 54–85 years) without sexual dysfunction before TURP (IIEF-5: 25.6 ± 3.0), 11 (10.7%) complained of ED (IIEF-5: 10.2 ± 3.1, after TURP), and the IIEF for the other 92 patients was 25.1 ± 3.0 after TURP. Of the 103 patients, seven had DM, of whom two (28.6%) had ED after TURP. Capsular perforation was found in eight patients, of whom four (50.0%) had ED. Capsular perforation was determined by the surgeon through visual inspection during TURP and recorded in the operation note. The patients with ED after TURP had higher incidence rates of DM and capsular perforation than those without ED. Of the eight patients with BNC after TURP, two (25%) had ED, which was higher than the total incidence (10.7%).

Patients with BPH who had ED after TURP had significantly lower PCAR, RIP, MHA and PSV than those who did not have ED after TURP (Table 1). There was no significant difference in age between the patients with or without ED after TURP (Table 1). Of the 103 patients, 58 (56.3%) had retrograde ejaculation and six had premature ejaculation (5.8%) after TURP. All the 64 patients with ejaculatory dysfunction after TURP did not have ED. The patients with retrograde ejaculation after TURP had significantly higher PCAR than those without (Table 1); however there were no significant differences in age, RIP, MHA and PSV. The patients with premature ejaculation after TURP had lower MHA than those without premature ejaculation (Table 1). There were no significant differences in age, PCAR, RIP and PSV between the patients with or without premature ejaculation after TURP.

There were no significant differences in PCAR, RIP, MHA, PSV and age before TURP between the patients with or without ED or ejaculatory dysfunction after TURP (Table 1). Comparing the parameters between baseline and after TURP, PCAR, RIP, and MHA decreased significantly in the patients with sexual dysfunction, but no significant differences were noted in the patients without sexual dysfunction after TURP (Table 1). PSV decreased significantly in the patients with ED after TURP, but no significant difference was noted in the patients with ejaculatory dysfunction after TURP (Table 1). LUTS improved in all of the patients 12 months after TURP (IPSS: 19.7 ± 4.2 before TURP vs. 2.9 ± 0.8 after TURP). Patients who had sexual dysfunction after TURP had a lower IPSS than those without sexual dysfunction, but the difference was not statistically significant (Table 1).

Discussion

Ten to 20% of men over 40 years of age have LUTS due to BPH, and TURP is currently the treatment of choice for these patients with a success rate of 85 to 90% [2–4]. Estimating the prostate volume before surgery is important because most patients with BPH are older and may not be able to tolerate a prolonged operation. However, a DRE, retrograde urethrography, urethrocystoscopy and urethral pressure profile may not accurately estimate prostate volume, especially for moderate and large prostates [10, 15]. Tewari et al. reported that transrectal ultrasound more accurate in estimating prostate volume than MRI [16], and Terris et al. suggested that the prolate spheroid formula could most accurately estimate the prostate weight, especially for a prostate of < 80 g [17]. In this study, we used the Eq. (0.52 × L x W x H) to measure prostate volume and calculate PCAR.

The principle of electrosurgery was evaluated by Mclean [18]. A conventional TURP resectoscope uses an electric current with a cutting loop to cut the prostatic adenoma, and bleeding is controlled by cauterization. However, some complications may occur, including BNC, ED, incontinence and ejaculatory dysfunction, and the reported rate of ED after TURP is about 3.5 to 8.3% [3, 5, 19–23]. Favilla et al. reported that patients older than 65 years had a higher risk of developing ED after TURP [24]. Corona et al. suggested that PSV (< 13 cm/s) measured in the flaccid penis by CDU can be used to diagnose ED with an accuracy higher than 80% [25]. Therefore, we used PSV in this study to detect penis blood flow. However, other reports have suggested that TURP does not have a negative influence on erectile function [6, 7]. Tuncel et al. found RI of neurovascular bundle decreased in patients with ED after prostate biopsy and suggested ED following biopsy of prostate might have an organic basis [26]. In this study, the ED rate was 10.7% after TURP. Furthermore, we demonstrated that the patients who had ED after TURP had significantly lower PCAR, RIP, MHA and PSV than those without ED. In addition, the patients with ED also had significantly lower PCAR, RIP, MHA and PSV after TURP compared to baseline.

Table 1 PCAR, RIP, MHA, PSV, IPSS and IIEF-5 before and 12 months after TURP in difference age groups with respect to sexual dysfunction

	ED (+), N = 11	ED (−), N = 92	p
PCAR[b]	0.89 ± 0.07	0.87 ± 0.08	0.31
PCAR[a]	0.67 ± 0.04	0.83 ± 0.06	0.03*
p	0.02*	0.19	0.21
RIP (ml/s)[b]	0.81 ± 0.05	0.84 ± 0.08	
RIP (ml/s)[a]	0.59 ± 0.04	0.77 ± 0.08	0.02*
p	0.01*	0.06	0.21
MHA (cm^2)[b]	7.8 ± 1.8	8.0 ± 2.2	
MHA (cm^2)[a]	4.7 ± 1.5	7.5 ± 2.3	0.01*
p	0.01*	0.09	0.27
PSV (cm/s)[b]	14.3 ± 1.9	14.7 ± 2.0	0.01*
PSV (cm/s)[a]	9.1 ± 1.6	14.4 ± 2.1	0.27
p	0.01*	0.27	0.08
IPSS[b]	20.9 ± 4.6	19.6 ± 4.2	
IPSS[a]	2.6 ± 0.7	2.9 ± 0.8	
p	0.01*	0.01*	
IIEF-5[b]	25.9 ± 3.1	25.6 ± 2.9	0.26
IIEF−5[a]	10.2 ± 3.1	25.1 ± 3.0	0.01*
p	0.01*	0.29	
Age (years)	71.5 ± 8.1	68.8 ± 8.7	0.06
PV (cm^3)	69.1 ± 10.5	68.4 ± 10.2	0.15
RW (gm)	52.9 ± 8.2	52.5 ± 7.9	0.22

	Retrograde ejaculation (+), N = 58	Retrograde ejaculation (−), N = 45	p
PCAR[b]	0.88 ± 0.09	0.86 ± 0.07	0.21
PCAR[a]	0.79 ± 0.05	0.84 ± 0.06	0.04*
p	0.04*	0.21	0.11
RIP (ml/s)[b]	0.82 ± 0.08	0.86 ± 0.11	
RIP (ml/s)[a]	0.70 ± 0.08	0.80 ± 0.11	0.07
p	0.04*	0.06	0.07
MHA (cm^2)[b]	8.2 ± 2.2	7.7 ± 1.8	
MHA (cm^2)[a]	7.1 ± 2.1	7.3 ± 1.9	0.15
p	0.04*	0.07	0.15
PSV (cm/s)[b]	14.1 ± 1.9	15.3 ± 2.3	0.14
PSV (cm/s)[a]	13.1 ± 2.2	14.8 ± 2.1	0.31
p	0.07	0.08	0.07
IPSS[b]	19.9 ± 4.1	19.5 ± 4.4	
IPSS[a]	2.6 ± 0.5	3.2 ± 1.2	
P	0.01*	0.01*	
IIEF-5[b]	25.8 ± 3.0	25.3 ± 2.8	0.26
IIEF-5[a]	23.1 ± 2.4	24.0 ± 2.7	0.22
P	0.18	0.19	
Age (years)	69.8 ± 9.3	70.1 ± 9.7	0.36
PV (cm^3)	68.6 ± 10.3	68.3 ± 10.1	0.26
RW (gm)	52.7 ± 8.0	52.2 ± 7.8	0.24

	Premature ejaculation (+), N = 6	Premature ejaculation (−), N = 97	p
PCAR[b]	0.88 ± 0.08	0.87 ± 0.07	0.28
PCAR[a]	0.80 ± 0.05	0.81 ± 0.06	0.13
p	0.04*	0.06	0.21
RIP (ml/s)[b]	0.83 ± 0.09	0.84 ± 0.11	
RIP (ml/s)[a]	0.74 ± 0.09	0.77 ± 0.09	0.09
p	0.03*	0.06	0.21
MHA (cm^2)[b]	7.9 ± 1.3	8.0 ± 2.4	

Table 1 (continued)

	Premature ejaculation (+), N=6	Premature ejaculation (−), N=97	p
MHA (cm^2)^a	4.1 ± 1.3	7.7 ± 2.4	0.01*
p	0.02*	0.09	0.19
PSV (cm/s)^b	15.1 ± 2.4	14.6 ± 2.0	0.09
PSV (cm/s)^a	12.9 ± 1.7	13.9 ± 1.9	
p	0.06	0.07	
IPSS^b	19.5 ± 4.0	19.8 ± 4.3	0.31
IPSS^a	2.7 ± 0.8	2.9 ± 0.8	0.11
p	0.01*	0.01*	
IIEF-5^b	25.7 ± 3.0	25.6 ± 2.9	0.28
IIEF-5^a	20.9 ± 2.6	23.7 ± 2.7	0.19
p	0.06	0.14	
Age (years)	70.3 ± 9.9	70.0 ± 8.9	0.38
PV(cm^3)	68.8 ± 10.4	68.5 ± 10.2	0.29
RW (gm)	52.8 ± 8.1	52.5 ± 7.8	0.31

PCAR: presumed circle area ratio of the prostate; RIP: resistive index in the prostate; MHA: maximal horizontal area of seminal vesicles; PSV: peak systolic velocity in the flaccid penis; IPSS: international prostate symptom score; IIEF-5: the five-item version of the International Index of Erectile Function; PV: prostate volume; RW: resected prostatic weight; N: patient number; ^{b}: before TURP; ^{a}:12 months after TURP; *$p < 0.05$ indicates a significant difference; Data are expressed as mean ± SD; The Mann–Whitney U test was used for statistical analysis.

A possible explanation is that more extended TURP may cause lower PCAR, and reduce the blood flow in the prostate and penis, which may then cause ED. Tuncel et al. and Zisman et al. suggested prostate biopsy induced ED may happen by direct damage to neurovascular bundle or secondary trauma to nerve by compression of hematoma or edema [26, 27]. Patients with lower PCAR after more extended TURP may lead to more indirect nerve injury; especially all the patients underwent monopolar TURP in this study. Reductions in RIP and MHA after TURP may be a consequence of low sexual activity due to ED rather than the co-effect of ED; however all of the patients in this study wanted to be sexually active after TURP. Although no significant difference in age was noted in this study even in patients > 70 years compared with those < 70 years, further studies are needed to clarify this issue. It would have been better to assess psychological impact of surgery on ED (libido/IIEF-15 questionnaire) as patients included in the study had wide range of age (54–85 years).

Ejaculation is a complicated process involving the emission and expulsion of semen, and includes somatic, sympathetic and parasympathetic pathways, and factors which interfere the balance between sympathetic and parasympathetic nerves can induce ejaculatory dysfunction [28]. Retrograde ejaculation is permitted by a pathologically open internal vesical sphincter or bladder neck and painful ejaculation may be induced by an abnormal sensation and inflammation of the prostate [1, 29]. Ejaculatory dysfunction has been reported in 65% of patients after TURP, with a retrograde ejaculation rate of about 50% after TURP [1, 24]. Bladder neck resection during TURP may lead to retrograde ejaculation and we routinely preformed this procedure for every patient in this study. The incidence of retrograde ejaculation in this study was 56.3%, which is higher than in other reports, and we first noticed that it occurred more frequently in the patients with lower PCAR after TURP. This may be because the wider prostatic fossa after TURP may decrease resistance of the bladder neck and increase the rate of retrograde ejaculation. We hypothesize that decreased blood flow in the prostate and neurovascular bundle may compromise the contractility of ejaculation-related muscles, and therefore greater contractility will be needed which may cause retrograde ejaculation. Side effect of α-blocker treatment is retrograde ejaculation, but no patients receive α-blocker after TURP in this study. However, further studies are needed to clarify the mechanism. The incidence of premature ejaculation after TURP is low and the incidence is 5.8% in this study. Patients who had premature ejaculation had lower MHA than those without premature ejaculation and a possible explanation is that decreased volume of seminal vesicle after TURP might increase the pressure and sensitivity of seminal vesicle which may induce premature ejaculation. MHA can change before and after ejaculation and a volume of seminal vesicle might be influenced by the timing of ejaculation, but we did not consider ejaculation timing in this study. The impact of blood flow in the penis on ejaculatory dysfunction is unclear. The patients with ejaculatory dysfunction had lower PSV after TURP than those without in this study. However, more studies are needed to evaluate these issues.

Wasson et al. concluded that more older men are now receiving TURP compared to the 1980s, and that the outcomes for men older than 65 years are good [30]. Symptoms of moderate to severe ejaculatory dysfunction increase with age [1, 31]. A possible explanation is that the older patients may have had a lower testosterone level, lower volume of semen and lower contractility of ejaculation-related muscles, which may have become more severe after TURP. However, in this study, there was no significant difference of age between patients with ejaculatory dysfunction or without ejaculatory dysfunction after TURP, which was different from the previous studies. Therefore, further studies are needed to evaluate these complicated issues.

We found that the patients who complained of sexual dysfunction 12 months after TURP had better surgical outcomes than those without sexual dysfunction (lower IPSS after TURP); however the difference was not statistically significant. The reason might be that more extended TURP will improve LUTS, but will induce a higher incidence of sexual dysfunction. However, more studies are needed to evaluate this issue. The limitations of this study are as follows. First: this is a retrospective study and some patients were excluded because they had ED before TURP or incomplete data. Second: the case number is relatively small. Third: there was no specific control group for comparison. Fourth: TURP was performed by different urologists, and so inter-operator bias might exist. Fifth: none of the patients received bipolar or laser TURP in this study. Sixth: the diagnosis of sexual dysfunction was according to the IIEF-5 scores and chart record.

Conclusions

More extended TURP may cause lower PCAR, RIP, MHA and PSV, which may compromise the blood supply in the penis and prostate, then induce a higher incidence of ED or retrograde ejaculation in BPH patients without ED 12 months after TURP. Patients with a lower volume of seminal vesicles 12 months after TURP may have a higher incidence of premature ejaculation.

Abbreviations

BPH: Benign prostatic hyperplasia; TURP: Transurethral resection of the prostate; CDU: Color Doppler ultrasound (CDU); PCAR: Presumed circle area ratio; MHA: Maximal horizontal area of seminal vesicles; RIP: Resistive index of the prostate; PSV: Peak systolic velocity in the flaccid penis; IPSS: The international prostate symptom score; LUTS: Lower urinary tract symptoms; IIEF-5: The five-item version of the International Index of Erectile Function; ED: Erectile dysfunction.

Acknowledgements

Thanks for statistical assistance from Department of Research and Teaching, Taipei city hospital

Authors' contributions

LKC: analysis and collect of data and paper writing. YWL: related paper searching and analysis of data. LPC: collect and analysis of data. SSC: study design and supervision and paper writing. All authors read and approved the final manuscript.

Author details

[1] Department of Anesthesiology, China Medical University, Taichung City, Taiwan. [2] Department of Anesthesiology, China Medical University Hospital, Taichung City, Taiwan. [3] Division of Urology, Taipei City Hospital Ren Ai Branch, Taipei, Taiwan. [4] Department of Urology, National Yang-Ming University School of Medicine, Taipei, Taiwan. [5] Division of Urology, Taipei City Hospital Chushing Branch, Taipei, Taiwan. [6] General Education Center, University of Taipei, Taipei, Taiwan. [7] Division of Urology, Taipei City Hospital Zhong Xiao Branch, Taipei, Taiwan. [8] Commission for General Education, College of Applied Science, National Taiwan University of Science and Technology, Taipei, Taiwan.

References

1. Delay KJ, Nutt M, McVary KT. Ejaculatory dysfunction in the treatment of lower urinary tract symptoms. Trans Androl Urol. 2016;5:450–9.
2. Mebust WK, Holtgrewe HL, Cockett AT, Peters PC. Transurethral prostatectomy: immediate and post-operative complications. A cooperative study of 13 participating institutions evaluating 3885 patients. J Urol 1989;141:243–247.
3. Holtgrewe HL, Mebust WK, Dowd JB, Cockett AT, Peters PC, Proctor C. Transurethral prostatectomy: practice aspects of the dominant operation in American urology. J Urol. 1989;141:248–53.
4. Mayer EK, Kroeze SG, Chopra S, Bottle A, Patel A. Examining the 'gold standard': a comparative critical analysis of three consecutive decades of monopolar transurethral resection of the prostate (TURP) outcomes. BJU Int. 2012;110:1595–601.
5. Roos NP, Wennberg JE, Malenka DJ, Fisher ES, McPherson K, Andersen TF, et al. Mortality and reoperation after open and transurethral resection of the prostate for benign prostatic hyperplasia. New Eng J Med. 1989;320:1120–4.
6. Pavone C, Abbadessa D, Scaduto G, Caruana G, Gesolfo CS, Fontana D, et al. Sexual dysfunction after transurethral resection of the prostate (TURP): evidence from a retrospective study on 264 patients. Arch Ital Urol Androl. 2015;87:8–13.
7. Muntener M, Aelig S, Kuettel R, Gehrlach C, Sulser T, Strebel RT. Sexual function after transurethral resection of the prostate (TURP): results of an independent prospective multicenter assessment of outcome. Eur Urol. 2007;52:510–6.
8. Thumann RC Jr. Estimation of the weight of the hyperplasia prostate from the cystourethrogram. Am J Roentgenol Radium Ther. 1951;65(4):593–4.
9. Kaplan SA, Te AE, Pressler LB, Olsson CA. Transition zone index as a method of assessing benign prostatic hyperplasia: correlation with symptoms, urine flow and detrusor pressure. J Urol. 1995;154:1764–9.
10. Watanabe H, Igari D, Tanahashi Y, Harada K, Saitoh M. Measurements of size and weight of prostate by means of transrectal ultrasonotomography. Tokohu J Exp Med. 1974;114:277.
11. Watanabe H. New concept of BPH: PCAR theory. Prostate. 1998;37:116–25.
12. Matsugasumi T, Fujihara A, Ushijima S, Kanazawa M, Yamada Y, Shiraishi T, et al. Morphometric analysis of prostate zonal anatomy using magnetic resonance imaging: impact on age-related changes in patients in Japan and the USA. BJU Int. 2017;120:497–504.
13. Hastak SM, Gammelgaard J, Holm HH. Transrectal ultrasonic volume determination of the prostate- a preoperative and postoperative study. J Urol. 1982;127:1115–58.
14. Chen SS, Hong JG, Hsiao YJ, Chang LS. The correlation between clinical outcome and residual prostatic weight ratio after transurethral resection of the prostate for benign prostatic hyperplasia. BJU Int. 2000;85:79–82.
15. Watanabe H, Kaiho H, Tanaka M, Terasaya Y. Diagnostic application of ultrasonotomography to the prostate. Invest Urol. 1971;8:548–59.
16. Tewari A, Indudhara R, Shinohara K, Schalow E, Woods M, Lee RTR, et al. Comparison of transrectal ultrasound prostatic volume estimation with magnetic resonance imaging volume estimation and surgical specimen weight in patients with benign prostatic hyperplasia. J Clin Ultra. 1996;24:169–74.

17. Terris MK, Stamey TA. Determination of prostate volume by ultrasound. J Urol. 1991;145:984–7.

18. Mclean AJ. The bovine electrosurgical current generator: some underlying principles and results. Arch Surg. 1929;18:1863–7.

19. Chiu AW, Chen MT, Chang LS, Huang JK, Chen KK, Lin AT, et al. Prophylactic bladder neck incision in the treatment of small benign prostatic hyperplasia. Chin Med J. 1990;45(1):22–5.

20. Lu CC, Chen KK, Chen MT, Lin ATL, Chang LS. The clinical presentation of patients with contracture of the bladder neck after transurethral resection of the prostate. J Urol ROC. 1994;5:8–11. https://doi.org/10.70204/JUAROC.199403.0008.

21. Tscholl R, Largo M, Poppinghaus E, Recker F, Subotic B. Incidence of erectile impotence secondary to transurethral resection of benign prostatic hyperplasia, assessed by preoperative and postoperative snap gauge tests. J Urol. 1995;153:1491–3.

22. Marshall FF, editor. Textbook of operative urology. Philadelphia: WB Saunders; 1996. p. 13p.

23. McVary KT, Roehrborn CG, Avins AL, Barry MJ, Bruskewitz RC, Donnell RF, et al. Update on AUA Guideline on the Management of Benign Prostatic Hyperplasia. J Urol. 2011;185:1793–803.

24. Favilla V, Comino S, Salamone C, Fragala E, Madibua M, Condorelli R, et al. Risk factors of sexual dysfunction after transurethral resection of the prostate (TURP): a 12 months follow-up. J Endocrinol Invest. 2013;36:1094–8.

25. Corona G, Fagioli G, Mannucci E, Romeo A, Lotti F, Sforza A, et al. Penile Doppler ultrasound in patients with erectile dysfunction (ED): role of peak systolic velocity measured in the flaccid state in predicting arterigenic ED and silent coronary artery disease. J Sex Med 2008;5:2623–2624.

26. Tuncel A, Toprak U, Balci M, Koseoglu E, Aksoy Y, Karademir A, Atan A. Impact of transrectal prostate needle biopsy on erectile function: results of power Doppler ultrasonography of the prostate. Kaoshing J Med Sci. 2014;30:194–9.

27. Zisman A, Leibovici D, Kleinmann J, Siegel YI, Lindher A. The impact of prostate biopsy on patients well being: a prospective study of pain, anxiety and erectile dysfunction. J Urol. 2001;165:445–54.

28. Hellstrom WJ, Giuliano F, Rosen RC. Ejaculatory dysfunction and its association with lower urinary tract symptoms of benign prostatic hyperplasia and BPH treatment. Urology. 2009;74:15–21.

29. Fedder J, Kaspersen MD, Brandslund I, Hojgaard A. Retrograde ejaculation and sexual dysfunction in men with diabetes mellitus: a prospective, controlled study. Andrology. 2013;1:602–6.

30. Wasson JH, Bubolz TA, Lu-Yao GL, Walker-Corkery E, Hammond CS, Barry MJ. Transurethral resection of the prostate among medicare beneficiaries: 1984 to. For the patient outcomes research team for prostatic diseases. J Urol. 1997;2000(164):1212–5.

31. Rosen R, Altwein J, Boyle P, Kirby RS, Lukacs B, Meuleman E, et al. Lower urinary tract symptoms and male sexual dysfunction: the multinational survey of the aging male (MSAM-7). Eur Urol. 2003;44:637–49.

Permissions

List of Contributors

Chun-Hsuan Lin
Department of Urology, Kaohsiung Medical University Hospital, Kaohsiung Medical University, No. 100, Tzyou 1st Road, Kaohsiung 807, Taiwan

Wen-Jeng Wu, Ching-Chia Li and Sheng-Chen Wen
Department of Urology, Kaohsiung Medical University Hospital, Kaohsiung Medical University, No. 100, Tzyou 1st Road, Kaohsiung 807, Taiwan
Department of Urology, School of Medicine, College of Medicine, Kaohsiung Medical University, Kaohsiung, Taiwan
Graduate Institute of Clinical Medicine, College of Medicine, Kaohsiung Medical University, Kaohsiung, Taiwan

Miriam Gahl and René Fahrner
Department of General, Visceral and Thoracic Surgery, Bürgerspital Solothurn, Schöngrünstrasse 42, 4500 Solothurn, Switzerland

Thomas Stöckli
Department of Internal Medicine, Bürgerspital Solothurn, Schöngrünstrasse 42, 4500 Solothurn, Switzerland

Tairo Kashihara, Koji Inaba, Hiroki Nakayama, Kotaro Iijima, Shie Nishioka, Hiroyuki Okamoto, Satoshi Shima, Satoshi Nakamura, Ayaka Takahashi, Kana Takahashi, Kae Okuma, Naoya Murakami, Hiroshi Igaki, Yuko Nakayama and Jun Itami
Department of Radiation Therapy, National Cancer Center Hospital, Tsukiji 5-1-1, Chuo-ku, Tokyo, Japan

Motokiyo Komiyama, Arinobu Fukunaga, Yoshiyuki Matsui and Hiroyuki Fujimoto
Department of Urological Oncology, National Cancer Center Hospital, Tokyo, Japan

Nao Kikkawa and Yuko Kubo
Department of Radiology, National Cancer Center Hospital, Tokyo, Japan

Hideyuki Minagawa and Katsuhiro Makino
Department of Urology, Ome Municipal General Hospital, 4-16-5, Higashiome Ome, Ome, Tokyo 1980042, Japan
Department of Urology, Graduate School of Medicine, The University of Tokyo, 7-3-1, Hongo, Bunkyo-ku, Tokyo 1138655, Japan

Takashi Murata
Department of Urology, Ome Municipal General Hospital, 4-16-5, Higashiome Ome, Ome, Tokyo 1980042, Japan

Taketo Kawai, Akihiko Matsumoto, Yusuke Sato, Yuta Yamada, Masaki Nakamura, Daisuke Yamada, Motofumi Suzuki and Haruki Kume
Department of Urology, Graduate School of Medicine, The University of Tokyo, 7-3-1, Hongo, Bunkyo-ku, Tokyo 1138655, Japan

Kenji Nagasaka, Masami Tokura and Nao Tanaka
Department of Rheumatology, Ome Municipal General Hospital, 4-16-5, Higashiome Ome, Ome, Tokyo 1980042, Japan

Eisaku Ito
Department of Pathology, Ome Municipal General Hospital, 4-16-5, Higashiome Ome, Ome, Tokyo 1980042, Japan

Shunichiro Nomura, Yuka Toyama, Jun Akatsuka, Yuki Endo, Ryoji Kimata, Yasutomo Suzuki, Tsutomu Hamasaki, Go Kimura and Yukihiro Kondo
Department of Urology, Nippon Medical School, 1-1-5 Sendagi, Bunkyo-ku, Tokyo 113-8603, Japan

Yechen Wu, Yiping Zhang, Jinxin Hu, Jun Zhu and Tinghu Cao
Department of Urology, Baoshan Branch, Shuguang Hospital Affiliated to Shanghai University of Traditional Chinese Medicine, Shanghai 201900, People's Republic of China

Xi Chen and Qiang Wu
Department of Urology, Tongji Hospital, Tongji University School of Medicine, Shanghai 200065, People's Republic of China

Duocheng Qian
Department of Urology, Shanghai Forth People's Hospital Affiliated to Tongji University School of Medicine, Shanghai 200434, People's Republic of China

Wei Wang
Department of Urology, Tongji Hospital, Tongji University School of Medicine, Shanghai 200065, People's Republic of China
The First Affiliated Hospital, Zhejiang University School of Medicine, Hangzhou 310003, Zhejiang Province, China

Lijuan Wang, Shucheng Pan, Binbin Zhu and Zhenliang Yu
The First Affiliated Hospital, Zhejiang University School of Medicine, Hangzhou 310003, Zhejiang Province, China

Giorgio Bozzini
Department of Urology, ASST Valle Olona, Via Arnaldo da Brescia, 21052 Busto Arsizio, VA, Italy
ESUT, European Section for UroTechnology, Arnhem, Italy

Umberto Besana, Albert Calori and Carlo Buizza
Department of Urology, ASST Valle Olona, Via Arnaldo da Brescia, 21052 Busto Arsizio, VA, Italy

Matteo Maltagliati and Lorenzo Berti
Department of Urology, ASST Valle Olona, Via Arnaldo da Brescia, 21052 Busto Arsizio, VA, Italy
Department of Urology, Ospedale Policlinico e Nuovo Ospedale Civile S. Agostino Estense, University of Modena and Reggio Emilia, Modena, Italy

Maria Chiara Sighinolfi
Department of Urology, Ospedale Policlinico e Nuovo Ospedale Civile S. Agostino Estense, University of Modena and Reggio Emilia, Modena, Italy

Salvatore Micali and Bernardo Rocco
ESUT, European Section for UroTechnology, Arnhem, Italy
Department of Urology, Ospedale Policlinico e Nuovo Ospedale Civile S. Agostino Estense, University of Modena and Reggio Emilia, Modena, Italy

Jean Baptiste Roche
Department of Urology, Clinique Saint Augustin, Bordeaux, France

Ali Gozen
Department of Urology, SLK Kliniken, Heilbron, Germany

Alexander Mueller
Department of Urology, Spital Limmattal, Schlieren, Switzerland

Dimitry Pushkar
Department of Urology, Moscow State University, Moscow, Russia

Evangelos Liatsikos
Department of Urology, University of Patras, Patras, Greece

Marco Boldini
Department of Urology, Clinica Sant'Anna, Lugano, Switzerland

Claudia Carolina Cruz-Gálvez and Martha E. Cancino-Marentes
Doctorado en Farmacología, Centro Universitario de Ciencias de la Salud, Universidad de Guadalajara, Guadalajara, Jalisco, México

Georgina Hernández-Flores, Pablo Cesar Ortiz-Lazareno, María Martha Villaseñor-García, Eduardo Orozco-Alonso and Raúl Antonio Solís-Martínez
División de Inmunología, Centro de Investigación Biomédica de Occidente del IMSS, Sierra Mojada 800, Col. Independencia, CP 44340 Guadalajara, Jalisco, México

Erick Sierra-Díaz
Servicio de Urología, Hospital de Especialidades, CMNO-IMSS, Guadalajara, Jalisco, México

Alejandro Bravo-Cuellar
División de Inmunología, Centro de Investigación Biomédica de Occidente del IMSS, Sierra Mojada 800, Col. Independencia, CP 44340 Guadalajara, Jalisco, México
Centro Universitario de los Altos, Universidad de Guadalajara, Tepatitlán de Morelos, Jalisco, México

Jinguo Wang, Sheng Xie, Jun Liu, Tao Li, Wanrong Wang and Ziping Xie
Department of Andrology, Renmin Hospital, Hubei University of Medicine, No. 39 Chaoyang Middle Road, Maojian District, Shiyan 442000, Hubei, People's Republic of China

Jong Jin Oh, Seok-Soo Byun and Sung Kyu Hong
Department of Urology, Seoul National University Bundang Hospital, Seongnam, Korea
Department of Urology, Seoul National University College of Medicine, Seoul, Korea

Sangchul Lee and Hakmin Lee
Department of Urology, Seoul National University Bundang Hospital, Seongnam, Korea

Hyungwoo Ahn and Sung Il Hwang
Department of Radiology, Seoul National University Bundang Hospital, Seongnam, Korea

Hak Jong Lee
Department of Radiology, Seoul National University Bundang Hospital, Seongnam, Korea
Department of Radiology, Seoul National University College of Medicine, Seoul, Korea

Gheeyoung Choe
Department of Pathology, Seoul National University Bundang Hospital, Seongnam, Korea

Yuliang Chen, Zhien Zhou, Yi Zhou, Xingcheng Wu, Zhigang Ji, Hanzhong Li and Weigang Yan
The Department of Urology, Peking Union Medical College Hospital, Chinese Academy of Medical Sciences, No. 1 Shuaifuyuan, Dongcheng District, Beijing 100730, China

Yu Xiao
The Department of Pathology, Peking Union Medical College Hospital, Chinese Academy of Medical Sciences, No. 1 Shuaifuyuan, Dongcheng District, Beijing 100730, China

Xuepei Zhang
Department of Urology, The First Affiliated Hospital of Zhengzhou University, No. 1 Jianshe East Road, Zhengzhou 450052, China
Key Laboratory of Precision Diagnosis and Treatment for Chronic Kidney Disease in Henan Province, Zhengzhou 450052, China

Shuanbao Yu, Jin Tao, Biao Dong, Yafeng Fan, Haopeng Du, Haotian Deng, Jinshan Cui and Guodong Hong
Department of Urology, The First Affiliated Hospital of Zhengzhou University, No. 1 Jianshe East Road, Zhengzhou 450052, China

Becky A. S. Bibby, Lingjian Yang, Elisabet More, Ananya Choudhury and Catharine M. L. West
Translational Radiobiology Group, Division of Cancer Science, School of Medical Sciences, Faculty of Biology, Medicine and Health, University of Manchester, Manchester Academic Health Sciences Centre, The Christie NHS Foundation Trust, Wilmslow Road, Manchester M20 4BX, UK

Niluja Thiruthaneeswaran
Translational Radiobiology Group, Division of Cancer Science, School of Medical Sciences, Faculty of Biology, Medicine and Health, University of Manchester, Manchester Academic Health Sciences Centre, The Christie NHS Foundation Trust, Wilmslow Road, Manchester M20 4BX, UK
Sydney Medical School, University of Sydney, Camperdown, Australia

Ronnie R. Pereira and Robert G. Bristow
Translational Radiobiology Group, Division of Cancer Science, School of Medical Sciences, Faculty of Biology, Medicine and Health, University of Manchester, Manchester Academic Health Sciences Centre, The Christie NHS Foundation Trust, Wilmslow Road, Manchester M20 4BX, UK
Translational Oncogenomics, CRUK Manchester Institute and CRUK Manchester Centre, Manchester, UK

Darragh G. McArt and Paul O'Reilly
Centre for Cancer Research and Cell Biology, Queen's University Belfast, Belfast, UK

Kaye J. Williams
School of Pharmacy and Pharmaceutical Sciences, University of Manchester, Manchester, UK

Yuhei Miyasaka, Hidemasa Kawamura, Hiro Sato, Nobuteru Kubo and Tatsuya Ohno
Department of Radiation Oncology, Gunma University Graduate School of Medicine, 3-39-22, Showa-machi, Maebashi, Gunma 371–8511, Japan
Gunma University Heavy Ion Medical Center, Maebashi, Japan

Tatsuji Mizukami
Department of Radiation Oncology, Gunma University Graduate School of Medicine, 3-39-22, Showa-machi, Maebashi, Gunma 371–8511, Japan
Division of Radiation Oncology, Department of Radiology, Faculty of Medicine, Academic Assembly, University of Toyama, Toyama, Japan

Hiroshi Matsui and Kazuhiro Suzuki
Gunma University Heavy Ion Medical Center, Maebashi, Japan
Department of Urology, Gunma University Graduate School of Medicine, Maebashi, Japan

Yoshiyuki Miyazawa
Department of Urology, Gunma University Graduate School of Medicine, Maebashi, Japan

Kazuto Ito
Department of Urology, Gunma University Graduate School of Medicine, Maebashi, Japan
Kurosawa Hospital, Takasaki, Japan

Takashi Nakano
Department of Radiation Oncology, Gunma University Graduate School of Medicine, 3-39-22, Showa-machi, Maebashi, Gunma 371–8511, Japan
Quantum Medical Science Directorate, National Institutes for Quantum and Radiological Science and Technology, Chiba, Japan

Jae Yoon Kim, Ji Hyeong Yu, Luck Hee Sung and Dae Yeon Cho
Department of Urology, Sanggye Paik Hospital, Inje University College of Medicine, 1342 Dongil-ro, Nowon-gu, Seoul 01757, Republic of Korea

Hyun-Jung Kim
Department of Pathology, Sanggye Paik Hospital, Inje University College of Medicine, 1342 Dongil-ro, Nowon-gu, Seoul 01757, Republic of Korea

Soo Jin Yoo
Department of Laboratory Medicine, Sanggye Paik Hospital, Inje University College of Medicine, 1342 Dongil-ro, Nowon-gu, Seoul 01757, Republic of Korea

Jeong Woo Yoo, Kyo Chul Koo, Byung Ha Chung and Kwang Suk Lee
Department of Urology, Gangnam Severance Hospital, Yonsei University College of Medicine, 211 Eonju-ro, Gangnam-gu, Seoul 06273, Republic of Korea

María García-Flores
Laboratory of Molecular Biology, Fundación Instituto Valenciano de Oncología, 46009 Valencia, Spain
IVO-CIPF Joint Research Unit of Cancer, Príncipe Felipe Research Center (CIPF), 46012 Valencia, Spain

Marta Ramírez-Calvo and Antonio Fernández-Serra
Laboratory of Molecular Biology, Fundación Instituto Valenciano de Oncología, 46009 Valencia, Spain

Christian M. Sánchez-López and Antonio Marcilla
Àrea de Parasitologia, Departament de Farmàcia i Tecnologia Farmacèutica i Parasitologia, Universitat de València, 46000 Burjassot, Valencia, Spain
Joint Research Unit on Endocrinology, Nutrition and Clinical Dietetics, Health Research Institute La Fe, Universitat de Valencia, 46100 Valencia, Spain

José Antonio López-Guerrero
Laboratory of Molecular Biology, Fundación Instituto Valenciano de Oncología, 46009 Valencia, Spain
IVO-CIPF Joint Research Unit of Cancer, Príncipe Felipe Research Center (CIPF), 46012 Valencia, Spain
Department of Pathology, School of Medicine, Catholic University of Valencia "San Vicente Mártir", 46001 Valencia, Spain

Chiaki Kawada, Hideo Fukuhara, Satoshi Fukata, Kenji Tamura, Takashi Karashima, Keiji Inoue and Shingo Ashida
Department of Urology, Kochi Medical School, Nankoku, Kochi 783-8505, Japan

Ichiro Yamasaki
Department of Urology, Kubokawa Hospital, Takaoka-gun, Kochi 786-0002, Japan

Taro Shuin
Kochi Medical School Hospital, Nankoku, Kochi 783-8505, Japan

Po-Fan Hsieh
Department of Urology, China Medical University Hospital, No. 2, Yu-Der Rd, Taichung 40447, Taiwan
School of Medicine, China Medical University, Taichung 40402, Taiwan

Graduate Institute of Biomedical Sciences, School of Medicine, China Medical University, Taichung 40402, Taiwan

Tzung-Ruei Li, Chao-Hsiang Chang, Chi-Rei Yang and Chin-Chung Yeh
Department of Urology, China Medical University Hospital, No. 2, Yu-Der Rd, Taichung 40447, Taiwan

Wei-Ching Lin
School of Medicine, China Medical University, Taichung 40402, Taiwan
Department of Radiology, China Medical University Hospital, Taichung 40447, Taiwan

Chi-Ping Huang
Department of Urology, China Medical University Hospital, No. 2, Yu-Der Rd, Taichung 40447, Taiwan
School of Medicine, China Medical University, Taichung 40402, Taiwan

Wen-Chin Huang
Graduate Institute of Biomedical Sciences, School of Medicine, China Medical University, Taichung 40402, Taiwan

Han Chang
Department of Pathology, China Medical University Hospital, Taichung 40447, Taiwan

Hsi-Chin Wu
Department of Urology, China Medical University Hospital, No. 2, Yu-Der Rd, Taichung 40447, Taiwan
School of Medicine, China Medical University, Taichung 40402, Taiwan
Department of Urology, China Medical University Beigang Hospital, Beigang, Yunlin 651012, Taiwan

Barak Rosenzweig
Department of Urology, Chaim Sheba Medical Center, 5262080 Ramat Gan, Israel
The Sackler Faculty of Medicine, Tel Aviv University, Tel Aviv, Israel
The Talpiot Medical Leadership Program, Chaim Sheba Medical Center, Tel Hashomer, Ramat Gan, Israel

Tomer Drori, Jacob Ramon, Zohar A. Dotan, Gil Goldinger and Dorit E. Zilberman
Department of Urology, Chaim Sheba Medical Center, 5262080 Ramat Gan, Israel
The Sackler Faculty of Medicine, Tel Aviv University, Tel Aviv, Israel

Orit Raz
Assuta Ashdod University Hospital, Ashdod, Israel

Gadi Shlomai
The Sackler Faculty of Medicine, Tel Aviv University, Tel Aviv, Israel
The Talpiot Medical Leadership Program, Chaim Sheba Medical Center, Tel Hashomer, Ramat Gan, Israel
Department of Internal Medicine D and the Hypertension Unit, Chaim Sheba Medical Center, Tel Hashomer, Ramat Gan, Israel

Moshe Shechtman
The Sackler Faculty of Medicine, Tel Aviv University, Tel Aviv, Israel
Department of Anesthesiology, Chaim Sheba Medical Center, Ramat Gan, Israel

Orith Portnoy
The Sackler Faculty of Medicine, Tel Aviv University, Tel Aviv, Israel
Department of Diagnostic Imaging, Chaim Sheba Medical Center, Ramat Gan, Israel

Fei Wang, Tong Chen, Meng Wang, Hanbing Chen, Caishan Wang, Peiqing Liu, Songtao Liu, Jing Luo and Qi Ma
Department of Ultrasound, The Second Affiliated Hospital of Soochow University, 1055 Sanxiang Road, Suzhou, Jiangsu, China

Lijun Xu
Department of Urology, The Second Affiliated Hospital of Soochow University, 1055 Sanxiang Road, Suzhou, Jiangsu, China

Jing Chen, Di Niu, Hu Li, Kun Wei, Li Zhang and Shuiping Yin
Department of Urology, The First Affiliated Hospital of Anhui Medical University, Hefei, People's Republic of China
The Institute of Urology, Anhui Medical University, Hefei, People's Republic of China

Haomin Zhang
The Second Clinical College of Anhui Medical University, Hefei, Anhui, People's Republic of China

Longfei Liu
Department of Urology, b Reproductive Medicine Center, Xiangya Hospital, Central South University, Changsha, People's Republic of China

Xiansheng Zhang and Chaozhao Liang
Department of Urology, The First Affiliated Hospital of Anhui Medical University, Hefei, People's Republic of China
The Institute of Urology, Anhui Medical University, Hefei, People's Republic of China

Anhui Province Key Laboratory of Genitourinary Diseases, Anhui Medical University, Hefei, People's Republic of China

Meng Zhang
Department of Urology, The First Affiliated Hospital of Anhui Medical University, Hefei, People's Republic of China
The Institute of Urology, Anhui Medical University, Hefei, People's Republic of China
Anhui Province Key Laboratory of Genitourinary Diseases, Anhui Medical University, Hefei, People's Republic of China
Institute of Urology of Shenzhen University, The Third Affiliated Hospital of Shenzhen University, Shenzhen Luohu Hospital Group, Shenzhen, People's Republic of China

Saira Khan
Epidemiology Program, College of Health Sciences, University of Delaware, 100 Discovery Blvd., 7th floor, Newark, DE 19713, USA

K. Y. Wolin
Coeus Health, 222 W Merchandise Mart Plaza, Chicago, IL 60654, USA

R. Pakpahan, G. A. Colditz and S. Sutcliffe
Division of Public Health Sciences, Department of Surgery, Washington University in St. Louis School of Medicine, 660 S. Euclid Ave., Campus Box 8100, St. Louis, MO 63110, USA

R. L. Grubb
Department of Urology, Medical University of South Carolina, 135 Rutledge Ave, Charleston, SC 29425, USA

L. Ragard
Westat, 1600 Research Blvd, Rockville, MD 20850, USA

J. Mabie
Information Management Services, Inc., 1455 Research Blvd, Suite 315 , Rockville, MD 20850, USA

B. N. Breyer
Departments of Urology and Epidemiology and Biostatistics, University of California - San Francisco, 400 Parnassus Ave # 610, San Francisco, CA 94143, USA

G. L. Andriole
Division of Urologic Surgery, Department of Surgery, Washington University in St. Louis School of Medicine, 4921 Parkway Place, St. Louis, MO 63110, USA

Toby Page, Rajan Veeratterapillay and Julie Burn
The Newcastle Upon Tyne Hospitals NHS Foundation Trust, Newcastle upon Tyne, UK

Kim Keltie and Andrew Sims
The Newcastle Upon Tyne Hospitals NHS Foundation Trust, Newcastle upon Tyne, UK
Faculty of Medical Sciences, Translational and Clinical Research Institute, University of Newcastle Upon Tyne, Newcastle upon Tyne, UK

Nikan Zerafatjou
Department of Urology, School of Medicine, Hamadan University of Medical Sciences, Hamadan, Iran

Mohammadali Amirzargar
Urology and Nephrology Research Center, Hamadan University of Medical Sciences, Hamadan, Iran

Mahdi Biglarkhani
Department of Persian Medicine, School of Medicine, Hamadan University of Medical Sciences, Hamadan, Iran

Farzaneh Shobeirian
Department of Radiology, School of Medicine, Guilan University of Medical Sciences, Rasht, Iran

Ghazal Zoghi
Endocrinology and Metabolism Research Center, Hormozgan University of Medical Sciences, Bandar Abbas, Iran

Zhiyong Su and Hongming Liu
Department of Urology, The Affiliated Hospital of Guizhou Medical University, Guiyang, China

Ye Tian, Guangheng Luo, Yong Ban, Zhen Wang and Zhaolin Sun
Department of Urology, Guizhou Provincial People's Hospital, Guiyang, China

Zrinka Lulic and Marianne Cunnington
GlaxoSmithKline, Brentford, Middlesex, UK

Hwancheol Son
Department of Urology, Seoul National University College of Medicine, Boramae Hospital, Seoul, Korea

Sang-Bae Yoo
GlaxoSmithKline, Seoul, Korea

Pratiksha Kapse
GlaxoSmithKline, Mumbai, India

Diane Miller
GlaxoSmithKline, Collegeville, PA, USA

Vanessa Cortes
GlaxoSmithKline, Bogotá, Colombia

Suna Park, Rachel H. Bhak and Mei Sheng Duh
Analysis Group, Inc., Boston, MA, USA

Li K. Chen
Department of Anesthesiology, China Medical University, Taichung City, Taiwan
Department of Anesthesiology, China Medical University Hospital, Taichung City, Taiwan

Yu W. Lai
Division of Urology, Taipei City Hospital Ren Ai Branch, Taipei, Taiwan
Department of Urology, National Yang-Ming University School of Medicine, Taipei, Taiwan

Li P. Chiu
Division of Urology, Taipei City Hospital Chushing Branch, Taipei, Taiwan
General Education Center, University of Taipei, Taipei, Taiwan

Saint Shiou-Sheng Chen
Department of Urology, National Yang-Ming University School of Medicine, Taipei, Taiwan
General Education Center, University of Taipei, Taipei, Taiwan
Division of Urology, Taipei City Hospital Zhong Xiao Branch, Taipei, Taiwan
Commission for General Education, College of Applied Science, National Taiwan University of Science and Technology, Taipei, Taiwan

Index

Prostate Cancer, 3, 12-18, 20-22, 24, 28-41, 44-46, 54-56, 58, 60-63, 71-73, 75, 78-86, 89-92, 94-99, 102-105, 108-111, 114-116, 118-123, 126-127, 135, 137-139, 141-146, 148-153, 156, 158-161, 163, 166-167, 169, 175-176, 186-187, 194, 201, 203, 214-216, 218-219

Prostate Gland, 6, 101, 112, 121, 150, 196, 200

Prostate Health Index, 84, 111-119, 144, 147-148, 150-151

Prostate Volume, 2-6, 23, 51, 74-77, 81-82, 85, 87-90, 119, 121, 123, 162, 165, 176, 178-179, 181-183, 185-187, 198-200, 203, 205-209, 217, 221-222, 224, 226

Prostate Weight, 2-3, 222

Prostate-specific Antigen, 3, 15, 81, 85, 89, 92, 107, 110, 112-117, 121, 126, 139, 142-143, 152, 154, 161-162, 165-166, 176, 178, 187, 195-196, 199, 205, 208

Prostatectomy, 1, 6-7, 15, 48, 52, 73-75, 77-79, 84-85, 92-93, 105, 110, 118, 144-146, 148-151, 167, 177-178, 207, 209, 225

Prostatic Urethral Lift, 188, 193-194

Pumpkin Seed Oil, 195-196, 198-201

R

Radiation Therapy, 12, 15-16, 104, 106, 110

Radiotherapy, 12-16, 29-30, 45, 55, 64, 94-95, 100, 102-110, 119

Randomized Clinical Trials, 52, 139

S

Saturation, 23, 84, 165, 167

Senescence, 54-55, 57, 60-62

Sexual Dysfunction, 169, 218, 220-223, 225-226

Sphincter, 2, 51, 149, 224

Spondylodiscitis, 22, 24-27

Surgical Efficacy, 202-208

Systematic Biopsy, 84, 147, 149-150, 160-161, 163, 165-167

T

Tamsulosin, 187, 195-201, 210-219

Targeted Biopsy, 84, 147, 149-150, 158, 160-163, 165-167

Transurethral Resection, 1, 6-8, 10, 22-23, 25, 47, 53, 178, 194, 202-203, 208-209, 220-221, 225-226

Tumor Diameter, 144-151

Tumors, 15, 20, 54-55, 68, 74-75, 87, 95, 105-106, 108, 165

U

Ultracentrifugation, 127-129, 136-137

Urinary Incontinence, 51, 53, 145, 196, 227

Urinary Retention, 2-4, 22, 120, 123, 161, 172, 188, 190, 192, 194, 203, 211

Urinary Tract Symptoms, 7, 47, 52, 172, 176, 186-189, 193-194, 196, 200-201, 208-209, 211, 214, 218, 225-226

Printed in the USA
CPSIA information can be obtained
at www.ICGtesting.com
JSHW050846251023
50683JS00018B/89